# THE NEW LANGUAGE OF CHANGE

# THE NEW LANGUAGE OF CHANGE

## Constructive Collaboration in Psychotherapy

STEVEN FRIEDMAN
*Editor*

Foreword by Kenneth J. Gergen

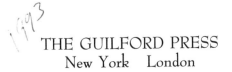

THE GUILFORD PRESS
New York   London

*To Donna with love . . .*
*and to the gang from Brooklyn*

© **1993 The Guilford Press**
A Division of Guilford Publications, Inc.
72 Spring Street, New York, NY 10012

Tables 4.1 and 7.1 are reproduced from *Expanding Therapeutic Possibilities:
Getting Results in Brief Psychotherapy* by S. Friedman and M. T. Fanger, 1991,
New York: Lexington Books. Copyright © 1991 by Lexington Books/
Macmillan, Inc. Reprinted by permission.

Chapter 8 is reprinted from *The New York Times Magazine*. Copyright ©
1986 by the New York Times Company. Reprinted by permission.

Illustrations by Sarah Friedman.

Printed in the United States of America

This book is printed on acid-free paper.

Last digit is print number:   9   8   7   6   5   4   3   2   1


**Library of Congress Cataloging-in-Publication Data**

The new language of change : constructive collaboration in psychotherapy /
    edited by Steven Friedman.
        p.   cm.
    Includes bibliographical references and index.
    ISBN 0-89862-145-3
    1. Family psychotherapy.   2. Solution-focused therapy.
3. Personal construct therapy.      I. Friedman, Steven, 1945–
    [DNLM: 1. Family Therapy—methods.   2. Family Therapy—trends.
WM 430.5.F2 L287]
RC488.5.L353   1993
616.89'156—dc20
DNLM/DLC
for Library of Congress                                         92-49093
                                                                    CIP

Our prevailing narratives provide the vocabulary that sets our realities. Our destinies are opened or closed in terms of the stories we construct to understand our experiences.

—*Harry Goolishian*

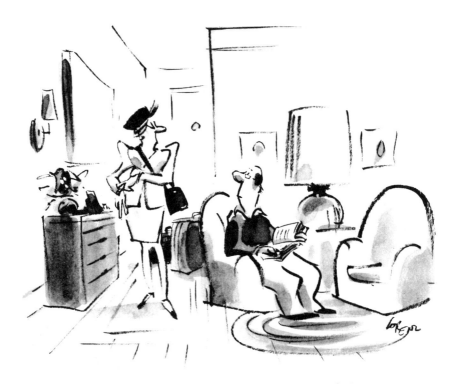

"*I'm sorry, Herbert, but you're no longer part of the story I want to tell about myself.*"

# Contributors

**Tom Andersen,** University of Tromsö, Tromsö, Norway.

**Harlene Anderson,** Houston Galveston Institute, Houston, Texas.

**Insoo Kim Berg,** Brief Family Therapy Center, Milwaukee, Wisconsin.

**Sally Brecher,** Harvard Community Health Plan, Braintree, Massachusetts.

**P. Lynn Caesar,** private practice, Arlington and Salem, Massachusetts.

**Judith Davis,** Center for Counseling and Academic Development, University of Massachusetts, Amherst, Massachusetts

**Steve de Shazer,** Brief Family Therapy Center, Milwaukee, Wisconsin.

**Victoria C. Dickerson,** Bay Area Family Therapy Training Associates, Cupertino, California.

**Michael Durrant,** Eastwood Family Therapy Centre, Sydney, Australia.

**Margot Taylor Fanger,** Harvard Community Health Plan, Cambridge, Massachusetts, and Cambridge Hospital/Harvard Medical School.

**Jennifer C. Freeman,** private practice, Berkeley, California.

**Steven Friedman,** Harvard Community Health Plan, Braintree, Massachusetts, and Innovative Training Systems, Boston, Massachusetts.

**Lynn Hoffman-Hennessy,** Brattleboro Family Institute, Brattleboro, Vermont.

**Kate M. Kowalski,** University of Wisconsin, Milwaukee, Wisconsin.

**Frank Langella,** Tony Award–winning actor.

**Eve Lipchik,** ICF Consultants, Inc., Milwaukee, Wisconsin.

**Dean Lobovits,** Graduate School of Professional Psychology, John F. Kennedy University, Orinda, California.

**Cynthia M. Mittelmeier,** Harvard Community Health Plan, Braintree, Massachusetts, and Lesley College Graduate School, Cambridge, Massachusetts.

**William Hudson O'Hanlon,** The Hudson Center for Brief Therapy, Omaha, Nebraska.

**Thomas Alan Parry,** Family Therapy Program, University of Calgary Faculty of Medicine, Calgary, Alberta, Canada.

**D. Donald Sawatzky,** Department of Educational Psychology, University of Alberta, Edmonton, Alberta, Canada.

**Matthew D. Selekman,** private practice and Consultation Services, Chicago, Illinois.

**Jeffrey L. Zimmerman,** Bay Area Family Therapy Training Associates, Cupertino, California.

# *Foreword*

There is something crackling fresh about these essays: they have an invigorating, effervescent quality. These are not features that jar the senses—no shrill chirping or incandescent flares—rather, they evoke the kind of excitement that accompanies periods of bold exploration, of unleashed creative energies. How are we to describe this formidable change of seas? Surely these essays are far removed from the belief of 19th-century romantics, as well as 20th-century psychiatrists, in deep and mysterious psychic forces—blocked impulses and unconscious dramas—governing human action. And they are less than respectful of the medical model that has come to dominate the mental health professions for the better part of the present century.

These chapters also demonstrate a remarkable disinterest in most of the central features of what we now see as the modernist orientation to human problems. They are little concerned, for example, with the cognitive dispositions, emotional incapacities, personality traits, and family structures that have long served as the chief focus of many therapies. They are disrespectful as well of the barriers traditionally set between therapist and client: that sacred distance between objectivity, neutrality, and reason on one side, and subjectivity, bias, and passion on the other. And there is a distinct absence of an overarching theory—conceptual distinctions, process models, systemic diagrams—from which therapeutic procedures and insights are supposed to emanate, and which should properly stand or fall depending on treatment outcomes. In effect, there are important respects in which these contributions represent a significant disjunction with the past century of therapeutic writing.

Again, how are we to characterize the broad movement of which these chapters are manifestations, and what account can we give of its origins? If there is one essential concern of the present volume, it is with language. Removed is the traditional emphasis on language as an outward expression of inner thoughts and feelings. Rather, the emphasis here is on language as it shapes and is shaped by human relationships. The analytic lens is turned outward onto language in use, away from the individual client and onto social relatedness, away from the "within" and onto the "between." Of focal concern is the way in which language frames the world, establishing the ontology and the array of values in which people invest their lives.

With language and relationships thus foregrounded, two major suspicions are generated. The first is the suspicion of all reality posits. The various accounts brought to therapy by the client—tales of misery, oppression, failures, and the like—serve not as approximations to the truth, perhaps biased by desires or cognitive incapacities, but as life constructions, made up of narratives, metaphors, cultural logics, and the like. They are more like musical or poetic accompaniments than mirrors or maps. And their major significance lies not in their relative validity, but in their social utility. In this context a major aim of therapy becomes one of freeing the client from a particular kind of account and opening the way to alternatives of greater promise. These chapters outline numerous means of achieving this kind of reconstruction: scaling questions, reflecting teams, positive reframing, solution talk, problem redefinition, self-perception questions, exception-oriented questions, goal enactment, externalizing conversation, artistic expressions, and metaphorical explorations among them. In each case the attempt is to shake loose the taken-for-granted world and to open new linguistic spaces. These spaces offer new options for action.

This suspicion of the taken for granted is coupled with a related distrust of the authoritative voice. So often the therapist–theorist fastens on a theoretical position, and then proceeds to elaborate, support, and defend it ad infinitum et nauseam, in the scarcely hidden hope that this will be the final voice. Yet, in the present volume, the suspicion of "words as truth telling" is everywhere in evidence and deeply colors the stance taken toward therapeutic writing. There is a subtle recognition that there is no authoritative voice, grand solution, or final answer. Rather, there is genuine dialogue: a sensitive listening to other therapists, even to clients and scholars. And the conclusions are often tentative, open to emendation, and sometimes nonexistent. There is a paucity of systematically contained theory, grand solutions, complex modeling, and unusable jargon.

Most important, this same stance is taken toward the client. There is little attempt by the therapist in these encounters to establish authority, to claim "the essential insight," objectivity, or conclusions based on established knowledge. Rather, the therapist typically engages in a form of conversation that deeply respects the lived validity of the client's account, while simultaneously enabling the dialogue to become dialogic. The therapist does not stand independent of the client, but joins him or her as a responsible co-constructor of realities. This stance gives rise to novel turns in many of the chapters, with clients and colleagues invited to write about the case at hand.

Yet, in spite of the historical disjunction between the present essays and the major therapeutic traditions, these renderings scarcely stand outside of history. This transformation in sensibility is not an anomalous event but, as I see it, richly wedded to a movement of far greater scope. Just beneath these chapters lies an enormous movement—a wave of scholarly writings that span the humanities as well as the sciences. These writings make their way both directly and indirectly into many of the chapters of this book. Such writings go under such varying labels as poststructuralism, postempiricism, interpretivism, and, perhaps most integratively, social constructionism. In general these writings represent a general skepticism toward the longstanding view that scientific language (or any other kind) furnishes objective or accurate reflections of the world. In place of this view, they search for alternative means of accounting for our modes of description and explanation. They look to the effects of literary traditions, social conditions, cultural values, and, most centrally, social processes. As these alternatives are explored new questions are everywhere in evidence, concerning, for example, the nature of science, education, moral discourse, individual functioning, and the possibilities for a pluralistic society.

As I have tried to describe in *The Saturated Self* (1991), I also see these movements closely tied to more general shifts within the culture, shifts often adumbrated by the term *postmodern*. Although there is much to be said about this more general transformation, special attention should be given to the technological revolution of the present century. With the mushrooming of communication technologies the stage was set for a vast proliferation of voices. We are saturated by a profusion of opinions, factual claims, theories, critiques, and hypotheses—often conflicting—from around the globe. In effect, we inhabit increasingly a multivocal world, and living viably in this world virtually demands a form of multilingualism—an ability to shuttle among the domains of intelligibility, to see, and reflexively to see, the peculiarities of one's seeing. It is in just these directions that I feel the present essays lead us.

No, I do not see these contributions as forming the apex or termination of a long discussion. Rather, they are significant entries into a dialogue that must, by its very definition, seek dynamic continuation with other colleagues, clients, scholars, and active participants in cultural life. Many important questions remain to be addressed, broad questions concerning, for example, the cultural effects of redefining therapy, cure, and therapist; the viability of DSM categories, the possibility of politically committed therapy; and the nature of therapeutic research. There are also specific issues, such as the goal of theory, whether the language of the therapeutic relationship can be usefully transported from the office, negative ripple effects of "re-storying," and the utility of deep beliefs. However, I do not see these issues as threats to the present work. These chapters mark not the end of a line of thought, but beginnings of conversations of enormous significance not only for the profession but the culture as a whole.

Kenneth J. Gergen
*Swarthmore, PA*

# Acknowledgments

I wish to thank Sally Brecher, Cynthia Mittelmeier, Ethan Kisch, Edward Bauman, and Madeline Dynsza, the members of my family therapy team at Harvard Community Health Plan in Braintree, for providing a supportive and collegial context that enables my clinical work to grow and expand. Several postdoctoral fellows who have joined the team over the past several years have also stimulated my thinking and brought fresh perspectives: Brian Meyer, Jacqueline Lapidus, Jonathan Simmons, and Amy Mayer. My colleagues Vicki Beggs, Rose Catalanotti, Stan Cole, Lauren Corbett, Ellen Frishman, Dan Gadish, Marge Lavin, Ted Powers, Rob Schneider, and Ronnie Tilles have made my eight years at the Braintree Center of the Harvard Community Health Plan a very special and rewarding experience. In addition, I want to thank my colleague Simon Budman for the original idea of using the format of a dialogue between editor and author.

I would like to give special thanks to Sarah Friedman, who created the illustrations for this book, and to the authors, whose responsiveness and dedication resulted in the completion of this book ahead of schedule. I am also indebted to Seymour Weingarten, editor-in-chief at the Guilford Press, who believed in this book and supported it from the start and to Anna Brackett and the production staff at Guilford, who put it all together.

# *Preface*

We live in a world abuzz with change: New technologies are rapidly impacting on our lives, immersing us in a constantly shifting ocean of opinions, values, and ideas (Gergen, 1991). These forces, while increasing confusion and complexity in our lives, also provide increased options and choices for defining self. In fact, we can no longer talk about a self, but rather a panoply of possible selves, all capable of emerging as contextual conditions permit. Our worlds, rather than reflecting a fixed objective reality, are constructed and defined contextually in social and community discourse. We no longer live in a coherent social world with a consistent set of "truths." Within this postmodern chaos is an opportunity for us as therapists to bring forth those alternative voices, embodied in our clients, that enable them to feel empowered and liberated from oppressive and constraining forces in their lives (Gergen, 1992). In this way, the therapy process can be conceived as a journey of liberation from oppressive constraints to new possibilities.

In this book the reader will be exposed to a new set of developments in the changing terrain of family therapy. The approaches presented reflect a move away from theoretical certainties and toward a critical respect for differences and a collaborative, respectful, hopeful, and socially responsive therapy. The primacy of human relationships and the benefits of nonpathologizing approaches to the therapeutic process are emphasized. As meaning is co-constructed in conversation, options and possibilities emerge.

We appear to be entering a new era in family therapy, marked by a respect for the client's self-authoring capacities as well as an emphasis on meaning and on the importance of language as a medium for change. The biologic, positivist analogies of the modern era are giving way to an emphasis on stories and conversation. The narrative metaphor is already a part of our daily cultural experience (see, for example, the cartoon by L. Lorenz that appears a few pages back). Several authors in this book creatively incorporate the narrative metaphor in their work.

My goal for this book was to bring together a group of innovative clinicians who would not only share their perspectives and ideas about the psychotherapy process but illustrate how their thinking directly translates into clinical practice. The authors whose work is presented here are swimming against a tide of established thinking and practice. It takes courage and stamina to swim against the strong currents that still hold sway in the field of psychotherapy. With this in mind, the authors should be applauded not only for their innovations but also for their willingness to present their ideas in such transparent form. This book is an attempt to acknowledge and highlight those innovative ideas that are transforming the field of psychotherapy as well as to provide illustrations of their usefulness in day-to-day clinical practice.

My hope is that this will be a practical book, one that offers the reader useful insights into and illustrations of the new ideas percolating in the field of psychotherapy. To make the material interactive and personal, each chapter ends with a series of questions asked by the editor of the author(s). Thus the author(s) have an opportunity to comment on and amplify the ideas presented in their chapters.

Although the authors all ask the question, How do I provide the context that will enable the client to see a world of expanding options rather than a world of limitations and constraints?, the reader will note many differences in how this goal is achieved. These differences are reflected in the therapists' styles, in the way interviews are organized and structured, in the use of behind-the-mirror teams, and in therapists' emphasis on outcome. While some authors view rapid solution development as a goal, others find brevity to be simply a beneficial side effect of the conversational process. Although chapters are grouped together in this book to represent solution-focused, narrative, or reflexive approaches, the reader will notice significant cross-fertilization of thinking and methods across these organizational distinctions.

In keeping with the postmodern tradition, this book is made up of many diverse elements. My hope is that, taken together, these contrasting and pluralistic melodies will converge in a symphony of liberating possibilities.

Steven Friedman
*Hingham, MA*

## REFERENCES

Gergen, K. (1991). *The saturated self: Dilemmas of identity in contemporary life.* New York: Basic Books.

Gergen, K. (1992, March). *The polymorphous perversity of the postmodern era.* Paper presented at the Family Therapy Network Symposium, Washington, DC.

# Contents

## II. NARRATIVES OF LIBERATION

## III. REFLEXIVE CONVERSATIONS

## IV. THE POSTMODERN ERA: A UNIVERSE OF STORIES

# Organization
# of the Book

This book is divided into four sections. In the first section, Paths to Solution, the authors engage in therapeutic conversations that shift attention away from the client's problem-saturated reality and emphasize "exceptions" and client resources. In Chapter 1, Berg and de Shazer look at therapy as conversation and give an overview on the nature of language and reality. They emphasize the benefits of staying simple in therapy and illustrate their thinking with the use of "scaling" questions. In the second chapter Lipchik shows us how to be both persistent and flexible in shifting gears to match the client's position and how to tactfully navigate around potential dead ends in the therapy process. She generates questions that help the client develop a "both/and," rather than an "either/or," perspective. In Chapter 3, O'Hanlon illustrates his therapy model in a single-session clinical consultation with a depressed woman. Getting a video description of the complaint allows him to develop stories and introduce ideas that free the client from her fixed views. In Chapter 4, Fanger integrates Ericksonian ideas, neurolinguistic programming, and solution-focused thinking in her clinical work. She persistently, humorously, and effectively directs the client's attention to possibilities and opens the door for him to think (and act) differently about his plight. In Chapter 5, Durrant and Kowalski offer us a competency-based map for therapy that presupposes change and employs a language of alternative possibilities. The therapist's persistence in maintaining a focus on the future opens options and frees the client to see her life and the therapy process in new ways. Selekman, in Chapter 6, presents a model for effective therapy with "difficult" adolescents and their families. He emphasizes the need to join with the adolescent and uses humor and a task orientation to create a forum for change. In the final chapter in

*1*

this section Mittelmeier and Friedman apply the "possibility frame" in working with a mother and daughter who are experiencing intense conflict. The clients enact a positive future that defines their desired goal, and a metaphor-generating reflecting team adds their voices to the process.

In Section II, Narratives of Liberation, the authors help clients free themselves from those oppressive forces that have been dominating their lives and relationships. The oppressive forces are objectified and externalized in conversation, freeing the client to generate new, more preferred, stories. In Chapter 8, Langella tells us a wonderful little story of both his and his son's battles with "monsters in my head." In Chapter 9, Freeman and Lobovits creatively integrate the narrative perspective with expressive arts therapy. In Chapter 10, Dickerson and Zimmerman apply the narrative approach to a blended family and provide opportunities to bring forth descriptions that fit a new, emerging story of competence and control. In Chapter 11, Friedman presents a client's journey of liberation from an oppressive past dominated by self-pity and guilt to a present of self-love and freedom. In the final chapter in this section Brecher and Friedman look at the impact of poverty on the lives and relationships of an inner-city family. With the help of a reflecting team, the therapist supports the mother as a competent and nurturing caregiver and enables her to make a better life for the family.

In Section III, Reflexive Conversations, the authors listen carefully to their clients, creating space for them to be heard, and invite their clients to listen as they generate ideas that open space in a recursive interchange of talking and listening. In Chapter 13, Andersen offers us an inside view of his thinking as the therapy process unfolds. He emphasizes the need to pay attention both to one's inner dialogue and to the comments of family members. In Chapter 14, Anderson presents a clinical illustration of the collaborative language systems therapy that she and Harry Goolishian developed. In Chapter 15, Hoffman and Davis offer a personal view of the process of therapy and articulately outline their philosophic perspective. Using a reflecting team and providing an opportunity for the voices of all family members to be heard, they demonstrate the value of a collaborative model for therapy. And in the final chapter in the section, Caeser creatively applies the principles of the reflecting process to the challenge of couples therapy.

Section IV, The Postmodern Era: A Universe of Stories, reflects a departure from the previous chapters. In Chapter 17, Sawatzky and Parry have a conversation based on Sawatzky's visit to Russia to reconnect with his relatives. His story, as defined through Parry's questions, provides the reader with a powerful example of a family's determination to survive and grow in the face of great adversity. Chapter 18 is an essay by Parry that carefully elucidates the dilemmas of the postmodern era and examines these issues in the writings of Thomas Pynchon. He concludes his chapter with his view of therapy as a "revisioning of stories."

# I

## PATHS TO SOLUTION

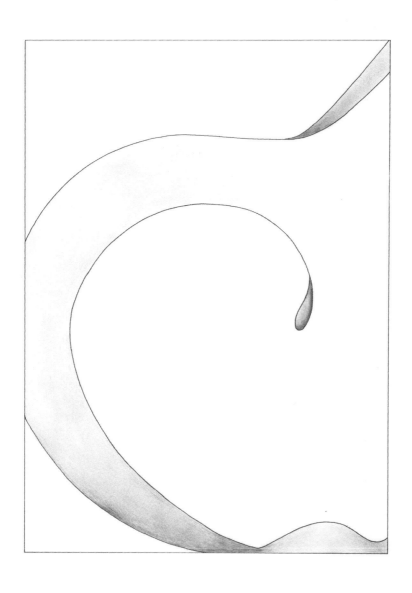

# 1

## Making Numbers Talk: Language in Therapy

INSOO KIM BERG
STEVE DE SHAZER

*Do you want to learn the sciences with ease? Begin by learning your own language.*

—ÉTIENNE CONDILLAC

The metaphor of therapy as conversation is simultaneously useful and dangerously misleading. The danger lies in what is probably an inevitable vowel shift from *a* to *i*, that is, from "therapy *as* conversation" to "therapy *is* conversation." The vowel shift marks a transformation from metaphor to metaphor disguised as concept.

Since conversation is a normal and natural activity for two or more people in the same place at the same time to do together, we automatically make the assumption that we know what we are talking about when we use the word *conversation*. It seems so simple and obvious that we do not even need to know anything about conversations to participate in them. With the inescapable vowel shift from *a* to *i* (which is already happening, at least in workshops and training sessions) a pronouncement develops—"Therapy is conversation"—and we reasonably begin thinking that therapy equals conversation. Thus, through a grammatical transformation we mistakenly and inadvertently lead ourselves into thinking that we know all there is to know about doing therapy, that it primarily requires the skills involved in maintaining a conversation or continuing a dialogue. We thus mistakenly think that it is the conversation itself that is the therapy, that talking together is the curative factor. Like the expression *therapeutic relationship*, which preceded it, the pronouncement "Therapy is conversation" seems to explain what therapy is all about and yet is so vague that it actually tells us nothing.

On the other hand, the fact that doing therapy can be seen as a conversation reminds us of the interactional aspects of the endeavor. First, for therapy to be seen as a conversation, it must involve two or more people. Second, conversations happen within language, and language is what we use to have conversations. Thus, the slogan points to Condillac's idea that we need to learn our own language in order to learn about therapy (and, in fact, to learn about conversations or any other human endeavor).

The notions developed from viewing therapy as a conversation, as an activity involving two or more people, tend to threaten or corrupt (or perhaps to counterbalance) the traditional meanings of the word *therapy* (from the Greek, meaning "to nurse, to cure"), which certainly can mislead us into thinking the therapist operates upon the patient or client. Consider, for instance, the following dictionary definition of *therapeutic:*

> serving to cure or heal; curative; concerned in discovering and applying remedies for diseases. That part of medical science which relates to the treatment and cure of diseases.

"Therapy as conversation" seems to be a useful contradiction in terms in that it leads us into seeing the doing of therapy and the using of the term *therapy* in ways that undermine and contaminate the usual dictionary definitions of therapy (which the term, unfortunately, automatically carries with it).

## LANGUAGE: FOUR VIEWS

Certainly, our readers, like Condillac's, believe they know their own language, and we as authors want to believe we have a similar understanding of our language. After all, we use it all the time, particularly when talking, listening, reading, and writing. Using one's own language seems to be a simple, uncomplicated thing.

All common sense relies on a naive view of language as transparent and true. The commonsense assumption that language is a transparent medium expressing already-existing facts implies that change does not come about in language. Language is assumed always to reflect changes that occur prior to the changes in language. Authors or speakers are seen as able to perceive the truth of reality and to express this experience through language, thus enabling the reader and listener to know exactly what they mean. However, it is not so simple. There are at least three other distinct ways to think about how language works.

In traditional Western thought (which is related to the commonsense view), language is usually viewed as somehow representing reality. This is based on the notion that there is a reality out there to be represented. Therefore, language can be studied by determining how well it re-presents that reality. This belief, of course, is based on the idea that language can represent "the truth," the revelation of which is the goal of traditional Western science. Furthermore, this belief leads to the idea that a science of meaning can be developed by looking behind and beneath the words, an approach usually called structuralism (Chomsky, 1968, 1980; Saussure, 1922), which was explicitly used by Bandler and Grinder (1975) to look at hypnotherapy and psychotherapy. The entire history of psychotherapy from Freud to Selvini Palazzoli to Minuchin involves structural thinking, that is, looking behind and beneath the surface of what is being investigated.

Buddhists, on the other hand, would say that language blocks our access to reality (Coward, 1990). Since they too think there is a reality out there, this point of view leads Buddhists to the practice of meditation, which they use to turn off language and put themselves in touch with reality.

There is yet another view, which is usually labeled *poststructuralism* (de Shazer, 1991; de Shazer & Berg, 1992; Harland, 1987), that suggests, simply, that language *is* reality. To put this in terms more familiar to therapists, this idea that our world *is* language suggests a view related to what is called *constructivism*. This way of thinking suggests that we need to look at how we have ordered the world in our language and how our language (which comes before us) has ordered our world. This view has led us to believe that we need to study language in order to study anything at all. That is, rather than looking behind and beneath the language that clients and therapists use, we think that the language they use is all that we have to go on. Neither authors (or speakers) nor readers (or listeners) can be assured that they can get at what the other meant with any certainty because they each bring to the encounter all of their previous (and unique) experiences. Meaning is arrived at through negotiation within a specific context. That is, messages are not sent but only received: this goes for the author as well as the reader (and, therefore, the author is only one of many readers). Contrary to the commonsense view, change is seen to happen within language: What we talk about and how we talk about it makes a difference, and it is these differences that can be used to make a difference (to the client).

Over the past 20 years our work with clients has led us from some version of the traditional Western view, through a version of the traditional Eastern view, to a poststructural view. That is, we have come to see that the meanings arrived at in a therapeutic conversation are developed through a process more like negotiation than the development of understanding or an uncovering of what it is that is "really" going on. Given the uncertainty regarding meanings involved during any conversation, misunderstanding is far more likely than understanding. As we see it, it is the therapist's job to use this misunderstanding creatively and, together with the client, to develop as useful a misunderstanding as is possible.

## PROBLEM TALK / SOLUTION TALK

> *All of the facts belong only to the problem, not to its solution.*
> —LUDWIG WITTGENSTEIN, *Tractatus Logico-Philosophicus*

For the sake of argument, we will use the terms *problem talk* and *solution talk* as a binary opposition,[1] which will allow us to follow Wittgenstein in setting up another expedient binary opposition between "facts" and their opposite, "non-facts." *Non-facts* is a conveniently broader term than the perhaps automatic term *fictions,* thus allowing us to include fantasies, hopes, fictions, plans, desires, and so forth, as the opposites of "facts."

### Problem Talk

As we listen to people describe their problems and search for an explanation, "fact" piles up upon "fact," and the problem becomes heavier and heavier. The whole situation can quickly become overwhelming, complicated, and perhaps even hopeless. This is, when a client's problem is explored in detail and he tells us more and more "facts" about his troubled life, he, as well as the therapist, is led to conclude, reasonably enough, that his could well be a difficult case. After all, these "facts" are what clients, as well as therapists, believe to be real and true. Such "problem talk," talking more about what is not working, is doing more of the same of something that has not worked; thus, problem talk belongs to the problem itself and is not part of the solution. Simply, the more clients and therapists talk about "facts," the greater the problem they jointly construct. This is the way language naturally works.

In general, problem talk appears as if it is based on the traditional Western view of truth and reality. As one "fact" follows another in the sequence of conversation, we start to feel forced to look behind and beneath them, forced to assume causal links and interconnections between them. This leads to the idea that the "underlying basic problem"—whatever is behind and beneath—must be worked on first, before the client can tackle other problems (which are on the surface).

However, a poststructural view suggests that the way we use language can and frequently does accidentally lead us astray. It is easy to forget that making a description has to be done in language and that the English language (at least) necessitates a sequential ordering of the words used in a description. Mistaking descriptions for causal explanations is a result of our being imposed upon or even duped by our language to the point that we forget how our notions developed from figures of speech (more formally, it can be said that we accidentally confuse ontology and grammar) and from the interactional process of therapist and client taking turns talking to-

---

[1]This is only a temporary expedient since the "inside/outside" of binary pairs cannot be guaranteed; the boundary is not a barrier.

gether, that is, asking for and being given a description. It is important to remember that neither therapist nor client is doing something wrong when this happens. Rather, the fault—if there is any—lies in language itself.

## Solution Talk

It seems quite clear that one cannot solve the problem with the same kind of thinking that has created the problem. Over the years we have learned from our clients that how they judge the effectiveness of therapy is far different from how therapists (and researchers) judge or measure success. Our clients have taught us that solutions involve a very different kind of thinking and talking, a kind of talking and thinking that is outside of the "facts," outside of the problem. It is this talking outside of the problem that we call "solution talk." As client and therapist talk more and more about the solution they want to construct together, they come to believe in the truth or reality of what they are talking about. This is the way language works, naturally.

## SCALING QUESTIONS

> *For a large class of cases—though not for all—in which we employ the word "meaning" it can be defined thus: the meaning of a word is its use . . .*
> —LUDWIG WITTGENSTEIN, *Philosophical Investigations*

### Questions as Therapeutic Tools

In recent years we have come to view questions as tools for therapeutic intervention. Unlike therapists who view themselves as the expert in solution finding, we have come to realize that it is the use of words, thoughts, events, and feelings that shapes the client's reality; perceptions and behaviors. Through the exchange of misreading and misunderstanding we help clients reconstruct and reshape their reality in a way that they see as helpful.

Berg and Miller (1992) have described five kinds of questions that are useful at various times during an interview: (1) questions that elicit descriptions of pre-session change; (2) "miracle questions," that is, those that help define the client's goal(s) and illuminate the hypothetical solutions (de Shazer, 1988, 1991), (3) exceptions-finding questions, (4) coping questions that highlight the often overlooked but critical survival strategies that clients use in even the most apparently hopeless circumstances; and (5) scaling questions. In this chapter we limit our focus to a discussion of scaling questions.

Of course, numbers, like words, can be magic, as anyone who has played around with numbers knows. As is our usual practice, we took a cue from our clients and developed ways to use numbers as a simple therapeutic tool. Unlike scales that are used to measure something based on normative standards (i.e., scales that measure and compare the client's functioning with that of the general population along a bell curve), the scales we use are designed to facilitate treatment. Our scales are used to "measure" the client's own perception, to motivate and encourage, and to elucidate the goals and anything else that is important to the individual client.

## Individual and Relationship Perspectives

As indicated elsewhere (de Shazer & Berg, 1992), all the questions the therapist asks a client are attempts to elicit the following information: (1) the client's views of the problem and of solutions to it, including his or her opinions and the degree of upset, hopefulness, and willingness to work hard to solve problems, and (2) the client's perception both of important persons in his or her life and of their perception of the client. As George Herbert Mead's (1934) perceptive observations suggest, our view of ourselves is, at least in large part, dependent upon our view of how other people see us; thus, questions that help the therapist get some idea about the client's perception of his or her relationship with important people provide useful information, particularly when the client's goal is vague or treatment is mandated.

Scaling questions are used to discuss the individual client's perspective, the client's view of others, and the client's impression of others' view of him or her. (It goes without saying that the therapist asks many other types of questions that are related to scales.)

## Clinical Illustration I

The following dialogues between client (C) therapist (T) are verbatim extracts from a first session.

T:[2] How confident are you that you can stick with this? Let's say ten means you're confident that you're going to carry this out, that a year from now you'll look back and say, "I did what I set out to do." Okay? And one means you're going to back down from this. How confident are you, between ten and one?

C:  Seven.

T:  Seven?

C:  Yeah.

T:  Wow!

C:  I don't have a choice.

T:  That's true. That's true. What do you suppose Charlie's mother would say? About the same question, what do you think she would say?

[2] Insoo Kim Berg.

C: She'd give me a lower one.

T: Probably . . .

C: She'd say we never stick to what we say we are going to do.

T: How low? What would she say between ten and one?

C: Four or five.

T: Four or five?

C: Yeah.

T: Okay. What if I asked Charlie about . . .

C: Me?

T: Yeah, about Joan. What would he say? Where would he say you were at? How confident would he say he is that you're going to carry this out?

C: Three or four.

T: Three or four?

C: Yeah.

T: Lower than his mother. What about your mother? What would she say?

C: My mom would give me a one. She doesn't let me think anything.

[While both Joan and her therapist know what they mean when they each use the word "confidence," neither knows for sure what the other means when she uses that word (or any other word, for that matter). Similarly, we as authors cannot be certain that we know what our readers mean when they use the term "confidence"; nor can they be certain that they know what we mean. Each of us brings to the use of the word our entire experience with that word. While there is bound to be some similarity, some overlap in what we mean, there is naturally also a vast difference in meaning that may come into play in the conversation. Of course, the more dissimilar our experiences, the greater the chances for creative misunderstanding.

In our example the scales give the client and her therapist some idea of her degree of confidence in her ability to persist in therapy and provide them with a means of comparing it with the client's views of how other people in her life see her. This gives the therapist an opportunity to compliment the client.]

T: Somehow you have learned to disagree with all of them.

C: Uh huh.

T: And you say your friends help you do this. What if I were to ask your friends, what would they say, on the same scale, about the same question?

C: They're not so worried that I'm going to be doing the things I want to be doing. They're just worried I'm going to take Charlie back again. So, for the "everything else" [life beyond the decision about Charlie] part, I'd probably get a seven too.

[The scales also help to give both client and therapist some idea of how much support the client gets from her friends. Clearly, from the client's point of view, her friends will be more useful to her in reaching her goals (vis-à-vis the "everything else" part) than will her mother, her husband's mother, or her estranged husband.

While the differences between 7 and 4 or 5, 7 and 3 or 4, and 7 and 1 leave room for us to wonder about how realistic the client's 7 might be, her friends' 7 does give it some support. Furthermore, the 7 within this context also suggests that the client believes herself to be more determined to do what she wants to do than others see her to be, and this comparison with other people may help to reinforce that determination.]

C: They'd probably say that I was going to take Charlie back.

T: So, they're worried about that.

C: Oh, yeah.

T: Oh, they are.

C: They've been calling me every five minutes. I have friends coming over this afternoon and everything because they always are going to say, "If he calls, you're going to talk to him or you're going to let him come over."

T: So, they think Charlie is no good for you?

C: Yeah.

T: They're convinced Charlie is not good for you?

C: Yeah. They hate him.

T: They hate him.

C: Yeah.

T: So, if I were to ask your friends "What are the chances that Joan is going to take Charlie back?" (*client laughs*) what would they say, on the same scale?

C: Ten to one.

[Client switches from scaling to giving odds perhaps in response to the therapist's asking about "chances" and the therapist follows.]

T: Ten to one.

C: Probably.

T: Really? They must be worried about you.

C: Yeah. I'm worried.

T: You're worried.

C: Yeah.

T: What chances do you give yourself?

C: Probably about the same.

T: Ten to one? So, you think not taking him back is good for you?

C: Yeah.

T: Really?

C: Right.

T: You're absolutely sure about that?

C: Positive.

T: Positive. So what do you need to do to increase the odds?

C: I don't know. I always think he's going to change, he's going to be better. He's always promising to do better. And then I sometimes think, well, okay. On the one hand, I am a decent person and this and that. And then on the other one, who's going to take me with three kids? Who's going to care about me, or want to care about them, or want to be with us?

T: So, what do you have to do to increase the odds that you're not going to take him back?

C: I have no idea. *(laughs)*

T: What would your friends tell you?

C: They always tell me that I should find somebody else and if I found somebody who was decent and did treat us decently, then I'd see the difference and wouldn't want him back.

T: That's what they'd say.

C: Yeah. Which makes some sense, but in the meantime . . . *(laughs)*

T: In the meantime . . .

C: I'm home all day, every day, twenty-four hours. And the phone is right there. And if he calls, I really don't have anything else.

T: That's it?

## Constructing Exceptions

C: Well, he called last night. He just made up an excuse . . . it was something about his insurance.

T: How come you didn't weaken last night when he called?

C: 'Cause I was busy. I was doing other things. *(laughs)* And I was watching a movie.

T: Why didn't you take him back yet last night?

C: He wasn't asking that. He was just trying to, you know, but I just talked to him like I talk to anyone.

T: So if he calls and asks you to take him back, is that when you're likely to weaken?

C: Yeah. *(laughs)*

T: So if he begs and he promises all this stuff, is that what's going to happen then?

C: Yeah.

T: I see. So that's when your odds are very low.

C: Yeah.

T: Okay. So, what do you have to do to increase your odds?

C: I don't know. *(laughs)* I don't know.

T: What would your friends tell you to do to increase the odds?

C: They don't know either. They just say I should do something and keep busy and once the baby gets here I'll be able to get out more and do more . . .

T: What is a small thing you can do to increase the odds, just a little bit?

C: I don't call him. I haven't called him and usually I would have by now.

T: Is that right?

C: Oh, yeah.

T: So,

C: Whenever he calls, like, it was quarter to eleven when he called . . .

T: Wow.

C: He sounded pretty shocked that I hadn't called him.

T: Wow.

C: So I was pretty proud of myself.

T: Wow.

C: I feel better. The more he thinks that I'm going to take him back . . . and the more he acts like that, the more I feel better, like "Ha, I didn't" you know, it's . . .

T: So, your not calling him, that helps. Is that right? And what else helped yesterday? Not give in or not ask him to come back?

C: Um . . .

T: Do you ask him to come back or does he beg you to take him back?

C: Both.

T: Both ways. Okay. So, I guess one thing you can do is to figure out how you're not going to ask him to come back.

[At this point some exceptions to Joan's view of herself as helpless against both Charlie's pleas or her own loneliness have been described; thus, both Joan and her therapist know that she knows how to avoid calling and asking Charlie back (which she would usually have already done by this point in a separation), and they know she now knows how to respond when he calls—by being "busy." Since she thinks that not taking him back is good for her, these acts in the direction of her goal (which were performed prior to therapy and are precursors to the goal) can be further constructed to increase the chances for Joan's success and to bolster her confidence that she can meet her goals. Furthermore, these behaviors can be the focus of a homework task that the therapist might suggest to help Joan increase her chances for success since Joan, of course, is capable of doing more of something she already knows how to do.]

T: Which is harder for you to do: Not ask him to come back or when he begs you to take him back, not to take him back? Which is going to be harder for you, do you think?

C: Well, he sits there and says, "Yeah, you just do this because you never cared about me" and this, that, and the other. And like, "Yeah, I just pick up any stranger off the street and stay with him for three years. And have my head beat in and have three kids for anybody." You know, and he'll sit there and say, "You don't love me," and he'll come back and he'll start crying and stuff and I'll say, "Well, I don't need it unless you're going to do this, this, and this." "Oh, I will, I will." That's the end; that's it. Because I want to believe him, I really do. There are times he can be a really nice person.

T: What is the likelihood that he is going to come back to you, promising that?

C: Pretty good.

T: Is It?

C: Basically, yeah.

T: So, he is not convinced that you mean business this time.

C: No. And you can't really blame him.

T: Yeah.

C: You know . . .

T: Your record isn't too good.

C: No, it's not!

T: Right. So this time you have to really do something different to indicate to him that you mean business.

C: And I don't know what.

T: Okay.

C: I mean, I've called the attorney and done all these other things. And that should be good . . . enough. And his mom had a fit.

T: I can imagine.

C: She started screaming . . .

T: I'm sure she was mad, sure.

C: "You can't keep my grandkids away from me."

T: But you didn't back down from that.

C: No.

[Going to the attorney's and not backing down with her children's grandmother can be constructed into useful exceptions since they too run counter to Joan's picture of herself as helpless. The therapist might use these examples as focal points for compliments to Joan about her strength and resourcefulness.]

T: Let me ask you a different kind of question. Let's say ten means you have every confidence that Charlie is going to change, to turn his life around, and one means, you know, the opposite.

C: I'd give him a two.

T: A two.

C: Nothing means enough to him. He'd rather be out drinking. Or he'd rather be out with some fourteen-year-old. And the kids are only good for show when there's a family event coming up or when there's a holiday . . . that's usually when he sits and he's really nice.

T: What do you have to do to stick to your guns this time?

C: I don't know. *(laughs)*

T: You don't know.

C: I've thought about just writing down all the things that he does and just keep looking at them . . . Every day I'll write down and say what there is good about him or what he's done good for us and what he hasn't, you know.

T: That will help you to remind yourself?

C: I thought it would.

[Joan's idea about writing down the good and the bad might prove to be a useful focal point for a homework task, particularly since it is her idea. Some clients find writing/reading tasks such as this quite useful for sorting things out when they are not clear about what they are going to do or how they are going to do what they want to do.]

T: You're saying the likelihood of him changing is about two. What do you have to see him do for you to say maybe three?

C: Take us seriously and put us as a priority. Right now his job is his priority. It's like he's embarrassed of me. He doesn't take me where he goes with his friends or out with his friends at all.

T: So what will he be doing different?

C: He would! He would not be ashamed of us. He would take us with him.

T: What's the likelihood of him doing that?

C: Two. *(laughs)*

T: *(laughs)* Not very high.

C: As a matter of fact, it could be a one because he's had three years to do it and he's never done it.

## Clinical Illustration II

Even seemingly concrete numbers can be fluid and changeable as a consequence of the changing perceptions resulting from the client–therapist conversation. In this case the family's view of the miracle was followed by the therapist's curiosity about whether or not any small pieces of this miracle had ever happened.

## Constructing Pre-session Change

During the conversation with the therapist the client may indicate that things are going a little bit better since the last session. In order to affirm, validate, and further query about what has to change in order for the client to feel like the therapy has been helpful, the therapist may find that scaling questions are useful.

The following transcript is from a therapy session with a family.

The first session with the family of three included the mother and her two daughters. The mother was about to be divorced from her second husband (the children's step-father). The family's view of the solution (obtained through the "miracle question") included the children observing their mother smiling more, being happier, and being able to end her phone conversation with their stepfather sooner and without getting upset. Both the mother's and the children's view of what the children would be like when the problem was solved included the children showing their increased happiness by repeating those rare but friendly and normal talks they used to have when the mother's marriage was going reasonably well.

In the course of the conversation it came out that the night before the first session the mother had acted differently on the phone with her estranged husband. The two girls described how their mother was able to "push the fussing aside" and just hang up on her husband and walk away, instead of "getting worked up pretty hard" about what he said. All three of them agreed that it was the first time she had been able to do it since the separation.

The timing of when to ask the scaling question is important. The following conversation between the therapist (T) and family (mother, M, and daughter, D) occurred after a fair amount of discussion concerning successes:

T: *(to mother)* Let's say ten stands for how you want your life to be when you don't need to come back to see me anymore and zero stands for the worst possible period in recent weeks when you were the most worried about your family. Where would you say you are right now?

M: I would say I'm at about halfway. About half, as far as I am concerned. I would say it's lower than that for the children, particularly when I'm with them.

T: What if you take the family as a whole?

M: I would say about three and a half or four. It's the children I'm concerned about, how this divorce affects them. If it wasn't for the kids, I would walk away from this marriage with no problem. It's the kids that make me caught up in the cycle.

T: How long would you say you've been at three and a half or four?

M: Last three or four months.

T: Wow. *(Therapist then turns to the older daughter.)* What about you? Ten stands for Mom taking everything in stride, like last night, and zero stands for when she was at the worst period about being able to walk away from getting upset.

D: I would say she is at seven or nine today.

T: So from your point of view Mom has come a long way. Wow. How about the family as a whole? Where would you say the family is, from zero to ten, today?

D: Five or six.

[The difference in perception between the mother and the daughter on how the mother and the family are doing needs to be highlighted as a change. The therapist decided to utilize this as the start of a solution-focused language game (de Shazer, 1991; de Shazer & Berg, 1992). Notice the emerging changes in the mother's perception of how she went about the recent changes and its impact on the children.]

T: *(to mother)* Are you surprised to hear this?

M: No. From their point of view I've come a long way because I held my ground last night.

T: How have you done that?

M: I didn't take him back.

T: So it's been good for you and your children not to take him back?

M: Yeah, they know now I will not take him back, and it's good for them to know that. It's a pretty certain thing for them now. I've gone through being mad at him and now I'm past that. I'm still not taking him back. I will be mad for a while and when I'm okay I'll take him back. I've been okay for a while and I haven't taken him back.

T: So it's a pretty certain thing that you won't take him back?

M: Year, I'm pretty certain.

T: *(to daughter)* What do you think, how does it help you?

D: When she is happier, she is more easygoing.

T: So you could tell when Mom is happier. How does that help you?

D: Yeah, when she is happier, it's better for us.

T: So when mom makes a decision and sticks with the decision, that makes Mom happier. When Mom is happier, it makes things better for you.

D: Yeah. *(Mother looks at her daughter and nods.)*

T: *(turning to mother)* Wow, how have you done this? That must have been very hard.

M: It's hard, very hard. But I noticed in our conversation that after eight and a half years he hasn't changed. He is not going to change. Getting back is not going to make things better.

T: You are convinced of that?

M: I am convinced of that. It's good for me to go on my own. It's also good for the children, too.

It is difficult to know exactly what the mother had in mind when she described herself as at 5 and the family as a whole at 3.5 or 4. It is also not very clear what the daughter meant when she put her mother at 7 or 9 and the family at 5 or 6. Whether or not the therapist knows is unimportant. However, it is important that mother and daughter each seem to know, as far as we can tell, what the other means.

Later in the conversation the mother was asked to describe what she would be doing when she had moved up one point on the scale. The daughters were also asked what differences they thought they would notice in their mother and how those differences would affect their lives.

## CONCLUSION

*How can I say what I know with words whose signification is multiple?*
—EDMOND JABÈS

Scales allow both therapist and client to use the way language works naturally by agreeing upon terms (i.e., numbers) and a concept (a scale where 10 stands for the goal and zero stands for an absence of progress toward that goal) that is obviously multiple and flexible. Since neither therapist nor client can be absolutely certain what the other means by the use of a particular word or concept, scaling questions allow them to jointly construct a way of talking about things that are hard to describe, including progress toward the client's goal(s). For instance, a young woman thought that she was halfway toward her goal and therefore gave herself a rating of 5. When asked what would be different when her rating was 6, she simply said, "I will feel more sixish." Of course, the therapist would have preferred a more concrete and specific description, but the client was unable to describe things concretely (even though she was sure she would know when she was at 6). Here the scales give us a way to creatively misunderstand by using numbers to describe the indescribable and yet have some confidence that we, as therapists, are doing the job the client hired us to do.

## EDITOR'S QUESTIONS

Q: *I am intrigued by your notion that the therapist's job is to creatively use the misunderstandings inherent in conversation to enable change to occur. Would you elaborate on this idea?*
A: Rather than saying the therapist enables change to occur, our view is that change is constantly occurring, stability is an illusion, and change cannot be prevented. The therapist's job is to use the misunderstandings inherent in conversation to help the client notice differences so that these noticed differences can be put to work. Then these noticed differences can make a difference.

Furthermore, rather than saying that misunderstandings are "inherent in conversation," our view is that misunderstandings constitute conversations and that, in fact, misunderstandings make conversation possible. That is, if we simply (radically) understood each other, we would have nothing to talk about.

For instance, if we could *understand* what clients mean when they say "I am depressed," there would be no reason to ask them any questions. We would know precisely and exactly the past, present, and future of their condition. Without saying a word, we could give them a prescription, chemical and/or behavioral, they would say "Thanks," and that would be all there was to it. Fortunately, even our field's most positivistic endeavors (such as the *DSM*) recognize that things are not that clear-cut. So we ask questions because we know that we do not understand what clients mean when they say they are depressed.

Depression is clearly not something simple. Clients' descriptions usually involve troublesome thoughts, feelings, behaviors, attitudes, and contexts, including other people. None of the words or concepts that clients include in their descriptions are simple; because we do not understand what they say, we are led to ask further questions. And, of course, none of our words and concepts are simple, and clients ask us questions because they do not understand us. All of this conversation is based on the belief that understanding, though perhaps improbable, is possible.

Of course, clients know what they mean (at that particular time), but we cannot know. Suppose you ask a client what she means by depression, and she starts by telling you that she has not been sleeping enough. Can you have any confidence whatsoever that her not sleeping enough has prompted her to choose the term *depressed*? Or was it your question that lead to her answer? Regardless, when she starts to make her private meaning public through talking to you about her depression, the meaning that develops is automatically interactional: In the therapeutic setting, meaning is a joint product of the conversation between therapist and client.

As therapist and client continue to talk about the client's "depression" and the therapist gets more and more details about what the client means by the term, what happens to the therapist? In our experience, after 30 to 45 minutes the therapist also starts to feel and act "depressed" and, if this talk goes on much longer, begins to feel just as hopeless as the client does. And thus the therapist accidentally joins the client in doing more of the same of something that has already failed to work, namely, searching for the meaning of the term *depression,* which in effect constructs its meaning and, at least sometimes, accidentally reinforces the feelings of depression.

In our view understanding, knowing exactly what is meant by the term *depression* is impossible: Behind and/or beneath every understanding or interpretation lurks another interpretation (see the second part of our answer to the next question). Therefore, searching for "the one true meaning" is useless (when it is not deleterious). As a result, we decided (radically, perhaps) to just accept the situation as it is and thus to use our misunderstanding toward helping the client construct a solution.

Since the meanings of words and concepts are variable, and at times even undecidable (there is no way to decide what they mean with any certainty), critics of our point of view frequently jump to the conclusion that we are saying anything goes, that, for example, *depression* could mean, absurdly, *tree*. However, logic, grammar, rhetoric (in a classical sense), use, context, and, importantly, the concept's opposite (non-depression) serve as constraints on the range of potential meanings. For example, what depression is not usefully limits the possible meanings of the term. Whatever might be attended to in non-depression we call "exceptions," "miracles," and so forth.

Talking with the client about what the problem/complaint is not (i.e., talking about non-depression) is one of our ways of using misunderstanding in a creative fashion. Focusing on non-depression allows therapist and client to construct a solution, or at least begin to construct a solution, based on the client's experiences that are outside the problem area. Thus, a solution is a joint product of therapist and client talking together about whatever it is that the problem/complaint is not. Of course, we do not and cannot understand what the complaint is not any better than we can understand what the complaint is. Fortunately, talking about whatever the complaint is not (and, again, this is not something simple) seems to be useful and valuable to most clients. As they continue to talk about the non-problem/non-complaint, they are doing something different, rather than more of the same of something that has not worked. The more they talk about exceptions, miracles, and so forth, the more "real" what they are talking about becomes.

Q: *Your approach in therapy has been described as "minimalist," and the material you present here certainly fits this description. I imagine your work evolved over time in this direction. Would you discuss this process and also comment on where you see your work evolving in the future. Also, what is required of the therapist in order to stay "simple"?*
A: As William of Ockham said, "What can be done with fewer means is done in vain with many." Indeed, our work has evolved, frequently in very unexpected ways, or at least ways we did not expect. Our clients have helped us—or, better, forced us—to continue to simplify our approach. Each step along the way we have always had the mistaken idea that (1) it (doing therapy) can't be this simple and that (2) this is as simple as it (doing therapy) can get. (Of course, just because the approach is simple does not mean that doing it is easy. Far from it.) Clients continue to surprise us, and thus we expect that one of these days a client, by doing something that surprises us more than usual and/or in a different way, will force us to simplify our approach once again. We have no idea in what specific direction this might take us.

Umberto Eco (1992), describing 2nd-century Gnostics' reading of Scripture, might almost be describing our structural urge (both yours and mine), that is, the search for truth:

Each and every word must be an allusion, an allegory. They [the words] are saying something other than what they appear to be saying. Each one of them contains a message that none of them will ever be able to reveal alone. . . . Secret knowledge is deep knowledge (because only what is lying under the surface can remain unknown for long). Thus truth becomes identified with what is not said or what is said obscurely and must be understood beyond or beneath the surface of a text. The gods speak . . . through hieroglyphic and enigmatic messages. (p. 30)

Eco goes on to say that "truth is secret and any questioning of the symbols and enigmas will never reveal ultimate truth but simply displace the secret elsewhere" (1992, p. 35), to somewhere further behind or deeper beneath the surface. The urge to look behind and beneath, to understand and explain, to find the hidden secret, leads to endless iteration because we can never be certain that digging yet another level deeper is not possible. The result, of course, is structural complexity.

However, the whole structural project falls flat on its face when some-one proposes the Wittgensteinian question "But what if there is nothing behind and beneath?" What if you've got what you've got and that's all there is? Once one simplifies and abandons theory (structural or any other grand design), one is stuck with accepting what one has, however con-tradictory and cryptic, as all there is to be had. Everything is there on the surface of things, where it has always been.

Simplicity takes a lot of self-discipline. For most of us it is not easy to put aside our highly valued urge to look behind and beneath, to understand and to explain things, and thus to just describe what happens. However, because of the way language works, we can (and all too frequently do) mistakenly think that descriptions are explanations, and a muddle develops.

Q: *How can the therapist assess where in the interview to engage the client in scaling questions? For which clinical situations are these questions most useful? What has been your experience using these questions with children and adolescents?*

A: Scaling questions were first developed to help both therapist and client talk about nonspecific topics such as depression or communication. All too frequently we talk about topics like these as if the experiences depicted by these terms were controlled by an on–off switch; that is, one is thought of as either depressed or not and couples are seen as able to communicate or not. However, fortunately, it is not that clear-cut. Even people who say that they have been depressed for years will usually be able to describe times (minutes, hours, days) when they were less depressed. By developing a scale, the range of depressed feelings, and thus the complaint, is broken down into more or less discrete steps. For instance, if a scale is set up on which 0 stands for the most depressed a client has felt in recent weeks (or for how the client felt at the time of the original phone call seeking therapy) and 10 stands for the feeling on the day after the miracle, which includes being free of depressed feelings (or, at least, not being aware of any depressed feelings and therefore feeling capable of doing something that now seems impossible), then any rating above 0 not only says that things are already better but it also says that progress is being made toward the goal. The goal in this situation, no matter how vaguely and nonspecifically described, is not just the absence of depressed feelings but, rather, the achievement of 10.

Similarly, a couple's perception of how well they communicate with each other varies for each of them from time to time. With 10 standing for communicating as well as is possible for a specific couple to communicate, their joint progress and their different perceptions are simply depicted through their ratings. We frequently ask each partner to guess the other's rating, which again simply depicts progress and differences in perception as well as implying that such differences are both normal and expectable. The question is not "Who is right?" but "what does the one giving the higher rating see that the other one does not?" Thus, no matter how vaguely and nonspecifically the clients describe their situation, scales can be used to develop a useful way for therapist and clients to talk together about constructing solutions.

Scales can also be quite useful in group therapy sessions when the members of the group tend to be somewhat guarded. Scales can be thought of as content-free since only the speaker knows what he or she means by a particular number; the other group members just have to accept this fact. The therapist can discuss how the client's life will be different when he or she moves up from, say 5 to 6. The natural follow-up to this question's response is to ask what the client needs to do to move from 5 to 6. Other questions include the following: "When you move from 5 to 6, who will be the first to notice the changes in you?" "What will your mother do differently when she notices the changes in you?"

Finally, we have found that scales can be used with small children, developmentally disabled adults, and even those who tend to be very concrete. Anyone who grasps the idea that 10 is greater than 0 or that 5 on this sort of scale is better than 4 can easily respond to scaling questions.

For example, an 8-year-old child was brought to therapy following molestation by a stranger in a shopping mall. During the fourth session the therapist drew an arrow between a *1* and a *10* on the blackboard, with 10 standing for the time when therapy was finished. The therapist asked the child to indicate how far she had come in therapy by drawing an *x* on this line. The child drew her *x* at about the 7 mark. She was next asked what she thought it would take to go from *x* to 10. After several minutes, during which time she shifted her weight from one foot to the other, she hit upon an idea and said, "I know what!" "What?" asked the therapist. The little girl replied in a rather somber voice, "We will burn the clothes I was wearing when it happened." The therapist, amazed at this creative idea, said, "That's a wonderful idea!" Soon after this session the child and her parents had a ritual burning and then went out to dinner in a fancy restaurant to mark the end of therapy.

## ACKNOWLEDGMENTS

The authors wish to thank their colleagues Larry Hopwood, Jane Kashnig, and Scott Miller for their contributions to this chapter. We thank Steven Friedman for his suggestion that we include the topic of therapy as conversation as part of our discussion of a poststructural approach to looking at therapy.

## REFERENCES

Bandler, R., & Grinder, J. (1975). *The structure of magic*. Palo Alto: Science & Behavior Books.

Berg, I. K., & Miller, S. D. (1992). *Working with the problem drinker: A solution-focused approach*. New York: Norton.

Chomsky, N. (1968). *Language and mind*. New York: Harcourt, Brace, Jovanovich.

Chomsky, N. (1980). *Rules and representations*. New York: Columbia University Press.

Condillac, E. (1947). Oeuvres philosophiques de Condillac. In G. Le Roy (Ed.), *Corpus général des philosophes Français*. Paris: Presses Universitaires de France. Cited in Derrida, J. (1980). *The archeology of the frivolous* (J. P. Leavey, Trans.). Lincoln: University of Nebraska Press.

Coward, H. (1990). *Derrida and Indian philosophy*. Albany: State University of New York Press.

de Shazer, S. (1988). *Clues: Investigating solutions in brief therapy*. New York: Norton.

de Shazer, S. (1991). *Putting difference to work*. New York: Norton.

de Shazer, S., & Berg, I. K. (1992). Doing therapy: A post-structural re-vision. *Journal of Marital and Family Therapy, 18,* 71–81.

Eco, U. (1992). *Interpretation and overinterpretation*. Cambridge, UK: Cambridge University Press.

Harland, R. (1987). *Superstructuralism: The philosophy of structuralism and post-structuralism*. London: Methuen.

Jabès, E. (1959). *Je bâtis ma demeure: Poèmes, 1943–1957*. Paris: Galimard. Translation cited in Derrida, J. (1978). *Writing and difference* (A. Bass, Trans.). Chicago: University of Chicago Press.

Mead, G. H. (1934). *Mind, self and society*. Chicago: University of Chicago Press.

Saussure, F. (1922). *Cours de linguistique générale*. Paris: Payot.

Wittgenstein, L. (1972). *Tractatus Logico-Philosophicus* (corrected 2nd ed.; D. F. Pears & B. F. McGuinness, Eds. and Trans.). London: Routledge.

Wittgenstein, L. (1968). *Philosophical Investigations* (3rd ed.; G. E. M. Anscombe, Trans.) New York: Macmillan.

# 2

## *"Both/And" Solutions*

### EVE LIPCHIK

It seems like only yesterday that I was sitting around with Steve de Shazer and Insoo Berg and the rest of the team (Jim Derks, Marilyn LaCourt, and Elam Nunnally) in Milwaukee brainstorming about the new therapeutic model we were going to develop. The work being done at the Brief Therapy Center at the Mental Research Institute in Palo Alto and by Palazzoli and her colleagues in Milan and the publications by Bateson and about Erickson served as our guidelines and inspiration. Now, nearly 15 years later, the solution-focused model that evolved has earned a place in the field of family therapy (de Shazer, 1985; de Shazer, 1988; de Shazer et al., 1986) and has become the foundation on which others base their work (Dolan, 1991; O'Hanlon & Weiner-Davis, 1989; Walter & Peller, 1992).

One of the most exciting things about working with this group was the constant change and growth. Our work was an ongoing recursive process in which practice informed theory and the testing of that theory affected practice. This process has continued for me in a different context since I left the Brief Family Therapy Center in Milwaukee in 1988. Undoubtedly, it has taken a different turn than it would have if I had stayed.

### THEORETICAL FOUNDATION

I don't know what to call what I do now. I think of it as an extension of the solution-focused model. The parts that I have developed since I left grew out of the questions that my trainees, colleagues who consult with me, and I had about what to do when things did not work as expected. It is also the further development of thoughts I have had for many years about interviewing (Lipchik & de Shazer, 1986; Lipchik, 1988a, 1988b) and solutions being a sense of rebalancing (Lipchik & Vega, 1985).

My present solution-focused model assumes clients come to therapy because they perceive themselves as stuck, usually in an "either/or" frame. The constraints of their perception of a totally negative frame make them experience their options as nonexistent or very limited and see solutions in unrealistically positive terms. The therapist operates on the assumptions that clients have inherent strengths and resources to find solutions and that, like most things in life, these solutions will be "both/and," (somewhere between the worst and the best scenarios) rather than "either/or." The process of solution construction occurs within the context of a therapeutic system that consists of the therapist and client(s). The participants interact in a recursive process (verbal and nonverbal) during which they all give and receive information on which they base their continuing responses. The therapist steers this process, which is actually directed by clients' goals. This is done first with questions and observations that help them define what they really want in a behaviorally recognizable manner and, secondly, by searching for, highlighting, and reinforcing exceptions to their perceived problem and both past and potential strengths. The perceptual and emotional shifts that occur for clients when their views are not only validated but expanded to include positives also generate hope. This hope is fanned by discussions of future options, rather than dampened by explanations of the problem or recitations of past failures.

Experience has taught me, however, that a positive focus on the future is often not enough to help clients achieve what they ultimately define as their goals. There are times when clients begin to experience positive changes toward their stated goals and yet behave as though they have not noticed this; they may consider their progress not good enough or may present with new problems. They appear to be in a quandry about whether to move forward toward something beyond their problem reality.

So I have begun to think of the search for exceptions and descriptions of hypothetical solutions in the future as only the first phase of construction. When clients choose not to use obvious strengths and exceptions as building blocks for solutions, we begin the second phase. This is when we talk about how to determine the right degree of balance between their "bad" presenting situation and their "good" stated goals.

A solution must have a unique fit for individuals in that it must represent a balance of good and bad that is acceptable to them at a particular time and in a particular situation. This means that problems and solutions are relative, not absolute, concepts and that neither therapist nor client should think of them as carved in stone. Talking about them as vacillations on the continuum of life seems much more useful for the therapeutic interaction.

I think of human systems as composed of individuals with a unique genetic and social heritage in interaction with each other. While these interactions take place on many levels (e.g., perceptual, emotional, cognitive, and behavioral), the quality of one's life is usually experienced and described in emotional terms. McKeel (personal communication, February 1992) suggested an interesting perspective when he said that it is easier and faster to think about changing emotional reactions than to think about solutions to problems.

I sense with all my clients (regardless of their origins, education, economic status, race, or color) the desire to be loved and affirmed by a significant other or others. This starts at birth, when emotional fulfillment is first triggered by physiological needs, and increases in complexity throughout life.

I think of the individuals, couples, and families who present with problems (not necessarily those who are referred involuntarily) as having reached a point of such personal discomfort in their relationships (or absence of relationships) that they no longer know what to do for relief. This discomfort may manifest itself or be expressed in various ways, depending on the individual, but I think of it as emotionally based. This leads me to think of my role in the therapeutic system as one that will generate new options for the family system to rebalance its individual, and therefore reciprocal emotional comfort levels (as long as these options are ethical and safe). I do not consider myself an expert on my clients' problems and their solutions. What I can offer is my philosophy and assumptions about helping people, my education, my intuition, and my experience. I can also create and maintain a climate in which my clients can feel safe, comfortable, accepted, and understood in interaction with me so that they can move on with their lives more comfortably. The clients' part of that systemic interaction is to contribute their understanding of their situation, their goals, and their unique way of seeing the world. The clients and I are not equals in that I, as a paid professional, have a responsibility to try to help them get unstuck somehow, but we are equal in the sense that neither they nor I can "know" how they can achieve greater emotional comfort.

I have found the interpersonal theory of Harry Stack Sullivan influential in developing these ideas. Except for the methodology, Sullivan's approach resonates with the systemic and constructivist ideas of today. In direct contrast to the biologically based theories of Freud, so popular in his day, Sullivan's thinking reflects our own current interest in the influence of fields such as anthropology, linguistics, communications, and social theories. In 1930 he wrote the following:

> The general science of psychiatry seems to me to cover the same field as that which is studied by social psychology, because scientific psychiatry has to be defined as the study of interpersonal relations, and this in the end calls for the use of the kind of conceptual framework that we now call *field theory*. From such a standpoint, personality is taken to be hypothetical. That which can be studied is the pattern of processes which characterize the interaction of personalities in particular recurrent situations or fields which "include" the observer. (Perry & Gawel, 1953, p. 368)

As for the process of therapy, Sullivan wrote that "with the utmost flexibility that you can muster, you must engage in a vibrant give-and-take dialogue with the patient. The direction of this dialogue is unpredictable. There are no guidelines, but only general principles, and human difficulties are too variable to allow dogmatic generalizations" (Chapman, 1976, p. 75). Indeed, "the therapist should never assume that he knows what the patient is talking about" (Chapman, 1976, p. 208).

What has been particularly meaningful to me in this, aside from reminding me that already-existing knowledge in our field may be a valuable resource on which to build new knowledge, is Sullivan's idea that all symptoms are "anxiety." This term is not to be thought of in the sense of today's DSM-III-R description but, rather, as emotional discomfort, a "tension in opposition to the tensions of needs and to actions appropriate to their relief" (Perry & Gawel, 1953, p. 44).

I have felt for years that the bottom line for human beings—regardless of race, color, nationality, culture, level of education, or wealth—is the internal state of comfort resulting from the affirmation or caring experienced in relation to others. So Sullivan's ideas serve as a useful underpinning for my own thinking about helping people regain emotional comfort by identifying the positives in relation to the negatives and defining a fitting balance between the two.

## CLINICAL PRACTICE

In translating all this to practice, I first start by asking clients about exceptions to problems, positive aspects of their lives, and possible future solutions. The answers may produce enough of a difference in the existing view of their situation to allow for solution construction. But if not, I ask as many questions as possible to help my clients perceive their situation from a perspective other than the "either/or" approach. This includes quantifying the complaint in relation to exceptions and possible solutions and translating these numbers into recognizable behaviors. It also means helping clients to consider possible options and to perceive the problem as "both/and" (the advantages as well as the so obvious disadvantages). This process substitutes a sense of control (choices clients were not aware of) for the emotional discomfort caused by perceived lack of control.

I always start out by telling clients about the one-way mirror in my room and the cameras. I invite them to meet the cotherapists behind the mirror, if there are any there, and explain that these people may call in questions during the session. Frequently, I do not work with a cotherapist. I also talk to clients about the purpose and confidentiality of taping sessions and the need for written permission for tapes to be used for purposes other than their therapy.

My sessions usually last an hour. After 45 minutes I break to consult with my partners or think by myself about the interview. While out of the room I compose a summation message, which I present to the client upon my return. This happens at the end of every session.

I have given much thought to how to integrate the solution-focused intervention message with my present theoretical stance, and I have decided to think of it more as a summation. The wording of this summation starts with "What I heard you say today was," which is followed by what I think the client was trying to tell me; the summation continues with "And my response to that is," followed by a repetition and reinforcement of those exceptions and positives that the clients mentioned or that I noticed. This part of the summary also includes normalizing statements, new information about stages of relationships or child development, and some ideas about things clients might want to do between sessions. This format is a better fit with my present concept of the simultaneous giving and receiving of information by all parts of the therapeutic system than the former one in which I came back more in the role of an expert who gave compliments and prescribed tasks.

I also believe that a break between interview and summary is useful for everyone. It provides an opportunity for a more detached review of the interview outside of each other's presence. For the clients the anticipation of the therapist's comments, including a message that assures them of the therapist's understanding and acceptance, results in an open mind, known as the "yes set" in Ericksonian hypnosis. Since this format also provides a good chance to rectify any misunderstanding before clients leave the session, it improves the chances that the response part of the therapist's summation will be received with as open a mind as possible. And this open-mindedness increases the likelihood that the therapist's comments will make a difference for the client between sessions.

Tasks, when given, are presented very casually and as a choice. I have found that the technique of using the customer, complainant, and visitor (de Shazer, 1988, pp. 87–89) categories to determine how to present tasks to the client, while useful as a guideline for the therapist, has a disadvantage. It may prevent the therapist from saying things to clients that could be useful for them. After all, clients will do only what they want to do, and often "visitors" decide they want to be "customers" or vice versa.

## CLINICAL EXAMPLE

Marilyn is a 30-year-old white female. She is married, has a 19-month-old child, and works part-time as a speech pathologist. I treated her 5 years ago for five sessions shortly after she was married. At the time, Marilyn, an adopted only child, was experiencing a great deal of stress with her father, a loving but controlling man whom she has tried to please all her life. Her mother has had periodic problems with alcohol abuse.

Marilyn married Jim, a nurturing, healthy man who was supportive of her relationship with her parents. He had won the struggle with Marilyn's father for acceptance as a future son-in-law with patience and understanding. He was, however, beginning to get tired of helping Marilyn deal with almost daily struggles over how to be both a good wife and a good daughter and had urged her to talk to someone. He was willing to participate in the treatment, if necessary.

Treatment centered around helping Marilyn think about how her father reacted when she did not conform to his demands, how she reacted to his reactions, and what options she had for feeling like a good daughter without doing all his bidding. Jim attended the first two sessions, and then Marilyn came alone to work on gaining control of the situation. She discovered that she was able to refuse her father's demands without feeling guilty as long as she also chose to do things she thought would please him. She had stopping doing that for some time because she had been so angry with him. This solution proved to work well for the young couple and for Marilyn's parents. For mother it had the benefit of reducing her need to drink, since father felt more secure in his daughter's love and was less critical and demanding of his wife.

About six months ago I had a call from Marilyn. She told me that she and Jim had decided it might be good for her to come in and talk to me about her "eating disorder." I asked if she thought Jim should come with her, and she said no.

The clinical work presented here took place over a period of 3 months and consisted of five individual sessions with the client. I worked alone except for the last session, when I had a team behind the mirror. (In the following dialogue C designates the client and T my comments as therapist.)

T: Well, so how have you been?
C: Pretty good.
T: *(looking at face sheet)* I see you have a little boy.
C: Yes, nineteen months.
T: Nice. Are you having fun with him?
C: Oh yes, he's lots of fun.
T: How's Jim?
C: He's good. He works second shift now, and I work mornings three times a week so it's really working out. We don't have to get a baby-sitter.
T: How are you doing with your father?
C: Not bad. He still makes comments here and now that I just let fly. I sometimes call my mom and complain to her about it, but I've avoided any arguments with him, so . . .
T: You must feel very proud of yourself.
C: Very . . . very . . . because that was a very big issue for me . . . a big problem.

T: Well, what brings you here today?

C: I've had a weight problem all my life and I am losing control more and more, you know, and putting on more and more weight and I just feel like there is some reason that I can't control that . . . my eating habits . . .

T: Was there a time when you could? [I immediately look for an exception.]

C: When I belonged to Weight Watchers. At that time I lost thirty pounds, but gradually I just went back to the old habits . . . and . . . you know . . . I don't know . . . my goals aren't to have the amount of weight loss I achieved at that time. You know at Weight Watchers they make you weigh and measure everything. Eating two teaspoons of margarine instead of one is not my problem. That's not what I want to do; it's the bingeing that's the problem.

[This is the first definition of the problem as bingeing. I also hear that the client does not want a solution that includes structure.]

T: Right . . . right . . . how often do you binge?

C: Daily.

T: What does that mean?

C: It means I go through the cabinets and the refrigerator and eat anything I find. If I don't find anything, I go to the basement, where we stock things, to find crackers or something.

T: How do you explain this to yourself . . . that you do this?

[I ask myself how I can best join her. I need to understand her meaning of this.]

C: It's a long-term thing. Ever since . . . probably I would say grade school or early high school . . .

T: Oh really? And daily?

C: Once in a while when I go on a diet . . . for a while . . . it stops . . . but, generally, yes.

T: Through the beginning of your marriage and everything?

C: Um. I try to analyze it, and it's just . . . I don't know . . . it's not necessarily when I'm depressed. I can't associate it with one emotion or another . . . I just can't explain it.

T: It's probably a habit by now.

[Since client spoke about eating as a "habit" twice, I join her in that thinking.]

C: Yeah, and it's so irrational, and while I'm eating like that I think, "This is ridiculous," and then I start getting depressed.

T: So the only time you don't do that is when you decide to go on a diet?

[Client starts on a negative tangent, and I go back to the exception to keep her on a positive track.]

C: Yes. When I was on Weight Watchers that was the longest time . . . probably four months . . . but then I go back into it, gradually, but now I'm up to when it was the worst ever.

[Client goes back to negative frame. I can't pursue the Weight Watchers exceptions and differences because she has already told me she doesn't want the structure of a diet but wants to develop the habit of self-control. Exceptions talk about this would be a difference that would not make a difference. I decide to explore the context.]

T: What does Jim think?

C: He . . . you know, I cry and say I have to get control . . . and when I join Weight Watchers he thinks it's a good idea but then he's had this attitude all along that I'm not going to maintain this way of eating. I like all the fatty foods. I've joined Weight Watchers three or four times since I lost all that weight and I never stick to it.

T: Yes . . . yes . . .

C: He's the only one I ever talk to about it because it's so embarrassing, but he's getting kind of tired of it.

[My impression at this time was that Jim may have shown signs of giving up on trying to be supportive around the eating issue, just as years before he had tired of dealing with the issue of his father-in-law. In response to questions about what she needed from her husband now Marilyn said that he wanted her to accept herself as she was and to stop struggling to lose weight but that she wanted to learn to control the eating.

We explored the details of Marilyn's stated goal, namely, not binge-ing. Apparently, she would start to look for food as soon as her husband left for work and would then eat for about an hour. Did she think it had anything to do with his leaving? She did not. What would she eat? In particular she liked lunch meats like bologna and liverwurst, crackers of all kinds, junk food, and peanut butter, which she would eat out of the jar like ice cream. Lately, she found herself eating cold leftovers from the refrigerator as well. She would eat a regular dinner around five-thirty and then binge again for about 20 minutes after putting the baby to bed at seven. She said she always ate in front of the TV, which was located in the kitchen. When she was busy she ate less, but she often found herself feeling too "lazy" to do the many projects around the house she could do. At those times she got stuck in front of the TV, felt angry at herself for being there, and then started to eat. Weekends were reported not to be as bad, although Marilyn would binge occasionally when her husband was out of the house. "I don't eat like that in front of anyone, even Jim," she said. Her perceptions of exceptions were un-predictable and vague no matter how I persisted: "When I am busier," was her reply.

I decided to talk with Marilyn about choices and options, as opposed to being totally out of control.]

T: If you were to choose to eliminate some of these snacks, which would they be? What would you miss the least?

C: Probably crackers.

T: Would you want to cut them out totally or just cut down?

C: I don't know how to approach this *with myself.*

[To me this means the client is thinking she has to make this change on her own, without Jim, and therefore I must help her make the choices that are best for her.]

Should I avoid totally or cut down?

T: What do you think is better for you?

C: I find that once I get started it is hard to stop; it's best not to start at all.

T: Is it realistic to expect not to snack at all when you are alone all afternoon and evening? Isn't that being too hard on yourself?

[The "either/or" frame changes to "both/and."]

C: No, if I could make it a planned snack—so many crackers, so much cheese—it might be fine, but once I start it's like a force coming over me. But no, it's not realistic not to snack at all.

T: So, ideally, if a miracle happened and you find you have control over the situation tomorrow, what will you be doing differently?

C: Probably I'll eat a little bit of chips . . . junk food, popcorn . . . and also I'll eat . . . if we have leftover spaghetti . . . I find myself eating that cold . . . that started recently. I would definitely not do that; that's like eating another dinner.

T: Ideally, then, when you are in control you will have a snack in the afternoon and after dinner, but you will choose . . . and it will preferably be junk food . . . maybe not all the time . . . maybe a specific amount of cheese and crackers.

[I try to keep the client in the future.]

C: Yes.

T: What do you imagine . . . how much . . . right now you feel like you are out of control . . . what percent of the time would you say that is?

[I work on finding a balance between total lack of control and what the client perceives as control.]

C: Ninety percent.

T: How much control do you think you would have to gain to feel comfortable?

C: At least seventy-five to eighty percent in control.

T: Okay and . . . well, that is not going to happen right away. Ninety percent out of control to seventy-five percent in control . . . big leap. How will you begin to see a five percent change? What will that look like to you?

[Small changes can be accomplished more easily and, when noticed, will give hope and motivation to keep on trying.]

C: Either stop sooner and have one or two days when I'm not . . . let's say five days, ten binges, eliminate one or two or five percent . . . something like that.

T: Which do you think is easier for you—stopping sooner or eliminating some?

[Choice!]

C: Probably eliminating one or at least change it to like a snack, you know, instead ot a binge . . . allowing myself something but not allowing myself to be out of control.

T: So when you choose a time and what to eat, when that happens, what do you imagine you will have to do to stick to that and not feel dissatisfied?

C: Probably do something . . .

T: Like?

C: I can be more in control when I keep myself busy.

[This is the exception she mentioned before, but she won't really elaborate. Next, we explored what Marilyn meant by keeping herself busy. She said she would have to be more conscious of the things she liked to do instead of getting in front of the TV and "shutting off." She felt a written list would not help because she did not like lists; if she made a list, she said, it would have to be a mental list. She also came up with another reason why she needed to have control: The people she worked with were all slim and diet-conscious, and she was afraid they all thought of her as a person who lacked control. Her husband thought this fear was ridiculous.

I decided to look for what I think of as the positive exceptions to the negatives in order to help Marilyn see things more "both/and."]

T: I know this question may sound strange to you. I want you to realize that I am hearing your stress and concern, but what would you say is the advantage of having this problem?

[I specifically word the question this way to let the client know I am not minimizing the extent of her problem and distress.]

C: That's a good question. I dont' really know . . . Well, I am finding that I don't go up to people I know, say in a restaurant. Maybe I use it as an excuse to do that. I don't know.

T: Why would you want to avoid that?

C: Because I feel fat.

T: Anything else?

C: I can eat as much as I want to and not think about it; that saves a lot of energy.

T: How can you have these advantages without having the problem you came in for?

[Options!]

C: Hm . . . stopping fighting with myself, I guess.

T: Fighting with yourself?

C: Oh, you know, telling myself I should not be eating so much but wanting to anyway.

T: Is that what happens when you binge?

C: Yes, that's really the problem, being angry at myself for wanting to eat.

T: Are there times when you don't do that?

[The client has now redefined the problem as being angry with herself so I seek an exception.]

C: Only when I keep busy, but I just can't keep busy all afternoon and evening.

[As I try to pursue why she is less angry with herself when she keeps busy, I experience the client as not wanting to engage in conversation about this or other positives. Therefore, I look to past solutions.]

T: What do you think made the difference for you when you came to see me after your marriage?

C: You gave me . . . I remember . . . ugh . . . you asked me what my options were in how to deal with my father, and I had never thought what *my* options were. One of them was not to have contact with my parents. That was one of the things I remember. [This was an "either/or" option.] I did not want that. You made me think of how I wanted to approach this and just asked me questions that gave me ideas.

T: What are your options now?

[Not "are there options" because I want to presuppose they exist.]

C: Either accepting things as they are or getting under control.

T: What are some of the options between those two?

[After we talked about various options to not fighting with herself about eating, Marilyn decided that it would help if she definitely stopped eating peanut butter out of the jar or ice cream out of the box. But she emphasized again that she did not really want to give up the enjoyment of eating, nor did she want a rigid structure around it. She also shared with me the fact that she had suffered an early miscarriage a few months earlier and was relieved in a way because she did not want to start a pregnancy so overweight. This made me think she had not committed herself to her goal and was still hoping for a miracle that would help her lose weight without effort.

Forty-five minutes had gone by, and it was time for me to take my break. Afterward, I presented my summation message to Marilyn.]

T: What I heard you say today is that you want to deal with a habit you have had since your high school days, late adolescence, fighting with yourself about eating what you want to eat and as much of it as you want to eat, and that it bothers you not only because of how it makes you feel about yourself but also what other people might think about you. You feel that at this time you want individual attention to get control over this problem, not a group program, and that you don't want an eating routine that is very structured and that you won't be able to keep up later. Your husband seems to be giving up on supporting your struggle and is trying to convince you to accept yourself the way you are, as he does.

I also heard you say you were very successful in keeping control of your relationship with your father since I saw you and that what helped you then was to think of options that you had. *(Client nods vigorously throughout.)*

My response is that your decision now makes a lot of sense since you are a person who when she makes up her mind to do something does it. If you chose this time to do it, there must be a good reason for it. You have a lot of understanding of what works for you and what doesn't, and since thinking through options worked for you before, that may work for you again.

C: Maybe I'm unrealistic to want to have it just happen just like that.

[The client is giving me new information, and I must give a new response.]

T: That may be. It may take a little time for you to figure out how you can best stop fighting and get the right amount of control you want, the options that you have. I am not sure, but maybe it would help to think of options for what type of snacking you want to do, at what times, what kinds of options you have for keeping busy. You might even want to try out some of these options by choosing in the morning how you want to snack and keep busy that day and see whether you like that or not.

[I mention the types of options she herself suggested during the session.]

C: Good, I'll do that. I just want to reach my prepregnancy weight and get a hold of myself.

[Client vacillates on goal again and suggests she wants weight control.]

## Second Session: Two Weeks Later

T: So what happened that you want to continue to have happen?

C: It was hard, very hard. Sometimes I wonder if it's even possible. I tried all the options religiously the first week, wrote it down, planned it, wrote it down. Then the second week I did it verbally . . . and didn't do so well.

T: Tell me about the first week and what worked.

[The client described being motivated the first week and then losing interest in the process. I questioned her in detail about the successful behaviors and learned that she had stopped eating peanut butter and ice cream and had substituted saltines for more fatty crackers. She did not take well to my enthusiasm about these changes and qualified her success by saying, "Well, some days it worked and some days it didn't." When I asked "But does that mean that overall you ate less the last two weeks than before?" she replied, "Oh, sure, much less overall, but I also know that I compensate for eating less in one area by overeating in another." This made me think that she was really not clear about what it was she wanted and that unless we were both clear about that our conversation would not go anywhere.]

T: I guess I'm not clear at this time what our focus is. You said last time you want to stop bingeing and have more control over your eating but now I think I hear you say you want to accept yourself more . . . even if you can't change your eating habits suddenly. Is that right? What do you want to work on first?

C: Maybe taking it a day at a time. There were a few days when I did not snack at all.

T: What did you do instead?

[The client's answer implies accepting the fact that change will go slowly, so I join her on that track.]

C: Well, Ash Wednesday was one day; that gave me a reason.

T: What did you do instead?

[It is important to make client think of substitute behaviors.]

C: Oh, I had it all written down, and I found things around the house to do instead. If I can do it one day or two, why can't I just *do* it?

[Client is rejecting the positive focus again.]

T: You sound so angry with yourself.

C: I am. The whole issue is a control issue. I know other people have the problem too, but I look at all my friends. They don't even have to think about it. Why can they and I can't? Maybe food just doesn't have the same meaning in their lives.

[I questioned the client about areas in her life in which she did accept herself and she described herself in positive terms as a mother, wife, daughter, professional, and friend but not in terms of control over her eating and body image. I wanted her to put this issue of eating into perspective and to view it with respect to the rest of her life.]

T: What percentage of your life as a whole does the eating part play?

C: Fifteen to twenty percent.

T: So about eighty percent of the time you feel in control?

C: Yes, but with the eating only I feel out of control almost all the time.

T: Do you think you can develop that control slowly or does it have to happen immediately?

C: Just having the support, individual support, and allowing myself to accept myself will help.

T: If things can only get better gradually, how will you keep yourself from being angry at yourself?

C: That's why I'm here.

T: Well, if there is nothing else you want to discuss today I will take a break and summarize what we talked about.

C: Okay.

T: What I heard you say today is that you realize that your goal for coming here is actually to stop being angry with yourself because of your eating habits and to accept your behavior and what you think others think about it, about controlling your eating, that is. You came in with the expectation to get immediate control. You say your husband says you are okay the way you are and you should accept yourself like he accepts you, but you think if you accept yourself you'll get heavier and heavier.

My response is that you seem to be on the right track by redefining your goal as self-acceptance. It seems to me that it is possible that the more you fight yourself the less energy you may have to find options that fit for you. I wonder what you think about changing the way you fight with yourself: Instead of doing it all day long, choose to fight and not fight on alternate days; one day you make sure you fight all day and the next you don't fight at all and accept yourself.

C: I don't know how I could stop it for a day.

T: But you told me you have done that already at times.

C: I don't think I could stop the internal argument.

T: How did you do it before?

C: Well, with a reason—like Lent or paying Weight Watchers. But I could try this. What should I do?

[She wants both to conform and not to.]

T: On the days you aren't supposed to fight, anytime you experience the struggle inside you, tell yourself you have to postpone it for tomorrow because today you can do anything you please. On the alternate days give yourself permission to find every possible opportunity to fight with yourself because the next day you won't be able to.

[The idea is to prescribe the same behavior but to change the pattern somehow.]

C: Okay, I'll try that. So what I am working toward is . . . ? I don't know if that part of me would shut off.

T: Would you be shutting if off or postponing it?

C: I think it would work better for me if I did it in smaller pieces. I think I would allow myself to argue with myself in the afternoon and leave the not arguing toward the end of the day when I am tired, when I have less energy to keep that argument going; work on it in the afternoon and allow myself to be myself in the evening. I can see that working better than a whole day at a time.

[Client chooses another option and asserts herself against someone else's control.]

T: Any way that you think it will work for you is fine. I just caution you not to expect too much too soon.

One might ask why I made suggestions for structured tasks when the client said she did not want structure. It was apparent to me that she was using the information from our sessions to allow herself to change gradually, but in her own way. She wanted suggestions from me and also needed to find her own way. I gave her both and then gradually challenged her view of the balance of things. This pattern is not unusual for people struggling with dependence–independence, and it plays itself out in therapy the same way: They ask for help but don't want to feel it helped them. This has to be pointed out eventually so that the client can take responsibility for committing to a direction for the future rather than becoming dependent on the therapist to keep reinforcing small changes that are never enough.

## Third Session: Two Weeks Later

From Marilyn's first comments it seemed as though she had not been at the second session at all. She reported that she was doing better in working toward the goal of bingeing less but had actually gained some weight and now wanted to work on losing weight. On closer questioning it became apparent that she had tried something different and that it was working. She was thinking much less about eating in the evenings, when she gave herself permission to "be herself" and not fight with herself. However, she insisted on clinging to the rationale that the change was due to the fact that her husband was around a little more and that she had had more things to do in general. She agreed that she was gaining control gradually but felt that it was not enough. She always seemed to find a reason not to be satisfied; for example, she said, "The thing that worries me though is that I'm just in a phase. I'll really work at something for a while and then lose interest. This is a lifetime thing and I'm not sure I'll ever get over it."

When she implied that she has a lifetime pattern of not maintaining changes I picked up on this. I wanted to remind her of an important exception: She had reported earlier that the resolution of her problem with her father had lasted 5 years. Marilyn agreed, but qualified it by saying that while she no longer lets her father interfere with her marriage she still feels she never was and never will be good enough for him. She admitted that his occasional criticism still bothered her in spite of the fact that she could honestly tell herself that she had always been and still is a good daughter who tried to please her father.

At the end of the session I chose this theme for the summation message. I said that I still heard her describing struggles within herself over whether to please her father or herself, and I suggested that she might find it helpful whenever she felt unaccepting of herself to ask herself whether that was her father's way of thinking about her or what she wanted to think of herself.

## Fourth Session: Three Weeks Later

Marilyn's first comment was that she might have been a little less angry at herself during the preceding three weeks. She said she was angry 50% of the time and that was "not good enough." She also reported that she had followed the suggestion I made at the end of the last session, and what had happened was that she began to feel as though there were a rebellious child inside her who was making her eat because that child had never been able to get her own way in the past, this behavior being her way of coming out and asserting herself. "It's like she's saying, 'This is what I really want to do and no one is going to stop me.' My line of questioning around this significant insight was about what Marilyn, as an adult who feels competent in all other areas except eating habits, could do to handle this rebellious child. She could not come up with answers that didn't echo the dilemma of choice, so I decided to confront the dilemma more directly in terms of how it played itself out in therapy. I asked Marilyn what her experience with therapy had been so far around this issue. She replied, "I always feel good about myself when I leave, [with] you the objective observer making me realize it's not logical, and then my objectivity gradually goes. I don't know how to change it. Maybe I'm lazy." I wondered whether there were other options.

C:  Maybe I should just concentrate on accepting myself.

   [Obviously, the client had not really committed to what we had redefined as the new goal until this time. What clients say may have different meanings for them at different stages in therapy, so it is important for therapists to repeat certain questions or themes throughout treatment.]
T:  How would that . . . what would that mean to you, accepting yourself? How could you both eat with enjoyment and accept yourself?
C:  I won't have these bad feelings about myself, and I think that the way they seem to come out is through the eating issue.
T:  That is the symptom of your feeling bad about yourself?
C:  Its my worst fault, the thing I'm most mad at myself for.
T:  Okay! So if that is what you want to accomplish here, how will you know you are accepting yourself more?

C: Not having bad feelings about myself again and not hearing that old tape "You have no control."

T: How did you learn to accept yourself in other situations?

C: I don't know. There aren't many other areas I don't accept myself in.

T: How about as a daughter?

C: I realized I was not a bad daughter; it wasn't my problem. It wasn't me bringing on the problem, but this situation is just me.

T: So if you were to think of yourself as both accepting and judgmental—critical, like you used to think of your father—how could you respond differently to yourself?

C: I let him say what he wants to say and do what I want.

T: So how could that translate to being critical of your eating habits?

C: I guess I'd have to tell that part to shut up.

T: That's not how you handle your father.

C: I ignore him.

T: Could you do that to your own criticism?

C: Yes, I think that's what I have been doing even without realizing when I feel better. I say this is what I choose to do right now.

T: Just the week after you come in here or later too?

C: It's better all the time, although it is much better right after I see you.

T: Would you say that as we are working together the percentage of your doing that has increased, that it's not either/or at this point? How much more accepting are you now than before?

[Quantifying feelings concretizes them and provides a much better measure of change.]

C: Thirty to forty percent more.

T: At the beginning you said that you were only ten percent okay, and now that is thirty to forty percent more. That puts it at fifty percent better.

C: Now my goal is different though. When I came in it was to lose weight; not anymore. My clothes didn't fit me, so I went out and bought new clothes. That's a sign of accepting myself.

T: How wonderful! That's great!

C: I know I could lose ten pounds in three weeks if I wanted to, but I just wouldn't. So I finally thought, Well, I'll buy clothes I feel attractive in," but then I wonder, "Am I just copping out?"

T: What is your answer to that?

C: That this is how I am right now. If I can accept myself the way I am now, maybe in a year I'll be lighter . . . or something else will happen . . . I want to get pregnant. I want to stop thinking of it as though it's either totally good or bad.

T: Right now how has that balance changed for you?

C: My feelings about my eating have changed so that I am much more accepting of my eating habits, but my eating is the same . . . well almost . . . sometimes better, sometimes worse.

T: Do you think you could accept making different choices for yourself at different times?

C: Hm, that's where I'm stuck.

T: Acceptance isn't being uncritical, but it's a perspective on your whole self . . . If one is not perfect in one area, one is not all bad; one also has to accept that at times one is better in certain areas than in others.

[At this point I wondered whether self-acceptance was possible as long as the client was coming to see me to work on changing herself.]

At the end of the session I presented the following summation:

T: I hear you saying you are making progress but it is not bringing you results quickly enough. I also heard you say that you are clear now that your main goal is to accept yourself, regardless of your eating habits.

My response is that I think you are on the right track, but the only way to be accepting of yourself is to stop trying to change yourself for a while and to let what happens happen, to stop and see how things go when you just let go of trying to change yourself . . . maybe for a month or so. Of course, you will still get the critical thoughts sometimes. Some people deal with them by setting aside ten minutes a day just for that purpose, for thinking all the critical thoughts they have during the rest of the day. I know you don't like to write things down. Some people find it useful to write down the critical thoughts at that time and then to tear them up and throw them away. You'll have to find other ways to dispose of them. See what happens!

## Fifth Session: Five Weeks Later

During this termination session I had a team behind the mirror. Marilyn came in reporting that she was feeling good because she had just found out that she was 5 weeks pregnant, which was beyond the time when she had her miscarriage last time. "So much has happened since I saw you last," she reported. Jim had taken her on a romantic weekend for two, which she interpreted as his way of trying to convince her that he accepted her as desirable just the way she was. She went on to say she was feeling better about everything because she was accepting herself and "looking at the good points as well as the bad." The pregnancy had changed her attitude about eating for the time being, but she said she was more in control there too. The major change reported was that she was not fighting with herself as much. "It's such a relief," she said, "just like when I finally stopped fighting with my dad." I asked how this new development affected her daily life, and she said that it kept her from getting depressed.

T: What was it about the way you ate—was it the weight that bothered you or the fact that you were doing something out of control—which affected you more?

C: It's hard to say; probably it's equal. No, the weight was secondary. What made me mad at myself was I was out of control.

T: When you came to see me about your father, was that the same or different? How would it compare?
   [I try to link this change to one that was permanent.]

C: Hm, I'm not sure I understand.

T: Is there something similar about having felt out of control in relationship to your father and with food? Did both make you feel angry at yourself because you felt you had no control?

C: I think so. I definitely felt I had no control and he had all; once I gained control, I felt relief.

T: Your behavior changed?

C: Yes, and that stuck.

T: Yes. So now you made the same realization about eating and fighting with *yourself* and being angry at yourself for not having control.

T: I don't fight with myself so much anymore.

T: You control it by allowing yourself to eat when you want to and what you want to.

C: Yes.

T: Two years from now . . . three years from now . . . how will this change you made now over control over accepting or not accepting yourself affect how you will eat in the future?

C: Hopefully, I won't fight with myself or think about it. I think if I give myself freedom to eat what I want to, I won't eat more. So I cannot see—unless my metabolism changes—that I'll gain a lot more weight than I have now, and I'll be comfortable with that.

Marilyn then told me that she had begun to notice that other people vary in size and shape, that some thin people don't always look better than heavier ones. She realized that most of her colleagues at work, who she imagined felt disdain toward her for not having control over her eating, either were single and looking for all the good things she already had or had superficial values, stressing materialism and physical appearance. She related how she and her husband carefully planned their lives for a balance between comfort in the present and security in the future and how satisfying that was compared to living "high on the hog" in the present. " I *really* like my life the way it is," she said. "I have a great husband and kid. Oh, my parents irritate me at times, but whose don't?"

Marilyn then related a recent story about her father. He had called to say that her mother had had a "spell" of some kind and that he was going to take her to the doctor again. Marilyn urged him once again to take her for psychotherapy, which she knows he does not value. He got angry, became rude, and hung up on her. She then did something she had never done before: She called him back and told him she did not deserve to be treated that way. Her father backed down quickly and ended up by telling her how much he loved and needed her. He admitted that he was trying hard not to interfere with things in her life he disagreed with because he did not want to lose her and her family. "Another thing that came out of that conversation," she said, "was that I said something about his not thinking I am a good person and he said, 'You are a very good person. I raised you to be one.' He took complete credit for how I am. He has no concept who I am, and here he is taking credit for it. It made me realize that I overcame that home situation to become the person I am more in spite of him . . . but on my own. Oh, he deserves some credit but just some. It was difficult the way I was raised and what I had to overcome."

I ended the session by asking her to scale for me the difference in her sense of acceptance of herself around eating, and she replied that eating was just part of the whole picture and overall she felt 80% to 85% in control as compared to 25% when she first came in. She decided that she hated structure around eating and had to find a balance between some eating and some restraint that worked for her. I reinforced this balanced position with the following questions:

> So if you no longer think you have to be thin all the time . . . or you can just totally let yourself go . . . if you find a balance, might there not be a different balance at different times depending on how relaxed or stressed you are? Is there some way you can always think of it in a broader sense, as "both/and" rather than *either* I am a totally bad person because I am out of control *or* I'm all good because I am in control?

My feeling was that the client had achieved what she had come for, and when I asked her where she was, she confirmed that. She said she did not think she needed more sessions at this time but would call if that changed. I then presented to her my final summation message:

T: I heard you say that you are feeling very good and that a lot of positive things have happened lately that have changed your perspective of yourself in relation to others. Overall, you have become more accepting of yourself, even with regard to your eating habits. [I listed all the good things the client said had happened with her father, how she thinks about colleagues, and so on. This is done in order to reinforce the client's own ideas about positive change.] My response is that you have come to terms with who you are and who you want to be and how not to fight yourself. You have stepped back and can see yourself as a good person overall—mother, wife, daughter, friend.

C: *(interrupts)* Everything is relative. Lots of people want instant self-gratification. Jim and I have our values in the right place. We think and plan for the future, and it work out for us. And we have a healthy well-adjusted baby.

T: So that made me think that your fight all along has been between an accepting self and a judgmental self, and what you are saying now is that you have confidence that you are okay and that you will be okay. We feel that you resolved your issues with your father some years ago, and this is the turning point of the resolution of the eating issue for you. But my team members wonder if you have as much confidence in yourself as we have in you?

C: I don't think I do, and that's realistic. It's so new.

T: And you will have to work on it and keep reinforcing the accepting self. One formula for doing that in the future . . . you know it's normal for self-acceptance and self-confidence to go up and down . . . eighty-five percent is great now, but it will take time to make it a habit to accept yourself more than less. So I was thinking so you don't feel disappointed if you don't feel at least eighty percent accepting of yourself, when you feel some slippage, think of what you have to do to adjust the balance between self-acceptance and self-judgment and how not to let yourself get torn between all negative or positive. Finally, since you and Jim plan so well for the future in other areas, think of how you can use that skill to plan ahead two, four, six years, as life moves one, so you can keep on accepting yourself overall, including eating, even if at times you are stronger in maintaining control in some areas than in others.

## Conclusion

This has been the story of my perception of the interaction between a particular client and me. I call it a story—my story—because it is a description of only my view of our interaction. I have no evidence that the changes the client reported occurred because of my intent and/or techniques.

As a participating observer in the process I worked hard at understanding what the client was really wanting and at deliberately choosing questions and responses that would fit with her needs. I started out hearing that she wanted one thing, to stop bingeing, and I chose the simplest route to helping her with that goal. But because I began to hear her uncertainty about whether or not she really wanted what she said she wanted, I then moved into what I call the second phase of treatment, in which I tried to construct a "both/and" frame with her instead of the "either/or" one she was stuck in. At that point she committed to a different goal: self-acceptance.

Marilyn's new goal seems to have connected her with her past problem with her father, which she had almost totally overcome. I suspect the goal also made a difference in her relationship with her husband, who had initiated the idea of therapy earlier when he could no longer handle Marilyn's struggle with her father (and may have done the same thing regarding her struggle with her body image). He seems to have become supportive in a meaningful way when Marilyn switched her goal from becoming thin to accepting herself, a change in priorities he had urged her to consider earlier. I don't doubt that his increased attentiveness, for example, the romantic weekend away he had arranged, contributed to the client's motivation to stop fighting with herself. One can also imagine that the pregnancy affirmed Marilyn in areas where she already felt successful and took her off the hook for a while in terms of a thin self-image.

I see the potential for lasting change in Marilyn's family system as well as in herself. Systemically, the different perceptions and behaviors on the part of her husband, her father and Marilyn herself, which in turn impinge on her mother, could reinforce each other recursively and lead to different, more satisfying interactions in the future, similar to those Marilyn reported following her past treatment. Marilyn's way of reacting to others (as demonstrated in the therapeutic interaction) was to conform on the surface to their expectations but to be angry about it and then to turn that anger against herself. This happened with her father until five years ago, when she gained some control over the situation, and in a less intense manner with her husband when he got tired of her diets. Her recent internal struggle—whether to accept her husband's idea of how she should be or her own—was more mature than the earlier one with her father. That struggle was evidenced in the therapeutic interaction around what her goals really were. While Marilyn's final commitment to self-acceptance could be interpreted as a capitulation to her husband's will rather than as an example of self-assertion, it is equally valid to see it as a shift in priorities from an emphasis on an ideal body image to a recognition of the importance of the whole self. Marilyn's choice just happened to be in agreement with her husband's loving view of her.

## EDITOR'S QUESTIONS

Q: *In the clinical material you present you continually and flexibly redirect your thinking and goals in an effort to match the client's shifting presentation. How were you able to avoid frustration and stay focused with this client? Would you also comment on the importance of having a specific goal for therapy and how you understood the goal(s) for therapy with this particular client?*

A: Your questions seems to assume that I have goals that are independent of the client's. That needs clarification! My thinking during the interview is directed by the client's responses to my questions and/or comments; that includes what they believe their goals to be. I don't have any goals other than that. Naturally, I am guided by my theoretical assumptions and beliefs in the choices I make around questions and responses. Thus, I will try to ask questions about positives and exceptions and how to build on those or how things could be rebalanced in a "both/and" manner, but the actual subject matter is determined by the client. I suppose we could say I guide a process that is defined by clients from their point of view. I often describe it to students by saying I let the clients decide which road to travel and then I steer.

I can stay patient and not get frustrated because I think of this process as the essence of what I think I have to contribute to solution construction. Moreover, keeping myself and the client as sharply focused as possible on where the client really wants to go is a crucial part of this process; in fact, it is the part that makes the therapy brief. This is never boring because I don't know what will happen next.

I do think it is essential for the therapist and client to agree on a goal for therapy, but what the client thinks of as a goal at the beginning of treatment often shifts greatly during the therapeutic process. In this clinical example I first heard the client say the goal for therapy was to deal with an eating disorder, specifically, to stop binge eating. When I pursued that goal with her, she discounted exceptions or made some positive changes and then said they were not good enough. So I continued to try to clarify what she really wanted. She then shifted to wanting not to fight with herself about eating and finally to the goal of accepting herself as she is (that is, not having to change at all). I think it is interesting how the interaction the client and I had around defining and redefining the goal reflected her progress from negative problem thinking to positive solution construction. She started out with the self-critical goal "I want to stop being the way I am" and ended up with a positive one: "I want to accept myself as I am." By the time she could articulate this she realized that she had already begun to do it.

Q: *Many times as therapists we harbor an unwarranted sense of our own importance in creating change, ignoring the contribution of many outside factors that impact on people's lives. You comment on this in a very humble way when you say, "I have no evidence the changes the client reported happened because of my intent and/or techniques." Would you discuss your ideas about how therapists can remain humble in the face of multiple impinging forces in people's lives and at the same time experience themselves as effective in helping to create change?*
A: This is an example of solutions being "both/and." If we have an unwarranted sense of our own importance in creating change, we lose out on empowering clients because we negate, or do not utilize, their inherent resources. If, on the other hand, we feel that what we do may be no more

effective than anything else that is going on in clients' lives, then we cannot
have much incentive to do what we do and it would be unethical to sell our
services and call ourselves professionals.

For me, the assumptions that clients have resources and past successes
go hand in hand with my acceptance of the fact that clients may suddenly
read something or talk to someone and feel that this provided them with
new information that helped them find their solution. If I fulfill what I
believe is my function—to talk with people in a manner that may help them
broaden their perspective and clarify their thinking about their situation and
to provide an accepting, respectful climate in which to do this—then I am
already giving my clients a different experience from what they came in
with. The effect of this will be different for different clients: For some it my
lead to direct solution construction; for others it may lay a foundation that
makes them respond differently to outside factors; and for still others it may
be an experience they do not make use of at the time but may utilize at a
later time—or maybe never. That is my way of feeling both helpful and not
omnipotent.

Q: *I was impressed with your use of questions with this client to help her
develop a "both/and" perspective. You also provide many opportunities for
her to make choices. What ideas can you suggest to others about how to
generate a "both/and" outlook in doing therapy?*
A: The best way to generate a "both/and" outlook in doing therapy is to
believe that problems are usually seen as "either/or" and solutions usually
turn out to be some degree of "both/and." Theory guides practice.

Q: *At the end of a session, you act like a one-person "reflecting team,"
presenting your understanding of what you heard the client say as well as
your own ideas. What guidelines do you use in developing your personal
statement response?*
A: My guidelines are first to repeat back to each person in the session what I
think I heard them say about what brought them in, what they see as their
goals, and *how they may be feeling about* their situation. I believe that making
an emotional connection with them at this point does a lot to generate hope
and motivation to do something different. The second part of the summary,
my response to what I heard them say, aims to reinforce past and present
positives to provide balance to their negatives and to add some new information to think about in the interim. The components of this part of the
summary are compliments, normalizations, reframes, or even educational
material (for example, about developmental issues in children, relationships, families), and these are followed by a suggestion or specific task
clients can choose to do if they wish. Tasks generally are designed to build
on already-existing positives and provide some new information about the
problem or exceptions. Frequently, tasks are intended to relieve the pressure clients put on themselves or to allow them to be patient with themselves as they try new things (for example, "Slow down!").

## REFERENCES

Chapman, A. H. (1976). *Harry Stack Sullivan: The man and his work*. New York: Putnam.

de Shazer, S. (1985). *Keys to solution in brief therapy*. New York: Norton.

de Shazer, S. (1988). *Clues: Investigating solutions in brief therapy*. New York: Norton.

de Shazer, S., Berg, I., Lipchik, E., Nunnally, E., Molnar, A., Gingerich, W., & Weiner-Davis, M. (1986). Brief therapy: Focused solution-development. *Family Process, 25,* 207–222.

Dolan, Y. M. (1991). *Resolving sexual abuse: Solution-focused therapy and Ericksonian hypnosis for adult survivors*. New York: Norton.

Lipchik, E. (1988a). Purposeful sequences for beginning the solution-focused interview. In E. Lipchik (Ed.), *Interviewing*. Rockville, MD: Aspen Publications.

Lipchik, E. (1988b). Interviewing with a constructive ear. *Dulwich Centre Newsletter,* Winter, 3–7.

Lipchik, E., & de Shazer, S. (1986). The purposeful interview. *Journal of Strategic and Systemic Therapies, 5*(1), 88–99.

Lipchik, E., & Vega, D. (1985). A case study from two perspectives. *Journal of Strategic and Systemic Therapies, 4*(3), 27–41.

O'Hanlon, W. H., & Weiner-Davis, M. (1989). *In search of solutions: A new direction in psychotherapy*. New York: Norton.

Perry, H. S., & Gawel, M. L. (Eds.). (1953). *Harry Stack Sullivan, M.D.: The interpersonal theory of psychiatry*. New York: Norton.

Walter, J. L., & Peller, J. E. (1992). *Becoming solution-focused in brief therapy*. New York: Brunner/Mazel.

# 3

## Take Two People and Call Them in the Morning: Brief Solution-Oriented Therapy with Depression

### WILLIAM HUDSON O'HANLON

Brief solution-oriented therapy is an approach that is based on two simple principles: (1) Therapists should avoid creating iatrogenic (therapist-caused) harm, invalidation, and discouragement. This means not doing or saying anything to clients that would physically harm them or bring them to harm, as well as not saying or doing anything that discourages the possibilities of change for them, invalidates them, blames them, or shows disrespect for them. (2) Therapists should engender health and healing and provide validation and encouragement.

The two main principles that guide the conversation during the therapeutic meeting are *acknowledgment* and *possibility*. Therapists must ensure that they have given clients the sense that they have been heard, validated, and respected. At the same time, the therapist must be careful not to crystallize the clients current sense of things (felt experience and points of view) but to introduce and keep open the possibilities for change and solution (O'Hanlon & Weiner-Davis, 1988; O'Hanlon & Wilk, 1987; Hudson & O'Hanlon, 1992).

Therapy is seen as a collaborative venture to which both client and therapist bring expertise. The client is the expert on his or her feelings and perceptions and has the essential descriptive data from which the therapist can construct a workable problem definition and solution frame and plan. The therapist is an expert at creating a collaborative solution-oriented dialogue and in noting and incorporating the clients responses to what is being discussed.

In this chapter I present a slightly condensed transcript, with commentary, of a one-session consultation with a depressed woman with whom the therapist felt stuck. The interview was done as part of a series of videotaped sessions and consultations while I was visiting a city some distance from my home. Ellie's therapist, Mickey, had come to see Ellie as having "characterological issues," probably narcissistic personality disorder. Therapy wasn't going anywhere, and Mickey was afraid that she would start to replicate some of Ellie's relationships, in which Ellie would get so needy and dependent that others would withdraw from her and the relationship would end. Mickey was fighting her own sense of despair and a feeling that Ellie was "sucking her blood."

Because the work that I do is fairly transparent, I have not provided a great deal of commentary for the following dialogue between the client (C) and me (T). I merely highlight some of the phases of the session and the therapeutic intent of some of my talk.

T: Because we have such a short time together and I can't know everything about you in this time, I just want to know a couple of things to orient me towards where you are and where you want to go.

C: Okay.

T: I've asked not to know anything about you; I guess I should say that first. So the question I have is "If we could wave a magic wand and everything was wonderful and terrific, how would you know when you get there and things are resolved and how would other people, if they were following you around in your life or making a videotape of Ellie's life, know that it's all resolved? That will help me understand where you are right now and where you want to go.

C: I feel like I need more self-confidence. I go through these patterns when I'm doing fine and I'm feeling great, but I get so that I feel like I can't handle everything and I can't cope. And I just kind of let go and quit my job or, you know, something like that, where I'm not coping with everything and I don't feel independent, and I really want to learn how to . . .

T: Make sure it's more consistent that . . .

C: Yeah.

T: Confidence that you have and that . . .

C: Right.

T: . . . independent feeling that you have . . .

C: Yeah.

T: So that you don't have these interruptions in the future . . .

C: Right.

T: Like, "Oh, here I go."

C: Yeah.

T: Two steps forward, two steps back.

C: Yeah.

T: Or three steps back.

C: *(laughs)* Yeah, it's been kind of this pattern, this cycle . . .

[When I hear this, I immediately know that there are times when she is feeling and doing better. She is speaking about the problem, and I am listening respectfully while at the same time making mental note of her saying that it is a pattern or a cycle.]

T: Um hm.

C: . . . where I get really depressed and can't seem to cope.

T: Um hm. Okay, but tell me about the competent and confident times when things are going pretty well. Give me like a typical day even during that time. If we could contrast the two, okay?

C: Um hm.

T: Unconfident, depresso times and the confident times. It's morning time, and you've been sleeping at night—or you haven't been sleeping at night, I don't know, that may be one of the differences. And it's time to get up and face the day. What's the difference between confident, competent times and depresso, no-fun times?

[In this exchange, I both reflect and shift her description of the problem. I incorporate her terms: "Depression" becomes "depresso times" and, later, "depresso-land," and "need more self-confidence" becomes "confident and competent times." This illustrates the two basic cornerstones of this approach: acknowledgment and possibility. I usually am doing both at the same time.

C: The confident times I, you know, get up and, um, I, like . . .

T: You get up any earlier?

C: Um, oh, definitely. *(laughs)* I get up on time. Yeah, I get up on time—it doesn't take me that long to get up—and . . . and I feel like I can handle the day. I think, you know, about what's coming ahead and . . . you know, I don't feel like I can't handle it. *(laughs)*

T: So, different feelings and different actions.

[Here I am acknowledging her focus on feelings and refocusing her on actions. I prefer action descriptions to help me to search for solutions and to contruct task assignments, as well as to deconstruct (cast a little doubt on the reality of) the concept of depression.]

C: Yeah.

T: You get up more quickly and get ready, and you know, go about your . . . you look forward to the day and think about what you've got to do?

C: Uh huh.

T: Okay, so that's the very beginning of the morning. But contrast the depresso feeling, incompetent and unconfident times. You would linger in bed more? You would turn off the alarm? You would what?

C: Oh yeah, go back to sleep. *(laughs)*

T: Okay, for how long? You know I used to be terrible at getting up in the morning. I couldn't sign up, I discovered after a couple of semesters in college, for any classes that started before eleven-thirty. *(Ellie laughs.)*

[Here I start to tell a little story, which has two purposes: One is to normalize having a hard time getting up in the morning, and the other is to steer her toward giving an action description of how she stays in bed or does not get up in the morning.]

T: Because I just . . . I had a snooze alarm thing.

C: Oh yeah.

T: And it went for ten minutes, and I would do this *(indicates pressing a snooze button)* for three hours.

C: Oh yeah.

T: Ten minutes, rrrrrring! Ten minutes, rrrrrrring!

C: Yep.

T: And I would do it for three hours. So, is it more like that? I mean, you would be sort of trying to get up or you would just go back to sleep? Or you would just say, "Forget it, I don't want to go in"—or that would never be true unless you hadn't quit your job—or have you sometimes flaked out on going to the job?

C: Oh yeah, I've called in sick and stuff.

T: Uh huh.

C: Yeah, and I just can't make it.

T: And how long would that last, maybe?

C: Oh, I'd sleep all morning.

T: Okay, all right.

C: You know, until, like noon or something.

T: So then why would you get up eventually? Why not stay in bed all day?

[Although she is telling me about the problem, again I am oriented to and orienting her toward change times and solutions. When I hear about a change, although she sees it as part of the depression, I highlight it and get an expanded description of that change.]

C: Ah . . . oh, I'd get up and sit in the living room. *(laughs)* So I'll be awake, so I won't be lying down the whole time.

T: I'm trying to understand the differences here. I've known some depressed people who just stay in bed all day.

C: Well, I have done that too.

T: But that's not typical for you.

[There is an invitation here from the client to explore and expand on the
problem description, but I refocus by guessing that staying in bed all
day is not part of her typical pattern of "depression."]

C: Yeah.

T: And what finally gets you out of bed, do you think?

C: Um, well, I think I should at least get up.

T: Um.

C: So, yeah, I feel like that around noon, I should at least get up. *(laughs)*

T: Um hm. Get dressed or maybe move to the living room. Do you get
dressed then or . . .

C: Not always. Sometimes.

T: All right. Okay, and then give me the rest of the day: the confident,
competent, doing pretty well, not depressed as opposed to the depresso
times.

C: You mean compare the . . .

T: Compare and contrast and go back to the confident time.

[This and the next few questions and statements could be viewed as
hypnotic suggestions for regression and retrieval of the sense of the
nondepressed times. I did not consciously intend that, but I do have a
background in hypnosis (O'Hanlon, 1987; O'Hanlon & Martin, 1992).]

C: Uh . . .

T: Okay, you've gotten up, gotten ready for your day, you typically go to
work.

C: Right.

T: You have a job at that time.

C: Right.

T: You typically go to work. You go to work, things go okay at the job,
things go hard, things are overwhelming, what? I mean, that could be
different days, but . . .

C: Yeah.

T: Typical day.

C: I do secretarial work and normally I can handle it fairly well, except
when it gets really busy and, you know, there's a lot of different things
happening, and I can't seem to handle, you know, too many things
happening at the same time.

T: There's those times you might be heading down the tubes into depresso-land, there's those times when things are pretty chaotic, difficult, busy at work, and yet somehow you handle it better.

C: I uh . . .

T: What's the difference between those days? Or those times?

C: Uh . . . I feel . I feel more cheerful or more . . . as long as I have people around me . . .

T: Um hm.

C: and I have some kind of a support system, like, you know, some friends or something that I can talk to.

T: And you can say, "Boy, it's been crazy at work."

C: Yeah.

T: Or whatever.

C: And just kind of, you know, just have some kind of an outlet, I seem to be okay. I seem to be able to handle it.

T: Uh huh.

C: And, um, and feel good about myself, that I can do it, that I can get through this day that's chaotic.

T: That's been crazy.

C: Yeah.

T: You know, it may even help you to have a stressful day if you've got the supports there and if . . .

C: Um hm.

T: . . . and if you're feeling cheerful, but especially if you've got the supports there, it may help you because it even strengthens, almost strengthens your [confidence] muscle, because . . .

C: Yeah.

T: Like, "Wow, I handled this day!"

C: Um hm.

T: "That must mean I'm doing pretty well. Okay!"

C: Yeah, and I can feel really good about myself.

[This is a reframing. I'm suggesting that successfully handling hard times can help build self-confidence. She agrees.]

T: All right, so you continue to go through the day, it's time to get off work, and then what, on those days when you're doing pretty well, confident, competent?

C: Uh . . .

T: You get off work, and then what do you do? Or do you do anything different during lunch? During those days?

C: I would go out with some friends of mine.

T: Okay. And if you're on the depresso slide but you're still at work, what would you do that's different?

C: I would probably go alone.

T: Ah.

C: And get myself even more depressed . . .

T: Right. Uh huh . . .

*(talking at once)*

C: . . . or get really bummed out and, I mean, can't even talk to anyone about it. Yeah.

T: Okay. So, good times, confident, you get off work, and what happens when you get off work, where do you go, what do you do?

C: I'm tired, I usually just go home.

T: Um hm.

C: And if it's . . . if I was really busy and I'm tired, I'd take a nap or something.

T: And then what would you do in the evening?

C: Oh, sometimes I like to call friends or just watch TV or, um, I like to do artwork occasionally too.

T: Um hm. Okay, now it's noon, you've gotten up finally from your bed, it's depresso time, and you move to the living room but you're still in depresso mode. You may not be dressed, you may be dressed, but you're in the living room. What do you do? Are you watching TV?

C: Yeah, sometimes I watch TV, but sometimes I can't even do that. Like it doesn't make any sense to me.

T: What else would you be doing?

C: I usually just kind of sit around, maybe listen to music.

T: Basically sit around.

C: Basically I can't . . .

T: You know, I used to major in depression in college; this was my thing. I was a really depressed person, and I almost killed myself at one time.

[Again I tell a little story about myself to normalize and equalize the relationship a bit, as well as to elicit a description of her process when she is depressed. This also has the effect of reframing depression as a process rather than being thing-like. I am also indirectly checking for suicidal ideation or impulses by mentioning it offhandedly. She does not seem to respond to the suicidal part of the story or to later indirect probes, reassuring me that suicide is probably not an immediate danger. Follow-up contact confirmed this impression.]

C: Um.

T: So I know how to do a good depression, because I used to do it so well.

C: Um hm.

T: And . . . and so . . . I need to tell you how I did it a little and ask you how you do it. What I used to do was sit around and think, and here's the kind of thinking I would do: "I've always felt this way, I'll always feel this way." You know, "this is forever" kind of thing.

C: Um hm.

T: And I would get myself into this "This is the only way I've ever been, I'm hopeless" or whatever.

C: Um hm.

T: And I would compare myself to other people and lose by the comparison. I'd think they were more mentally healthy or less depressed or smarter or—you know, I was a real skinny guy, so they were, you know, physically nicer, or better looking than I am, and this and that. I would compare myself to other people and lose by the comparison, and that would be a good way for me to do a depression. And I . . . the way I did my depression is I would sit in a chair and read books about self-help, books about depression, is how I would do it.

C: Uh huh.

T: I would never do anything about what I read, I would just read these books about . . .

C: Um hm.

T: . . . how I might help myself. And that was a good way to do a depression. But so what do you do when you're sitting there? What kind of thinking? Like, if you were going to teach me the Ellie way to get depressed. *(Ellie laughs.)* I want to know the Ellie method of . . . for depresso thinking.

C: Ah, yeah!

T: How, how could I do it? Give me the typical kinds of thoughts that Ellie would think.

C: I have gone the self-help book route before, but . . .

T: But it's not what you're specializing in these days.

C: Yeah, uh, yeah, I don't do that now. Sometimes I . . . I read books that are like, um, fantasy, science fiction, to totally remove myself from, you know, what, um, is going on and . . .

T: And does that help?

C: No.

T: So, sometimes the reading, but if you're sitting there thinking, what are you thinking? Just sort of blank? Or?

C: No, I think about, you know, how I've been through the same pattern and . . .

T: Yeah the same pattern.

C: Yeah, it's the same feeling of hopelessness and like, you know, "Am I going to have to go back home to live with my dad." or something or, you know, like, . . .

[This could have been an invitation to explore family relationship patterns, but I do not take that route as it seems a distraction from the main path we are on toward solution. I note it mentally in case I need it later, however.]

T: "Here I go again."

C: Yeah, "Here I go again."

T: "What's wrong with me?"

C: Oh definitely, yeah. Like I feel like I'm even closer to the edge of not being able to cope at all than I ever have been before.

T: Because this time is another one that . . .

C: Yep, um hm.

T: "I thought I'd moved out of this, but here I go again, I guess."

C: Right.

T: "Maybe I'm more hopeless than I thought."

C: Um hm.

[Here I'm using a technique that I never knew I used until someone did a dissertation on my work (Gale, 1991). I talk for my clients at times. I do this to acknowledge what they are feeling and thinking and to subtly restate their feelings and points of view so that they are more open to the possibility of change and solution. As long as clients agree that it is an accurate enough reflection of their experience, this technique can save a great deal of time and trouble.]

T: Okay. So how long would you sit there either reading or doing that, typically?

C: Um.

T: Typical depresso day.

C: Uh.

T: When you're in the midst of it

C: Pretty most of the day . . . most of the day, yeah. Um.

T: Would you eat anything?

C: I'd eat a little bit. Just like breakfast kind of stuff.

T: Okay, so it's now late afternoon, early evening. What's happening?

C: Uh, I decide I need to take a shower.

T: Uh huh.

C: So I take a shower and get dressed. Around like seven o'clock or so.

T: Okay, and then, in the midst of that, does it help a little?

C: It helps a little bit.

T: Okay, all right, and then what?

C: And then I start thinking of friends that I can call. I've been doing that a lot lately.

T: Uh huh.

C: Calling girlfriends and . . .

T: Does that help? I mean, does that alleviate it a little? Or a lot? Or . . .

C: It alleviates it a little bit. Only when I'm talking with, you know, only when I'm talking with . . .

T: Okay, would you ever go out during those depresso times, like go out with friends or do anything? Would you ever do art? Would you . . . what?

C: I've done a minimal amount of art. Um, and I have a really close friend that I go see sometimes—my friend Steve.

T: Only when you're depressed?

C: That's the only one I feel comfortable with.

T: Only the . . . he's the only one who . . . the only one you typically see when you're that depressed?

C: Um hm.

T: Because he understands and he's okay with that? He knows about . . .

C: He knows what's going on.

T: But the other ones you feel it would be too much of a burden on or you feel like, "Oh, they don't ca——— . . .

C: Basically, I don't have the energy to even explain, you know, what's going on. So, ah, I generally don't see anyone.

T: Okay, and then theres something I'm real curious about. You've been in depresso land, you're living there for a while, and then somehow you come out, back into confidence and competence land.

[Here again I am emphasizing and gathering information about a time when things changed this time the end of the larger pattern of depression.]

C: Um hm.

T: Because you've gone through cycles.

C: Um hm.

T: What makes a difference? What happens when the cycle is ending, different from in the middle of it, and what do you think makes the difference? You think some biological shift, something else? What makes the difference, how does it finally end? And also, I'm just real curious, anything under your influence that is it, changes it? Or do you just finally go, "Ah, I'm tired of just sitting here doing nothing; I'm going to go out and get another job"? I or "I'm disgusted"? Or "I'm going to try and kill myself, "and then when you get to that point, you scare yourself and get up and go? What? What!

[I'm searching for what she does to create the end of depression times. Im also probing about the likelihood of suicide. Again she does not respond, reassuring me.]

C: Um, well, I get to the point where I think, well, you know, I [think], "No one else is going to help me." You know, "Obviously no one wants to help me." *(laughs)* And, um, so I start getting a little bit bored of sitting around, and I finally start feeling like I can do something.

T: Um hm.

C: Like I can at least go out of the apartment and do something.

T: Um hm.

C: And once I start maybe going out and doing little things, then I start feeling a little bit better.

T: Um hm.

C: Like I . . . maybe I could handle, like, one step . . .

[She succinctly describes the solution to her problem. I follow with a few additions of my own to create a few new connections that she might not have come to on her own.]

T: Um hm.

C: And, um . . .

T: And that one step creates a little more energy, because . . .

C: Yeah.

T: . . . you're not stuck in your old pattern.

C: Yeah.

T: And then, from that, that makes . . . that leads to the next step, or you put yourself out a little more . . .

C: Yeah.

T: And then how do you finally get another job? What . . . what . . . when do you get to that point, in that . . . course?

C: Um, I might just do like one thing a week, you know, like one interview or something, you know, and, um, and then, like, tell myself, "Wow, that was really good," you know, that I could do it.

T: Yeah!

C: That I could do that one thing.

T: Yeah.

C: And then I'd start realizing that maybe I'm not so bad after all and, you know, and I'd try and, um, you know, feel good about what I have done in the past.

T: Okay.

C: But it takes a really long time.

T: Okay.

*(long pause)*

[Next I tell a story that mirrors many of the things she has told me about her depression and how she gets out of it. It also highlights some of the solutions that I am going to suggest she use. Notice that while earlier in the session I talked for her quite a bit, here she talks for me by finishing my sentences.]

T: I saw a woman once who was seeing another therapist—and the therapist was on vacation and she worked at my mental health center where I worked—and she came in depressed and, uh, I said, "Well, I really don't"—Louise was the name of the therapist—I said, "I really don't

know how Louise works and I just started working here and I don't
want to mess up anything you two might do, so tell me, how did you
and Louise work, you know, when you worked on depression." And
she said, "Well, I came in and I was in desperate, you know, I was
sleeping all day. I was, you know, really depressed. "And she dropped
out of college, and she, you know, she had lost her grants and scho-
larships, so she was in financial problems, and she would just sleep
pretty much all day, and, um, so she said, "Oh, I've been seeing Louise
for years," and she hadn't seen her for about eight months, and she
hadn't been in because she was doing better. And, um, I said, "Well,
what did you and Louise do that worked?" And she said, "Well, the first
thing was get me up by nine o'clock every morning, take a shower, and
get dressed, and I had to walk around the block one time. And it was
like . . ."

C: Hm.

T: ". . . torture to drag myself out . . ."

C: Um hm.

T: ". . . of the bed, get showered, get dressed, and walk around the block."
But she said, "When I walked around the block one time, I had a little
more energy, you know, just that little more energy."

C: Um hm.

T: "And then I would . . . I would . . . started, on my walks, I would stop
and get a paper, look for jobs, you know, that kind of thing." So she,
and you know, again, maybe just having walked around the block or
walked in the store to get the paper, she had a little more energy. She
could do the minimal kind of applying for jobs, she, um, started
walking around the block, two times, in the morning, three times. She
started increasing it to—it was weird because . . . she said, "It's weird,
because you're using energy to walk around the block, but the more I
walked around the block, the more energy I got." So she . . .

C: Wow!

T: . . . would get her energy up and . . .

C: Uh huh.

T: . . . she finally got a part-time job. She decided to go back part-time to
school, and what she did was curious—it reminded me, because you
were talking about it—is, she would recontact friends that she had when
she . . . before she was depressed and she just sort of let them drop out
because . . .

C: She didn't have any energy to deal with them . . .

T: Right.

T: And she would talk to this one person on the phone kind of thing—and
not even go over to their house—and she would just talk to one person

on the phone. And that was the only contact she had with anybody, and she was starting to drop back, kind of thing . . .

C: Uh huh.

T: . . . and she saw Louise. And so just getting up and coming to Louise's office was something, you know. She would look forward to it every week.

C: Um hm.

T: And that would be something she would organize herself around.

C: Um hm.

T: And then gradually she really got herself back into where she would go out with friends and she would, ah, you know, do all this kind of stuff. So she came in—and she was, uh, she was going to school part-time and working part-time—and she had gotten depressed again. And I said, "Well, what happened?" and she said, "Well, I met this guy at school, we moved in together, and things were going pretty well, but then he started to become real critical and real controlling and . . ."

C: Hm.

T: ". . . he was sort of smothering me, and I felt really good about myself because I stood up to him and I said, 'I don't want this relationship anymore, you're dominating my life, leave,' um hm, and it was my apartment and he left."

C: Um hm.

T: And, um, so she said, "I was feeling like . . ."

C: Powerful.

T: ". . . wow, I really did get a lot out of therapy." Yeah, powerful. "I did it . . ."

C: Yeah.

T: ". . . but now I'm depressed, and maybe I think I need a man to be okay." And I said, "Well, what are you doing? I mean," and she said, "Well, I'm sleeping all the time."

C: Oh no.

T: And she said, "It's funny, you know, as we're sitting here talking, you know, I realize I know exactly what to do not to be depressed. I need to get up . . ." *(laughs)*

C: Get up, walk around. *(laughs)*

T: ". . . walk around the block, call my friends *(Ellie laughs.)* go, make sure I don't call in sick to work, go to school." And she said, "Um, you know, it isn't that I need a man, it's just that I'm doing the same things I did when I was depressed before . . ."

C: Um hm.

T: ". . . and may . . . you know, I realize I know exactly what to do not to be depressed." And so it's like, "Okay, good. You know, I don't have to do any therapy *(Ellie laughs.)* with you if you already know." So, that's what I'm . . . I'm curious about with you. What *(pause)* Ellie already knows about the patterns.

C: Yeah.

T: You . . . you've memorized the . . . the patterns.

C: Yeah.

T: You've got them down . . . *(Ellie laughs.)* you've got them down to a science. I work with people with migraine headaches sometimes.

C: Uh huh.

T: And, um, I do hypnosis sometimes.

C: Uh huh.

T: And, um, with migraine headaches sometimes I'll say to people . . . I'll put them in trance and say, "Okay, you're an expert at getting rid of migraine headaches," and they'll go, "Wh— what does that mean?"

C: *(laughs)* What?

T: "No, I don't think so. That's why I came to see you." *(Ellie laughs.)* I say, "No, I've never had a migraine headache in my life, and I've never gotten rid of one. But you've gotten rid of hundreds of migraines."

C: Right.

T: "And you've told me that medications don't work for you."

C: Hm.

T: For some people medications work and they don't come in to see me, but for these people medications haven't helped them.

C: Um hm.

T: Somehow the migraines have gone away. So I say to them in trance, "Okay, fine, something in your body knows how to get rid of a migraine headache, maybe changes in blood chemistry, changes in breathing, changes in the muscles of your neck or the blood vessels. I don't know what it is, but your body knows. So let your body take care of it."

C: Um hm.

T: So with hypnosis it happens automatically, but I think the same thing about depression. So if Ellie already knows—and you've been able to teach me a little—

C: Um hm.

T: How . . . here's the patterns of going into a depression . . .

C: Um hm.

T: . . . or a discouragement time, or feeling unconfident time, and here's the patterns of getting out of it. What I'd be curious about is, could you try an experiment? I don't know what phase you're in now, but given that you're in, you know, in here . . .

C: I'm in a depression.

T: . . . you at least got out of bed today.

C: Yeah.

T: It's eleven o'clock in the morning and you're out of the house!

C: Yeah. *(laughs)*

T: So, maybe today's a little better.

C: Yeah.

T: But maybe, yeah, you're in the midst of one of those phases.

C: Um hm.

T: So what I would say is, okay, so let's design a program for Ellie to walk herself out of depression. Deliberately.

C: Um hm.

T: Different from the migraine headaches. Deliberately. Okay, so I would say tomorrow morning you set the alarm and no matter what you feel like—like, "Ah, I can't get up; no, I can't, I'm too depressed, I can't handle it, I'm overwhelmed"—you get up, you go take a shower at eight-thirty, nine o'clock, whatever it is, you know, eight or seven-thirty or whatever your usual wake-up time when you had a job or when you were in the midst of good times . . .

   [When I am negotiating a task assignment, I usually use multiple choice options (7:30, 8:00, 8:30, 9:00) and then note my clients verbal and nonverbal responses to each option. That gives me a better sense of which options fit for them and which they are more likely to follow through on.]

C: Um hm.

T: Or you may find a job this month, but, um, you get up, you get dressed, and you walk outside the house, and you go do something, I don't know what, you have . . . have breakfast, go get a cup of coffee . . .

C: Um hm.

T: . . . go get a paper, whatever it may be, go see a friend, ma——. . . make a breakfast date with a friend, you know, something that would be totally in the non-depresso pattern.

C: Yeah.

T: And then arrange two or three things in your day that would be non-depresso things.

C: Um hm.

T: And then force yourself—it would have to be force yourself to do it at that particular time—like maybe you had to force yourself to get up to get here. Maybe you didn't, maybe this had its own natural energy . . . or because of Mickey [Ellie's therapist] and that helped or whatever.

C: Yeah.

T: But somehow you got yourself up today.

C: Yeah.

T: Even if you're in the middle of a depresso pattern. So how'd you do that? How did you get yourself up today?

[I want both to highlight her ability to do the task and to find out how she got herself up during this depression time in order to build that into the assignment to increase the likelihood of success.]

C: 'Cause I . . . well, I didn't want to let Mickey down.

T: Somebody outside pulled you out to a certain extent.

C: Yeah.

T: So it wasn't you, you relating to you and thinking, "Who cares if I get up or not?" You had sort of an appointment or an expectation . . .

C: Right.

T: . . . from somebody else.

C: Right.

T: Okay, but . . . but so then you just . . . there was just no question, it was like, "Ahhh, I don't feel the energy to get up," but you got up, or did you feel more energy?

C: Um, well I set my alarm for, like, a quarter to eight, so I had plenty of time to lie there and think about getting up. *(Both laugh.)*

T: Uh huh.

C: So it took me almost an hour to get up. But I did it.

T: Yeah! And that's the curious part of it. I mean, there's, . . . that's the part that I always . . . that I home in on like a . . .

C: Uh huh.

T: You know, I'm a therapist and I love this. I go for change. So that's the moment that I'm real curious about. I mean, it's the . . .

C: Um hm.

T: . . . moment that the hour is up, it's a quarter to nine, um, or nine.

C: Um hm.

T: And you're thinking, "I really need to get up."

C: Right.

T: And you get yourself up

C: Go now.

T: "I've gotta go now."

C: Yeah.

T: And you get yourself up, different from those days that you're lying there thinking, "I *can't* get up."

C: Hm.

T: "I just *can't*."

C: Right.

T: Or "I don't want to."

C: Yes.

T: It may have been the same feeling this morning, the exact same feeling that you have in the midst of all the depressions, but something . . . you made a decision differently . . . you did something different inside, or you just had some external constraints . . .

C: Um hm.

T: . . . that said to you, "Get up!" I mean . . .

C: Yeah.

T: "You gotta get up."

C: Right.

T: "There's no . . . there's no choice about it, you just have to get up. You promised Mickey you'd be there."

C: Yeah.

T: "You gotta be there."

C: Yeah.

T: So I . . . I guess what I'm saying is, could you . . . could you . . . *would* you—I know you could—but would you make some sort of program to hasten the departure of discouragement and depression and un-confidence and that would involve breakfast dates . . . um . . . commitments to walk, uh, check in with Mickey, by getting up and going there even when you don't have an appointment, check in and go by her office at nine o'clock in the morning where she comes out from a client or she's just gotten up and she says, "Okay, Ellie, you have to be at my office at nine o'clock and check in with me"?

C: Yeah. *(laughs)*

T: You have to be dressed and you have to get here, and I'm expecting you every morning for the next week . . .

C: Uh huh.

T: . . . or until you get out of depression land.

C: Um hm.

T: Is . . . wha . . . uh . . . ah . . . Are you willing? Is that possible? What do you think about that?

C: That sounds really hard. I mean . . .

[She shows some signs of uncertainty. When I get that kind of response, I go back to acknowledgment. I take the response as a message that I've been emphasizing the change part of the acknowledgment and need to balance. Several times in the next few exchanges I acknowledge ("Very hard") and then I introduce the change piece again ("Not impossible") and balance it with acknowledgment again ("and hard, real hard")

T: Yeah.

C: . . . to do that.

T: Definitely hard.

C: Yeah. To get up the . . .

T: No question about it.

C: . . . to get up and see her.

T: Not impossible and hard, real hard.

C: Really hard.

T: Um hm.

C: Yeah.

T: Because that feeling of not wanting to cope is . . .

C: Is so strong.

T: . . . very strong.

C: Yeah.

T: And you had it yesterday. Yes?

C: Oh yeah.

T: And you had it this morning. To a certain extent.

C: Um hm. It did feel a little different today though, that . . .

[I seize upon this reported difference as evidence of the new frame of reference I am offering: If she has a commitment to get out of the house and see somebody in the morning, it not only changes her actions but it changes her feelings of depression.]

T: Yeah, but that's it.

C: Yeah.

T: You got something scheduled here.

C: Yeah.

T: And so you're in this slightly different frame of . . .

C: Um hm.

T: So it could just be a physiological thing, even neurological.

C: Still that scared kind of feeling.

T: Little bit scared.

C: But it wasn't strong.

T: But somehow it didn't dominate. *(both speaking at once)*

C: Yeah.

T: And I think that can pull you out of your depression quicker, I think.

C: Uh huh.

T: Then I think that in addition to that, there are some preventative things that you can do right in the middle of confidence time, when you hit a crisis point, like—you recognize this by now and you said it really well—if things are really stressful at work . . .

C: Um hm.

T: . . . and you go out to lunch alone, that's a danger, a warning sign.

C: Yeah.

T: So the next day, if you have one of those days, when you're feeling overwhelmed, "Oh God, I'm not going to be able to handle this, here I go again."

C: Yeah.

T: If you have that thought, the next day you make a promise to me, to Mickey, to whoever it might be, to Steve, whoever it matters to, whoever will keep you on track, and . . .

C: Right.

T: . . . won't let you slide out of it. *(Ellie laughs.)*

T: And not just to yourself, because you make it . . .

C: Flake out on it. *(laughs)*

T: . . . to somebody else, that you make a promise that the next day you'll make a lunch date with somebody.

C: Um hm.

T: That you would absolutely make a lunch date with somebody.

C: Um hm.

T: That you would go out for lunch with somebody, or you ma—— . . . and/or you may have to, and it may have to be a multi——, you know. *(both speak together)*

C: Two different people maybe.

T: That is, with two different people, and also that you would talk to one person on the phone about how overwhelmed you were feeling.

C: Um hm.

T: You know, one of those friends in addition to Steve.

C: Yeah.

T: That you would write these things down. Here's the prevention plan for going into depression and discouragement land, and here's the escape from depression land, um, program . . . and go write them down, because when you're in the midst of it and not sitting here talking to me—I know this because I've lived in depression land so long—I almost guarantee you won't be able to remember *(laughs)* or put them in play, those programs . . .

C: Um hm.

T: . . . consciously.

[I again shift the label just a bit to "discouragement" from "depression." I also want to ensure follow-through by having her write down what we work out for preventing her from becoming depressed and for her getting out of depression if she gets depressed in the future. This is another hypnotic suggestion. She will remember it consciously.]

T: I mean, you won't . . . you'll . . . you'll forget about it.

C: Right.

T: You'll . . . you'll say, . . .

C: Right.

T: . . . "What was I thinking? I couldn't do that!"

C: Yeah.

T: If you write it down, almost like a letter to yourself, saying, "Ellie, wake up," you know you're in depression land *(laughs)* or you're about to head to depression land. *(laughs)*

C: *(laughs)* Yeah.

T: And here's the program to prevent your going into it.

C: Steps.

T: Yeah. Now the action steps, things that, you know . . . because if . . . if you . . . if I said, "Okay, what's more likely to get you depressed, what's less likely to get you depressed?" you say, "Oh, it's rainy and I'm, . . . I'm more likely to be depressed, and when the sun's out I'm much less likely to be depressed," well, there's not much to do about that.

C: Ha.

T: But if you say, "Ah, when I get up and take a shower, I feel a little bit better."

C: Um hm.

T: That's something you can do something about. So on that action list . . . on that list would be only actions that you could do.

C: That would work.

T: Yeah, that were . . . that you've already found would work.

C: Uh huh.

T: So that's why I asked you so many questions about it.

C: Uh huh.

T: Because I want to find out in Ellie's ecology what are the natural things that occur in her ecology to get her out of depression or that help her a little when she's in discouragement or unconfidence land.

C: Oh, okay.

T: And then what I think happens is after a while you're flexing your muscle of confidence—because part of what discourages you now is that any moment you can go back into one of these and you're, . . . that's always sort of a like a wariness because even when you're doing well, it's like, "Yeah, I'm doing well now, but . . ."

C: "Who knows how long it will last."

T: ". . . who knows how long it will last." And that's somewhat discouraging in its own right, but in any case that's sort of the underlying thing. If you actually had tools that you knew could pull you out of it, it wouldn't be so intimidating to think, "Oh, my God, I might go into one of those, and that time I might not make it through."

C: Yeah.

T: So I'm thinking that these programs strengthen your confidence muscle.

C: Um hm.

T: Because when you have those days that you're overwhelmed at work and it's really bad but you make it through those days, you get a little more strong.

C: Um hm.

T: "I handled it!" I mean . . .

C: Um hm.

T: . . . wimpy Ellie, little, you know, wimpy Ellie, uh, handled it.

C: Did it! *(laughs)*

T: So that helps your confidence in the long run, the more experiences like that you get under your belt, the better it goes in the long run.

C: Um hm.

T: The more experiences that—but I think the one that you have to tackle that's much more difficult than being overwhelmed at work is starting to go into a depressing, discouraging episode or unconfident episode and actually by dint of your own effort, either avoiding it or getting out of it.

[Another subtle change is introduced here: the notion that these are episodes rather than depression as an internal disease or disorder.]

C: Um hm.

T: In your . . . in that muscle of being able to do it—because if you're just going to be a victim of it and say, "Oh jeeze, it may come over me again, and I don't know how long it will last," then it's pretty discouraging.

C: It . . . there's like no hope.

T: Right.

C: Because it's a pattern.

T: Because it could come on at any time, and you don't know how long it will last. I mean, you've gotten a sense of how long they . . . it will last.

C: A couple months. *(laughs)*

T: Now. But if you could cut the time short——now how long have you been in this one?

C: About a month and a half.

T: Okay, so maybe it wouldn't be quite so dramatic to . . . to get out now or in the next couple of days, but if you . . .

C: Usually about now is when I start getting out of it.

T: So, okay, but so, if you could make it a little quicker when you get out of it . . .

C: Yeah.

T: . . . maybe that would make a difference. But what would really make a difference, then, is the next time you either started to get in, and if you could prevent going in, when you say, . . .

C: Um.

T: "I can tell one is coming on . . ."

C: Um hm.

T: ". . . but somehow I didn't go into it!"

C: Um.

T: That would be real powerful.

C: Yeah.

T: And/or, if you actually went into one, that you got yourself out quicker than a month.

C: Yeah.

T: Or quicker than a week, you know, you could do it within a week if you could move yourself out of there, or you could even prevent the loss of a job, you know, the quitting of a job or whatever it may be.

C: Yeah.

T: That would be really great, I think.

C: Yeah!

T: It would make a difference.

C: Oh, it definitely would.

T: Okay.

C: Um hm.

T: So can you design that program? Have we talked specifically enough so you have a pretty good idea about, if you left right from here—and I . . . I wouldn't take too long to do it—if you left right from here and wrote down, "Here's the program of things that have worked to avoid going into depression and discouragement and unconfidence."

C: Um hm.

C: Um hm.

T: "And here's the things that have gotten me out of it, that can get me out of it a little when I'm in the midst of it or could get me out of it." And you could write down those two programs. Do you have enough specifics or enough ideas? Can you remember those from us talking, and do you know other ones that maybe we should talk about now?

C: Um, like the calling . . . calling friends, um, to go out to lunch or whatever.

T: Um hm.

C: That . . .

T: And this is on the prevention side.

C: And what you said about like getting up and taking a shower and going outside . . . that's the . . . that would be a big one for me.

T: Okay now, it ` . . . so who do you think can keep you on track about that?

C: *(laughs)* Well, Mickey.

[She participates in designing the task by filling in the name of the person when I ask her.]

T: You'd have to check with Mickey whether she'd have the time or how this would fit with her schedule, but if you actually . . . if you were in the midst of one of these depression things or started going into one, if you'd promised her that you'd get up and go over to her office or meet her for coffee wherever she's going to or, you know, again, whatever meets with her life and . . . and if you would promise her, again, she'd be a good one.

C: Um hm.

T: Be good just to get you out of the house, get you dressed, and get you onto that track.

C: Yeah.

T: So, all right, so that may be your prevention and also get you out of it. So what if I said, "Okay Ellie, here's your assignment, your assignment is to start this one, to get you out of it, for the next five days and the next week or whatever, every morning you have to get up by . . . you, you have to meet Mickey by anytime before ten o'clock that she says that she can meet, for two minutes, just to check in with her. And you have to be dressed, showered, um, and, uh . . ."

C: Ah.

T: ". . . have gotten yourself out of the house."

C: That would work.

T: Could you? Would you?

C: That would work.

T: All right.

C: If I had to meet her at a specific time.

T: Right. Would it be best to have the same time every morning?

C: Probably.

T: Okay, if she can work that out.

C: Yeah.

T: That would be best, and she's listening . . .

[Ellie's therapist, Mickey, was watching and listening through a video monitor in the next room.]

C: Um.

T: She can sort that out with you.

C: Um hm.

T: And . . . and that's the kind of thing that I'm talking about, because I think if you just make a commitment to yourself—"Oh yeah, I'll get up and walk every morning"—uh uh.

C: Might not work.

T: Uh uh.

C: No. *(laughs)*

T: Because I make all sorts of promises to myself that I don't keep. I keep some of them, but I don't keep some of them. If I promise somebody else, I'm a million times more likely to do it.

C: Oh, definitely.

T: So, promising her, promising Steve, promising other friends, and actually scheduling it in and making sure you can't get out of it kind of thing. Making sure you can't get out of it and even maybe tell them, "Don't let me get out of this one."

C: Oh, yeah, that would make a difference too.

T: Good.

C: Yeah.

T: So . . . so I'd say the first task then is to get you out of this phase or this slump of dep—— . . .

C: Um hm.

T: . . . um, or discouragement and unconfidence, and I think that that makes the confidence muscle go up, and gets you back. Have you got a job now or are you working on getting a job or are you not in that stage yet?

C: I'm working on getting a job.

T: Okay, and you're doing those minimal things, those once-a-week kind of things.

C: Um hm.

T: Okay, so if you could make that every day, that would be helpful, but in any case just the things to get you out of the house that I think first . . .

C: Yes.

T: . . . makes the difference. That makes the difference in the whole day, I think, because . . .

C: Um hm.

T: . . . you've gotten up. It's before noon, you've gotten out of the house, and it sort of sets the tone for the whole day.

C: Gives you a little more action, or . . .

T: That's right.

C: Yeah.

T: Gets you out and going.

C: I have a different feeling once I've gotten going.

T: That's right. Different feeling.

C: Um hm.

T: So what I'm saying is that you're trying to tip the balance between those scary, depressed, discouraged, unconfident feelings and the other ones, that crucial action in the morning can tip the balance that day.

C: Um hm.

T: I think it's that beginning of the day . . .

C: Beginning of the day.

T: . . . that's really crucial.

C: Yeah.

T: Very crucial.

C: Um hm, um hm.

T: Like getting up today, I think, and being here makes a difference in the rest of your day.

C: Um hm.

T: Also crucial is writing it down. I used to . . . this is . . . this is something that I sort of spontaneously discovered, because I would go in and out also. I would, uh, just not of depression always, but of muddle. I would just get to a place in my life where I'd just get muddled.

C: Um hm.

T: And I one time stumbled on the thought, and I did it, of writing a letter to myself when I was clear.

C: Um hm.

T: Like, "Bill, if you're ever muddled, read this." And I remember, uh, I kept it in one of my journals, and I would read it and think, "Ah yeah, now I remember." It was a letter to myself from a better time and a better part of myself to the petty, you know, stuck part of myself, and it was helpful to do that.

C: Um hm.

T: Because I . . . "Oh yeah, I'm not such a shit." You know? *(laughs)* "I'm not such a terrible person, and things aren't as bad as I thought."

C: Yeah.

T: So what I . . . what I'm focusing on there is to make sure you write this thing down . . .

C: Okay.

T: . . . because I'm afraid that in the midst of it you'd forget it.

C: That . . . it's very easy to forget. Uh. Yeah. I have written down, um, before.

T: Yeah, and that's useful in its own way. And this is an action plan.

C: Um hm.

T: Two action plans to write down. One action plan is how to prevent going into discouragement and unconfidence, and the other action plan is how to get out of discouragement and depression land.

C: Okay. Unconfidence.

T: All right, so that's what I have. Any other thoughts or ideas or questions that you have or things that I really haven't asked about that are probably pretty crucial that I should ask about?

C: Um, I tend to, like, make myself feel real confused or just like . . .

T: Um hm.

C: You know, I have all these issues going on, and I just get really confused and . . .

T: And what's the Ellie technique for confusion? I want to know. *(Ellie laughs.)* How would I do it if I were doing it like you?

C: Um, oh, just worry about all these different feelings and . . .

T: Um hm.

C: And, um, oh, I'll make myself feel bad because, you know, here I am, thirty-four, and you know, I shouldn't be like this now. You know?

T: Have it more together and . . .

C: Yeah.

T: . . . not be as confused and not be worrying about this kind of stuff?

C: Yeah.

T: Okay, so in addition to thinking these things and having these doubts and all this stuff, you've gotten down on yourself, saying, you know, "But I . . . and I shouldn't feel, shouldn't think these thoughts; I should have it more together than this." That kind of stuff?

C: Yeah.

T: Well, okay, so I, uh, you know, I have some ideas, but before we get to that, what helps then? I mean, you're in the midst of all these confusing thoughts and feelings, and then what happens? What's helped?

C: Um.

T: What gets you out of it? I mean, you're not there at this moment.

C: Probably being with other people makes a big difference.

T: So it stops going around the squirrel cage and starts coming out of the mouth?

C: Um hm.

T: Or do you focus on something else?

C: Yeah.

T: Yeah. I think it's a pretty crucial thing, and I, you know, I . . . like, I have this observation I made about myself and other people and life, and the observation seems to be that, um, in the . . . where . . . when I'm doing the worst, I do the worst things for myself. Like, when I'm doing the worst, I'll eat sugar. *(Ellie laughs.)* Which sends me into a sugar, you know, cycle, where I sort of go down.

[Here I tell another little thing about my struggles, which equalizes the relationship a bit and also introduces an idea that Im going to use to reinforce the task assignment.

C: Um hm.

T: If I'm doing the worst, I'll eat sugar. Like . . .

C: Yeah.

T: If somebody else is doing the worst, they do drugs, and that's their thing.

C: Um hm.

T: You know, they stop doing drugs, but then they start doing really badly. And then they do drugs, which in the short run, interimly, tastes good on my tongue, sugar, but in the long run makes things go downhill for me.

C: Um hm.

T: So I think, "Okay, you know in your worst moments that you have your tendency." Ellie's tendency is to withdraw. You may have other vices as well that we haven't heard about. *(Ellie laughs.)* But your tendency is to withdraw from people.

C: Um hm.

T: And in the short run it sort of seems to relieve you a little, to withdraw from people; in the long run, it's the worst thing you can do.

C: Right! Exactly!

T: So what I would say is, whenever you feel the worst—whenever I feel the worst, I should eat protein. *(laughs)* I should head for the protein.

C: Hm.

T: You know, when, even so, for the moment, I want sugar, sugar, sugar, I should head for the protein. Whenever you feel the worst, you should head for the people.

C: Um hm.

T: And be . . . it . . . it's like . . . here's the thing, okay. When Ellie feels bad, my prescription for you is take two people and call them in the morning.

C: *(laughs)* Yeah. In the morning. *(speaking together)*

T: Call Mickey in the morning.

C: Yeah.

T: Get together with other people.

C: Yeah.

T: Because your tendency when . . . when you're in confusion land, when you're in doubt, when you're in depression land, when you're in un-confidence, is to go back into yourself.

C: Yeah.

T: And there's certainly a time for that, I admit, but if you're doing the worst, that's not the time for it.

C: Right.

T: The time is to go out into the world and contact with other people. And then later you can spend time by yourself 'cause that's . . . there's nothing bad about that, that's the moment.

C: Um hm.

T: You know, later I can have sugar or once I've had proteins.

C: Right.

T: Then I can have carbohydrates, sugar. That's okay with me. But if I stay on that downward binge, it's not good for me.

C: Right.

T: So I think it's the same prescription. Get yourself out rather than in.

C: Um hm.

T: When things are going bad, if you go in you're likely to dwell in there for a while in a no-fun place. And I'm not saying avoid the issues you need to deal with. Go ahead and deal with them later, but not at that moment. That's not a good time to sort out where you're going in life or who you are. That's the worst time . . .

C: Um hm.

T: . . . to sort it out because all you do is go into doubt and discouragement and depressions.

C: Um hm.

T: Get out and be with other people, and then later come home and think, "Now where am I?" Then you're in a much better place to get in touch with it.

C: Yeah, yeah, a lot of times I think I need to do all this thinking all by myself.

T: Yeah.

C: And that's when it kind of spirals into . . .

T: Yeah.

C: . . . something worse.

T: Yeah, right. And then it doesn't ever get the first thing you wanted to sort out sorted out because you're into depression at that point . . .

C: Um hm.

T: . . . and you're not thinking very clearly.

C: Um hm.

T: I think it dovetails nicely with what we are talking about but, again, anything else . . . I sort of cut you off a little quickly here. Anything else that you think is important that we haven't talked about or covered at this point that's pretty crucial?

C: Um.

T: Have we covered the main points?

C: Um, I think you've covered the main points. Um, I have been feeling, um, more scared about totally, um, not being able to cope.

T: Uh . . .

C: More than, like I said, more than I ever have . . .

T: Than . . .

C: . . . before.

T: Then, then would you say that's just happened with each episode, that that's been somewhat true with each time when you've gotten discouraged? It's like, "Oh my God, it's even, you know, it's even worse this time." Would you say that's true, in general, that there's been a trend, and . . .

C: Yeah.

T: . . . it's even worse each time?

C: Yeah. Yeah.

T: And I attribute that to just the discouragement of "Here we go again."

C: Um hm.

T: That's, you know . . .

C: There's the pattern . . .

T: Yeah, and then, and then, the discouragement of, "Is this going to happen for the rest of my life? Am I not going to make it through? I mean, they're pretty terrible. I mean, am I not going to make it through?"

C: Yeah.

T: Or, "Am I going to kill myself?" Or, "Am I not going to last?" I, uh, you know, uh, I have a friend, a mentor, John Weakland, who's a brief therapist. He told me, "Bill, you know, you've got to be humble as a therapist, because you'll never fix people's lives forever, I mean, that's Utopia. Because its just like the old folk saying, you know, 'Life is just one damn thing after another.' "

C: Huh.

T: ". . . But for people who come into therapy, here's the discouraging thing, that life has become the same damn thing over and over again."

C: Um hm.

T: So I think that's what you're talking about . . .

C: Yeah.

T: . . . is that your life becomes the same damn thing over and over again, and each time it does, it's a little more discouraging.

C: Yeah.

T: So I'm concerned that if this keeps happening, you may not make it on this planet after a while. You may check out, and you may say, "It's not worth living like this anymore."

C: Um hm. Um hm.

T: At the times when you're doing better, and even at these times it's worth being around, but you forget about that during the midst of that and . . .

C: Right.

T: . . . and you have your doubts and fears and things like that. And I think it would be a real shame if you made that decision on one of these episodes because "Here we go again, here we go again."

C: Um hm.

T: So I think it's pretty crucial to have a sense of empowerment so that you can have a sense you can get out of these or prevent them. That . . .

C: That it's me that's doing it and . . .

T: Right.

C: Yeah.

T: Because that strengthens the confidence muscle.

C: Um hm.

T: And then you don't fear so much. It's, "Here we go again and I need to do the stuff that I need to do," but you won't feel like "I'm a victim of this and there's nothing I can do, I just have to ride through it, and I'm not sure I'm up to riding through it."

C: Um hm.

T: "I get so scared, I get so discouraged, I get so, you know, it disrupts my life. I'm not moving on because I keep having to interrupt my life for these things."

C: Right, right. But if I, like, have kind of these action plans on what to do, maybe it won't be so scary the next time.

T: If you put them into prac——. . . place. It . . . *(Ellie laughs.)* That's the crucial elements. *(Ellie laughs.)* You can have the plans, all the plans. *(Ellie laughs.)* You've actually got to put them into . . .

C: Oh yes, doing it.

T: And again, what I would say is "Be gentle with yourself." So maybe you're not perfect at putting them into place, but if you do a little more than you did before, . . .

C: Um hm.

T: . . . that's progress.

C: Yeah.

T: And then, ultimately, putting them into play so you just don't go into that same, uh, uh, month and a half, two months', three months' period; it's maybe a week, you know. Maybe you do have a physiology or a neurology that's more likely to get you depressed.

C: Um hm.

T: I thought I did but, to tell you the truth, over the years I just don't go into these depressions . . .

C: Hm.

T: . . . anymore. So for me it wasn't physiological or neurological, uh, it was pretty much emotional, psychological, and lifestyle kind of stuff.

C: Um hm.

T: For other people it might be more neurological, physiological, or whatever, but to me it hasn't been. What it will be for you if you actually put this action plan into play . . . when you put it in play, you'll find out, I think, whether you continue to, every once in a while, be plagued by the likelihood of going into these things or whether it just goes away once you settle it.

C: I think . . . I think it'll really help.

T: Um hm.

C: I do. It feels like it'll really help.

T: Great. *(Ellie laughs.)* Well, again, you have a possibility of getting a copy of this tape, and you can watch it again to remind yourself. And if you're in the midst of depression and you don't feel like watching soap operas, you could watch the tape.

C: *(laughs)* I think that would be great.

T: Any other questions or comments or concerns you have before we end?

C: Um, no. Thank you.

T: So I think that's all.

C: You're great.

T: Oh, well, thank you! Thats a nice thing to say.

When I called Ellie for a follow-up, I did not get her directly, so I left a message. She returned the call and left this message on my answering machine: "I'm doing fine. Meeting with you really made a difference. And it's helped me a lot." That's the short version of the follow-up.

During our subsequent conversation Ellie indicated that she had followed through on the plan of coming to her therapists office each day by 9:30 A.M. She met with the therapist three more times after the consultation. The therapist got her to write down and follow through on a "to do" list each day. Ellie got a temporary job and started going out more with friends. She restarted flute lessons and joined a quartet that meets regularly.

When asked to compare and contrast meeting with me and meeting with other therapists and to indicate what was helpful, Ellie said it was helpful to contrast and describe in detail the difference between depressed times and nondepressed times. She admitted that this was the first time she had felt that she could do something about the depression herself. She had always thought therapists would have to get her out of it. She mentioned that she thought we were able to accomplish so much in one session because she knew that I understood her depression: "You had been there too and that was good to know." She also indicated that having to describe what she did while she was depressed was hard but helpful. "Nobody had ever had me describe in such detail what I did while I was depressed. It was embarrassing." However, while describing what she did, she was able to see that there were things she could do to get herself out of her depression. She said, "Because of the way I get depressed, many therapists have problems with me. They get discouraged or stuck."

Without any prompting from me, Ellie gave me some history during the follow-up. She thought her trouble had started when her parents divorced. Father was cold and distant, mother was overinvolved and dependent on Ellie. When Ellie moved away it had upset the balance, and mother divorced father. She had run to Chicago to escape family problems and to establish her independence. She did both and then decided it was time to return and deal with her family. She returned to the area in which she had grown up and moved in with her father and stepmother, a very warm and friendly woman. Ellie grew close to both of them. She found a job and moved about an hour away from their home. In Chicago Ellie had had two long-term relationships that ended badly; the more recent one had been with a man who decided after several years that he did not want to commit.

Follow-up contact with Ellie's therapist, Mickey, indicated that Ellie had followed through with the suggested arrangement. She had checked in every morning before 9:30 A.M., between Mickey's clients, just for a minute. She came to Mickey for therapy only three times after meeting with me. Mickey and Ellie agreed to stop therapy, in part owing to money concerns and insurance hassles. Every once in a while in therapy Ellie would start on some of the old patterns, namely dwelling on family of origin issues and what was wrong with her. Mickey, citing Ellie's session with me, would then steer her into focusing on what was working during those sessions. Ellie appreciated being reminded and agreed with this new focus. Ellie called a few weeks after treatment ended to tell Mickey that she had a new boyfriend and that things were going well.

Because Mickey usually worked in a long-term, more psychodynamic, and functionally oriented way, I asked her what she thought of my session with Ellie. She told me that she did not think that this type of therapy would work for most of her patients but that it seemed to work quite well for Ellie. I asked her if she had any concerns that she did not think were dealt with in the consultation and she said that we had not dealt with a long-standing relationship pattern of Ellie's. As mentioned earlier, Mickey had the impression that in her relationships, especially romantic/sexual relationships with men, Ellie became too needy and dependent. Her partner would start to withdraw, and then Ellie would become even more clingy and dependent, which would ultimately sow the seeds for the dissolution of the relationship. Mickey said that she expected Ellie to continue to have those problems since the therapy and my consultation did not resolve those "core relationship and characterological issues." I explained that the way I would handle the issue of Ellie's relationship pattern, which Ellie had not brought up in our meeting, would be to tell Ellie that my door was open for return visits if she ever had any further concerns. On the basis of our relationship and her previous success in dealing with her depression, I assumed Ellie and I would have an easier time sorting out her relationship issues, but I indicated to Mickey that I would prefer to wait until Ellie was in a relationship to deal with those issues. That way we would have a chance to try some experiments to make a change from the old unworkable patterns, rather than just talk about or analyze them. That reassured Mickey that my approach did not simply dismiss or deny other issues.

I spoke to Ellie about Mickeys concern that we hadn't taken care of the core relationship issues. That led to a few minutes of discussion about the warning signs that would indicate that she was starting to go into "dependency patterns" in her new relationship with Bruce, a guy at work. Ellie thought that she would feel a helpless feeling, similar to the feeling of depression. We agreed that she should again seek out friends and spend time away from Bruce if she felt any warning signs and that she would also force herself to keep up her friendships while establishing the relationship with Bruce. I told her that I thought she had two good models for what she needed in order to achieve balance in her relationship with Bruce: Her mother had shown her how to get close to people, and her father had shown her how to keep a distance. Perhaps she could balance the two, since she had them both in her. I suggested that she might also use her new stepmother, who was pretty balanced in those areas, as a model and a consultant. She liked that idea.

## EDITOR'S QUESTIONS

Q: *There has been much debate recently about the use of power in therapy and about the therapist's role as expert. Some therapists take a nonexpert position, embrace a stance of not knowing, and see their role as facilitators or reflective listeners. Others believe the therapist cannot avoid an expert position and must assume responsibility as an active director of the therapy process. You talk about both the therapist and client bringing their unique expertise to the therapy encounter. What are your views on the issue of therapist control and power?*

A: I rarely use conceptions of power and control in thinking about or talking about therapy. If there is no physical coercion, both therapists and clients have power in the therapeutic relationship. Their power is in the fact that either can leave the room or terminate the relationship (even if the therapy is court ordered, the client is free to find another therapist). The other power issue is in determining the focus of the conversation. In this respect I think both therapist and client have an equal opportunity. That does not mean that they always equally determine the focus, just that they have an equal opportunity to determine it. I unabashedly use my influence to focus on those aspects of the conversation in which I find the possibilities for change and empowerment for the client.

Q: *Had Ellie been actively abusing alcohol or cocaine, what modifications would you have made in your approach?*
A: If Ellie had brought up such issues as concerns or if I had learned about them through the referral source, I would have asked about them and their relationship to her depression patterns. If we agreed that they were concerns to be included in the therapeutic goals, I would have taken an approach to dealing with them as problems similar to the one I used with the depression. The other difference would have been in the stories I would have told, which would have had a lot more reference to drug and alcohol problems.

Q: *You make use of self-disclosure in dealing with Ellie's episodic feelings of depression. David Epston talks about the importance of therapist "transparency." What guidelines do you use in deciding when and how much to share with the client? In the clinical situation presented, you tell Ellie about some very heavy circumstances in your own past history. What do you see as the benefits and potential risks of self-disclosure, and why did you decide to tell Ellie your story?*
A: I think it is important for the therapist to bring his or her humanity into the office. I accomplish that by telling some of my story when it is appropriate and relevant. During the therapy interview I feel as though I am one of those sculpture boards with pins through it: If you put your hand on the back side of it, the pins take on the shape of your hand on the front. During the interview the client's concerns and my undertandings of them begin to pull some stories and responses from me that arrange themselves into a shape unique to that client and interview. I trust that process. I do not share personal stories about which I still am greatly upset or am unfinished. I also do not share intimate sexual stories with female clients or male homosexual/bisexual clients, as those stories seem to me too much of an invitation to sexual intimacy.

Q: *In this interview your energy level seems to be very high. You talk more than the client and are working diligently to move the process toward a well-defined goal. How do you avoid overwhelming a client who may be quiet, depressed, or very passive? In what situations would you be more laid back, that is, less active and directive in the therapy process?*
A: I tend to be very energetic in general in therapy. I am passionate about

helping people find their possibilities and move through their pain and I think that comes across. I modify this in response to the client's responses. If he or she is indicating (verbally or nonverbally) a discomfort with my activity or energy level, I shift gears and meet more closely with the client nonverbally. The way I avoid running over clients is to attend to their verbal and nonverbal reponses and occasionally asking them if I am on the right track or if there is anything I have missed.

Q: *In your conversation with the client you seem to serve as an editor of the therapeutic narrative. You actively reframe parts of the client's story in such a way that the client develops a more hopeful view. You seem to make a conscious, decision to focus on certain aspects of the client's narrative and ignore others. By homing in so quickly, aren't you at risk for overlooking significant information?*

A: This question presupposes a view I do not subcribe to, namely that there is some information that is *really* the most significant. My view is that clients' narratives, positions, and significant issues can and usually do shift during the therapeutic conversation. If the client is satisfied and the problem is resolved, I feel that what I have emphasized has been adequate. If the client is dissatisfied and/or the problem hasn't been resolved, I then try to find a different emphasis. The only time I impose my bias is when I think there is a physical danger to the client or someone else (such as cases of domestic or sexual abuse, suicidal impulses or homicidal inclinations). If this information is not included, the results could be damaging or lethal.

## REFERENCES

Gale, J. (1991). *Conversation analysis of therapeutic discourse: Pursuit of a therapeutic agenda.* Norwood, NJ: Ablex.

Hudson, P., & O'Hanlon, W. H. (1992). *Rewriting love stories: Brief marital therapy.* New York: Norton

O'Hanlon, W. H. (1987). *Taproots: Underlying principles of Milton Erickson's therapy and hypnosis.* New York: Norton.

O'Hanlon, W. H., & Martin, M. (1992). *Solution-oriented hypnosis: An Ericksonian approach.* New York: Norton.

O'Hanlon, W. H., & Weiner-Davis, M. (1988). *In search of solutions: A new direction in psychotherapy.* New York: Norton.

O'Hanlon, W., & Wilk, J. (1987). *Shifting contexts: The generation of effective psychotherapy.* New York: Guilford Press.

# 4

## After the Shift: Time-Effective Treatment in the Possibility Frame

### MARGOT TAYLOR FANGER

*In treatment,* process *is what's important, content is a handmaiden. Your presence and connection evoke the healing. Results, not time spent, are what's important in treatment.*

—Virginia Satir

*The greatest discovery of my generation is that human beings, by changing the inner attitudes of their minds, can change the outer aspects of their lives. . . . It is too bad that more people will not accept this tremendous discovery and begin living it.*

—William James

Consider the client who requested help in passing the bar exam. He had taken it once, passed the essay part, but failed the multiple-choice. His distress was palpable as he described both his fear of failing again and his long history of stumbling through multiple-choice exams. He had brought a sample test with him, and I asked him to read a question to himself and choose the answer. He looked down at it, sighed, his shoulders slumped, and finally said, "Well, it's either A or D, I'm really not sure." At his work he was a popular manager and frequently had to make difficult choices. Reminding him of this fact, I asked him to recall a recent successful decision he had made and to go through that process again. His shoulders straightened as he looked up over my head, smiled, and recalled the decision process. I pointed out to him that answering multiple-choice questions also involved making decisions. I then asked him to read the multiple-choice question, look up over my head, and make a *decision* about the answer. He did so, then smiled as he quickly told me that he was confident that the answer was D. I invited him to practice this strategy at home, going through the entire booklet of sample questions, and reminded him once more that choosing an answer was the same as making a decision. A month later he called to say that he had passed the bar—which made this a one-session treatment (see Bandler, 1985; Bandler & Grinder, 1979, for a discussion of this and similar strategies).

This case illustrates time-effective treatment in the possibility frame. Let us first define that frame and differentiate it from the more traditional or problem frame. Simply put, in the problem frame you ask the client, "What is your problem?" or "What's wrong?" In the possibility frame (Friedman & Fanger, 1991) you ask the client, "What is your request?" or "What do you want?" This deceptively simple-sounding shift profoundly affects the entire shape and direction of the therapy that ensues (see Figure 4.1 for elements of this paradigm shift).

In the possibility frame a specific algorithm is used: The therapist *elicits* the specific request, *identifies* the stuck behavior pattern, and then *interrupts* this pattern with a "*reframe.*" When the *reframe* is effective, it generates

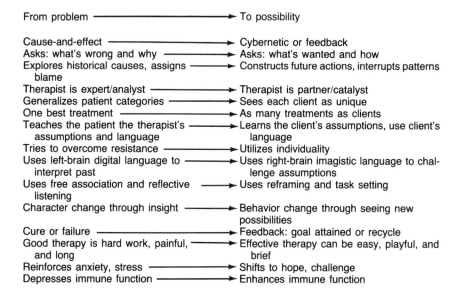

| From problem | To possibility |
|---|---|
| Cause-and-effect | Cybernetic or feedback |
| Asks: what's wrong and why | Asks: what's wanted and how |
| Explores historical causes, assigns blame | Constructs future actions, interrupts patterns |
| Therapist is expert/analyst | Therapist is partner/catalyst |
| Generalizes patient categories | Sees each client as unique |
| One best treatment | As many treatments as clients |
| Teaches the patient the therapist's assumptions and language | Learns the client's assumptions, use client's language |
| Tries to overcome resistance | Utilizes individuality |
| Uses left-brain digital language to interpret past | Uses right-brain imagistic language to challenge assumptions |
| Uses free association and reflective listening | Uses reframing and task setting |
| Character change through insight | Behavior change through seeing new possibilities |
| Cure or failure | Feedback: goal attained or recycle |
| Good therapy is hard work, painful, and long | Effective therapy can be easy, playful, and brief |
| Reinforces anxiety, stress | Shifts to hope, challenge |
| Depresses immune function | Enhances immune function |

**FIGURE 4.1.** Paradigm shift. From *Expanding Therapeutic Possibilities: Getting Results in Brief Psychotherapy* (p. 297) by S. Friedman and M. T. Fanger, 1991, New York: Lexington Books. Copyright 1991 by Macmillan, Inc. Reprinted by permission.

new behavior. Let us examine how this algorithm sequence applies to the treatment example above. I first *elicited* the client's request by asking, "How would you like your life to be different as a result of our talking together?" His request—to pass the bar exam—was both appropriate and well specified. (Had his request been more general, for example, "I'd like to feel like a good person," I would have encouraged him to clarify his request by asking him, "How would you know that you were a good person?") To *identify* the stuck behavior I asked the question "What stops you from doing that now?" In reply the client reported difficulty in taking multiple-choice exams. In keeping with the notion that the very solution attempted is the difficulty, I asked the client to behaviorally demonstrate his process of choice. His sigh, slumped shoulders, and downcast eyes seemed to show his unresourceful approach to the task at hand, an assessment borne out by his uncertain answer. I realized that in choosing a multiple-choice answer, you evaluate alternatives and then make a decision. Knowing that in his work this client frequently made successful decisions, I *interrupted* his stuck pattern with this new perspective or *"reframe"* of the process involved.

In other words, answering multiple-choice questions is simply a subcategory of decision making. Having offered the client this new point of view, I then asked him to test it out behaviorally by putting his body through his more resourceful decision-making sequence of motions (straightening his shoulders, looking up over my head). His smile and ready answer attested to the success of this trial. He saw new possibilities for effectively dealing with multiple-choice questions. I invited him to practice and thus reinforce this new skill pattern by doing it at home with all the sample questions. This, in essence, is the process of treatment in the possibility frame.

To summarize, then, you first elicit from the client the presenting request for some well-specified future action. Then you identify the unsuccessful attempt to reach that goal. Next you find a way to interrupt that unsuccessful pattern with a reframe—through words or tasks—that provides the client with a new, expanded perspective that may support new, effective action in his or her life.

Needless to say, this whole process does not always happen in one session. So what form does it take across several sessions—perhaps a number of sessions over a period of years? That is the subject explored and explicated in the case transcript material that follows, but first let me discuss other essential ingredients of the time-effective process.

While there is general agreement that providing time-effective treatment demands an *active* therapist who enables the client to define a *specific* goal, two other critical components are the therapist's *expectation* and *intention* to get results in a timely manner.

> The therapist's attitude about change and expectations and optimism about how swiftly a desired result can be obtained have significant impact on the

outcome of therapy. Studies suggest that clients will comply with the therapist's expectations about the length of treatment. In addition, no evidence
exists that more therapy is "better" or leads to more enduring outcomes. The
creation of a positive rather than negative self-fulfilling prophecy needs to
guide the therapy. This will usher the client toward the desired change.
(Friedman & Fanger, 1991, p. 111)

The immediate practical effect of directing your attention/intention
toward a desired result becomes apparent when you simply follow the
suggestion to "look around the room and find six items that contain circles.
With a circle mind-set, you'll find circles jumping out at you. . . . When you
set your attention to look for something, you almost always find it. You
just need to know what you are looking for. *What you pay attention to
determines what your world is like*" (Wujec, 1988, p. 45; emphasis added).
When we focus on problems the world is full of obstacles. Focus on requests
and the future springs to life. Focus on results and they become a beacon to
guide us. So when the therapist directs his or her intention to create
possibilities and to use therapeutic time efficiently, rapid results are more
surely reached. Keen attention to a future orientation also supports the
endeavor. *For learning to be the person you want to be is quite different—and often
less time consuming—than learning why you are the way you are.*

Time-effective therapy is further supported when the therapist sees a
client's individuality rather than a client's resistance. The concept of resistance is squarely in the problem frame, where the therapist/expert knows
best what the client should do. Resistance can then be regarded simply as
the client's not doing what the therapist thinks he or she should. The
therapist can neutralize the concept of resistance and join the client's reality
with the internal question "What has to be true for this person to be acting
this way?" Asking this question serves a double purpose: It gives invaluable
information about the client's world, and it allows the therapist to utilize
that world in discovering the client's request. After the therapist helps the
client to define his or her *own* (as opposed to the therapist's) goals, the
therapist is then a resource to help the client move toward these goals. If the
client resists the therapist's strategy, it may be time to find another
strategy—one that fits *the client* better. In this mode of thinking we see our
clients not as our adversaries but as our teachers.

Words themselves continue to be our basic tools of intention. We need
to use care in the choice and deployment of them. We also need to remember that as we interact with clients we are constant models of effective
communication; as such, we have the responsibility to teach our clients such
skills. We all shape both our moods and actions from what we hear from
others as well as from what we say to ourselves. Therefore, we need to be
cognizant not only of *what* effect we want to produce but of *how* we
produce it. When we work in the possibility frame, it is essential to both use
and elicit positive language unremittingly. This directs attention toward

hope and future prospects. When therapy is oriented in such a direction, even talking about past and current impediments takes place under the umbrella of possibility, which keeps the interaction away from the mire of unsolvable past problems that obscure the future.

We need to take particular care that our presuppositions—those assumptions subtly imbedded in our common speech—serve us and our clients well. Take, for example, the difference between a simple opening question in the problem frame—"How may I help you?"—and one in the possibility frame—"What would you like to have happen here today?" The assumptions in these two questions are totally different in terms of relationship (hierarchy vs. partnership), autonomy (therapist in charge vs. client choice) and immediacy (indefinite time frame vs. results today). Every statement that we make has its own set of presuppositions, and we need to be acutely alive to them so that they work for us and our clients.

Paul Watzlawick (1978) contends that the language that promotes or produces change needs to be the language of imagery. He believes that we all hold our assumptions about what is possible to do in the world in *internal images* (what is correct behavior, for example), and so we therapists need to find ways to challenge those limited images. We can do that by using either imagistic language or behavioral assignments or both. Whatever method is used, the goal of all treatment strategies is to help the client create new images that expand his or her horizon of possible behaviors. When the original limiting image is changed or enlarged, we say that the original image has been *"reframed";* in other words, the same sensory experience is seen in a new way. (This is what happened with the bar exam client in the case presented at the beginning of this chapter.) As Virginia Satir (1986) says, "Words don't have any energy unless they spark or trigger an image. The word in and of itself has nothing, nothing. One of the things I keep in touch with is, 'What are the words that trigger images for people?' Then people follow the feeling of the image."

During the course of treatment—of whatever length—the therapist needs to strive constantly to improve the client's mood to support new behaviors that are both intiated by the client and congruent with his or her life. The specific methods that the therapist uses include the following: continual reinforcement of positive statements; eliciting of specific language; and challenging negative assumptions through reframing, either with imagery or tasks. Sequenced behavioral assignments belong both in the sessions and between them. The therapist receives whatever the client says or does only as feedback, to be utilized to help move the client forward, by supporting positive results and discarding what doesn't work.

A great deal of attention has been lavished on the initial interview in time-effective treatment, so for a transcript example I have chosen a segment of treatment in a long-term intermittent therapy. In this example I hope to show in detail how the aforementioned principles play out from session to session in a well-established ongoing treatment.

The client in the transcripts had already been seen over a span of 7 years, during which there were some 36 sessions. Although the therapeutic relationship has been a long one, the actual number of sessions has been small, averaging about five sessions a year. The client has come through several developmental crises in treatment and is currently dealing with being laid off from work. (The earlier course of treatment is reported in Friedman & Fanger, 1991, chap. 10.)

The client, Mike, in his late thirties, lost his job as an assistant college baseball coach when the head coach took another job and Mike's application for the head coach job was rejected. Over a period of 6 months I saw Mike for five sessions with the goal of shifting his mood from that of inactive despair to active hope, which would support his job search. I worked with him in the possibility frame by eliciting his request, helping him to identify his specific experience in uncovering his current stuck patterns, challenging his limiting assumptions, and collaborating with him in the design of appropriate tasks.

In the transcripts that follow please note that I work toward a positive mood shift in each session as well as across the five sessions. I constantly search for the specifics of behavior that will support an improved mood as well as help the client shape a detailed plan of action, thus fostering his independence so that he feels supported and cared for when he initiates new actions. (The following transcripts are from sessions 37–41 of Mike's 8th year of therapy.)

## INITIAL SESSION OF CURRENT COURSE OF THERAPY

T: What would you like to have happen here today?

   [The therapist elicits the client's request.]

C: *(sigh)* I should have anticipated that question. Uh, today.

T: Today.

C: Uh. I feel kind of hopeless right now. I'm not feeling well in any part of my life, and somehow or other I'd like to get some help in finding some hope—you know, discovering if it's there already or mapping out strategy or sort of getting help for myself, you know. But I don't feel very good, and not feeling very good, you know, not feeling that I have much hope about, you know, anything . . .

   [Client identifies stuck pattern.]

T: Sounds awful.

C: It is awful . . . it sucks.

T: So . . .

C: But I mean it; my job thing is really hard for me.

T: What's the hardest thing about being laid off, Mike?

   [Therapist elicits specifics.]

C: Feeling like a failure. You know, I'm about to turn forty, and I've always felt like a failure. You know, I always felt like I wasn't doing what people had expected of me, and that's really hard. And I've always had this thing in the back of my head that I was going to be a street person someday, and I mean honestly, I feel sort of strangely drawn to that. I feel a kinship with those people, and, uh, it's just really frightening. I guess it's just the sense of a wasted life. It's like this life is passing me by, and, uh, it feels like a shame.

T: Yes. So exactly when did this happen?

C: January thirtieth, when I didn't get the job. Seems like a long time ago now. At that point it was like, "Well, I've got ten months until my paychecks stop." That's a frightening thought.

T: Um, do you think it would have been better if they hadn't given you the ten months?

C: In some ways. But then people say, "You must be lucky, it must be great."

T: So what plans have you made to get yourself another job?

[Note therapist's presuppositions in the question, namely, that the client has already made plans.]

C: So the plan now is, number one, stay in touch with those people who could hire me and, number two, who could help me get jobs, like uh . . .

T: And how do you do that?

[Therapist goes for specifics.]

C: Well, I go to games. Like that southern head coach's team will play here and I'll make sure I'm there to talk with him and his assistant and I'll send him a note very soon and say that it looks like his team is playing very well, wish him luck, and tell him I'll see him in June and also include in there that fact that I've been doing scouting, you know.

T: Good, good!

[Therapist reinforces positive statement.]

C: So he knows that I'm very involved.

T: So how do you spend your time these days?

C: Yup. I wonder that. I really wonder that. I had this idea a while ago. I mean I'm always saying to myself, "Tomorrow I'm going to start doing this."

T: What, for example, would you start doing? [Therapist again requests specifics.]

C: Meditate, exercise, take my vitamins, uh, spend a certain amount of time on this baseball networking thing—writing letters or making lists or calling people or going to practices—that kind of thing, uh . . .

T: Of course. So what would it take for you to fulfill your daily plan—your exercise and so forth?

C: I have no idea. I feel incapable of doing it.

T: So, Mike, what are you going to do if you don't get a baseball job?

C: *(pause)* No idea.

T: What kinds of things have you thought of?

C: I haven't thought about it much. I mean, I have thought about it some but without getting anywhere, you know. I mean, I could teach but I can't get a teaching job. That would be hard for me to get, perhaps even harder than a coaching job. The other thing is, I want to coach, dammit.

T: Yeah, okay. Let me tell you why I asked that. I have every faith that you'll get a coaching job. It has to do with the sense I get from you that feeds your feeling of despair—that if you don't get a coaching job, it's the end of the world, the end of your life, you're going to drop off the edge. That's the sense I get from you, and so if you have an alternative plan, you see, then life goes on. So what's the plan for today?

C: I'll probably go play handball. I haven't really exercised in the last three weeks. Actually, I had been pretty good about exercising until then. It's probably unfair to myself to say I haven't been doing it, but not doing it for three weeks probably contributes to my not feeling good.

T: Yes, it does. What is this "probably going to go?"?

C: Yeah, probably.

T: What's that word? *(Both laugh.)* So what's going to happen after you leave today?

C: Oh, you want me to go play handball?

T: Yes!

C: Oh, all right, I will then.

T: Great!

C: That helps. That helps.

T: I want you to go play handball every day! And certainly today. And what can you do to meditate? You say that you don't have a positive attitude; that is one of the single best things for it.

[Therapist reinforces positive behaviors.]

C: I know. I must not really want to have a positive attitude.

T: Oh no you don't!

C: I'm just trying to tell the truth.

T: Yes, I know, but you're weaseling out, because if you really don't want to have a positive attitude, then you don't have to meditate. *(laughs)* Don't you see? That's very tricky of you. *(pause)* And besides that I would like to see you exploring other volunteer coaching possibilities, perhaps in the high school. I expect you to do that.

C: Great. *(smiles)* I like when people say things like that.

T: Well, you know me, I do expect you to do this. And I would like to make another appointment with you so that I can check up on you.

C: I want to be checked up on. That's a funny thing, but it helps me. And I don't really enjoy being that way. I'd like to be able to just say to myself, "Do this," but if someone sort of encourages me, expecting me to do something . . .

T: Mike, are you objecting to being a human being?

C: Aw, I don't know.

T: Sounds like it to me.

## TWO WEEKS LATER

T: So, you know my question: What would you like today?

C: What would I like today?

T: Yeah.

C: *(sighs)* I've been thinking about that question and I've sort of come up with a list of things that I wanted but they sounded a little empty to me, probably since I've asked those questions before and, uh, I'm really stuck, you know, in the cycle of worrying about things all the time and not feeling healthy. Last two nights I swore that I wasn't going to be awake and alive in the morning. I had chest pain, you know, like I had before and, you know, just not being able to develop any kind of positive attitude about anything. Like there's not hope in terms of jobs or anything. I just feel like I'm facing toward a premature death, and I want to say, "Gee, Margot, I just want strategies to deal with that." And I guess I've said that before . . . I know what I should be doing to feel better, but I just don't . . . and I don't feel very well . . . Like last night I get these pains and I have them for about an hour and I can't fall asleep. I'm breathing and trying to relax . . .

T: Really deep breaths, belly breathing? Does it help?

C: Not really, although I eventually fell asleep.
   [Client then discusses possibilities of moving to get a job.]

T: Listen, if you wanted to get a high school coaching job, how would you do it?

C: You mean what would make me more attractive to them?

T: No, *how* would you do it? [Therapist asks for specifics.]

C: Well, I guess I'd have to find out where there were jobs.

T: How would you do that?

C: I guess there must be national organizations, like a teaching organization that puts out a weekly or monthly newsletter. Or if I found out there were jobs in New Mexico, I could get the out-of-town newspapers or maybe get in touch with someone I know in New Mexico and maybe find out about the opportunities there, I guess.

T: Or contact the state department of education.

C: Yeah, I mean I'm smart enough to figure how to do that.

T: *(smiles)* That's a relief! So I still have this question: *When* are you going to start making those contingency plans?

C: Well, I could make a schedule this afternoon.

T: Did you hear your verb?

C: I *can* start.

T: Yes, all right, and so is there a way that you can say it that would give it a little more energy?

C: I might start working?

T: Nooo!

C: That was a joke! I *will* start working.

T: Hey!!

C: I *will*. I haven't done that; I haven't structured things.

T: You see, one of the things I know—because I have known you so long—is that you have that little Mike . . . you know, the one we've talked about who used to climb up on his mother's bed and not understand her illness and not understand why his father divorced her . . . all that . . . and didn't understand really how his father could marry this woman who was so difficult . . . all this . . . that little boy is always there ready to say, "Oh my God, everything is going down the drain!" And when you have a real dislocation—that not getting that job is, Mike, that's a big one, a really big one—he naturally comes up again and says, "See, I told you so, it's all hopeless, let's not bother with anything, let's just die young and get it over with." [Therapist uses past experience to reframe present one.]

C: Yeah.

T: And all of this is perfectly normal and understandable, and the fact is that the way you have learned to deal with him is what you have to do again. And this will not be the only time you have to do it again. Life is full of "agains" of this sort. You have to pull yourself up by your bootstraps, as they say, and "get with the program"—*making your own program*—and get with it. Do it. He needs your help.

C: Good idea.

T: And the part of you that needs a kick in the rear to get going, he's going to feel better too. You're going to have to pull him kicking and screaming into feeling better, you know.

C: It's good to hear you say all that because I don't process that through my mind, you know, that part about the younger Mike. I didn't even put not getting the job in the same territory as those other losses, you know.

T: Not getting that job is a real loss, a *real loss*.

C: Yeah, it feels real. I guess it's a good time to do some planning.

T: Um hm, so I invite you to come up with ten different contingency plans so you don't think that you make one and you're stuck in that. One of the reasons that you don't do it is that you're afraid you'll make one and that you will be stuck with it. So make a list of ten different things, and make some of them things that you don't have the qualifications for but just something that if you could do anything you wanted, that would be it, besides coaching.

C: It sucks sitting home alone.

T: You bet, and this is about organizing yourself to dig yourself out. Also, keep looking in the paper to find some kind of part-time work because to have a regular commitment is helpful. [Therapist avoids becoming immersed in the client's problem-saturated view.]

C: Yeah.

[Client then discusses exploring various volunteer coaching possibilities, including one at the local high school, and decides that he needs to call the coach back.]

T: When are you going to call him?

C: I'm going to call him today, I suppose. . . .

T: Okay. Do you know his name?

C: Yes, I do. *(smiles)* Do I know where he lives? Yes, I do. Did he already tell me his name is in the phone book? Yes, he did.

T: *(laughs)* I like the way you're doing it. You don't even need me! So what time are you going to call him?

C: Uh, I'll probably call at ten of one. Of course, it's hard to do with all the other things I have to do—schedules and lists, plans and contingency plans, not to mention meditating and exercising. *(Both are smiling as client teases the therapist.)*

T: So when are you going to come back here and "report"?

C: In a month.

T: And you'll come back with schedules and everything?

C: I don't know, I can't promise.

## SIX WEEKS LATER

T: So, what's on your agenda? What are we going to do? You know, what would you like to have happen here?

C: Well, in the last couple days something new has come up for me, and, uh, that's . . . it's hit me, the inevitability of us moving. It seems as though we're going to be moving, and it feels like I'm going to get a job in baseball.

T: Great.

C: Yeah, it is great. But it feels like we're definitely going to move, and it makes me really sad . . .

T: Yes.

C: Yeah . . . and then I was actually feeling, "Well, I don't want to coach, I don't want to move more than I want to coach," but it didn't seem very real.

T: You also don't want to face what you have to do if you didn't coach.

C: Right.

T: *(smiles)* So that's a real trade-off, isn't it?

C: Yeah, I don't know what that would be. Uh, I mean, when I was here last time I was supposed to come up with ten contingency plans. I started out with one or two or three and the last thing you said was, "Ten." I did . . . I mean, I was investigating about ten things, but none of them—really, almost none of them—interested me, except for one thing sort of came to me. I saw an ad for the director of Project Open Hand, which obviously I'm not qualified for—you have to do a lot of things before you're qualified for that—but that really struck me. It was really interesting how I felt about that and . . .

T: What appeals to you about that?

C: It seems like, uh—other than the fact that it's a worthwhile cause and organization and that kind of thing—but also seems like the kind of thing that I could do. Not just do but be motivated to do, like get up in the morning and spend my time thinking about it.

T: So what is there about a cause like that that makes you feel that way?

C: No, I mean . . . I think I already said this, that it stirs some kind of passion in me, you know.

T: Stirs passion?

C: Yeah, you know, it makes me want to work, you know. Does that answer your question?

T: I want more specifics.

C: Yeah, you know, it's different from working at one of the schools I've worked at. It's on a broader scale, and it seems like I could affect things positively for more people.

T: Um hm, and it's good because it gives you a new area in which to think about possibilities.

C: I thought about writing to them to explore, or something else having to do with poverty—seeing as how I'm so close to it myself. *(Both laugh.)* I thought about writing them and say that I'm not applying for the job but I'd like to apply for the job ten years from now, like what are the kinds of things that you think that would make someone qualify for a position like that?

T: That's great! You should write that letter.

C: And also I thought about getting my master's in something that also might help me qualify for something—what a good plan! *(smiles)*

T: Yes. Now what has happened in relation to getting coaching jobs?

C: Well, I don't know, nothing definite. But it's funny, I feel optimistic. [Client then describes in detail various trips, interviews.]

C: Well, anyhow, I made a schedule and, uh, I tried to do what it said on the schedule and that was so hard for me—although one thing it did was it got me writing. I'm trying to write, like, a short story.

T: Great! [Therapist reinforces positive activities.]

C: I'm trying to just, like, make a finished thing. People told me so many times that I'm such a good writer and, uh, I started writing this story and, uh, I wrote a couple pages and I loved it! I loved reading it; it really made me laugh. And so then I wrote a couple more pages and I read, like, five pages and I find it, like, wildly entertaining, funny, and clever and all that kind of stuff. But that's an outgrowth of making my weekly schedule. I always start later than the schedule says because I have to drive my wife to work and uh . . .

T: So why don't you make a more realistic schedule?

C: Yeah.

T: Do it! You're setting yourself up not to do it by putting in times you can't actually meet!

C: *(laughs)* I'm aware of that but, anyhow, one of the sections on there was an hour and a half late afternoon, sort of after I've gone through all my things—baseball stuff, working out, doing whatever—of writing, you know, so it sort of got me into that.

T: Good!

C: I don't think I would have done it without the schedule.

T: Good! So what's your next step? [Therapist continues to press client to make efforts for change.]

C: Well . . . um . . . what's happening is, there are jobs opening up. There's one especially in the Midwest.

T: So how can you go after it?

C: Well, first of all, I have to find out who's up for it, and this is complicated . . . need to make some phone calls to find out the lay of the land so that I know what course to pursue. *(discusses many specific details of various teams and coaches)* I need to get all my letters out to everyone I know to remind them that I'm still looking for a job in coaching. So maybe I'll rewrite my schedule—how do you feel about me not working on contingency plans?

T: It sounds to me as though . . . the single thing I would like you to do about contingency plans is to write that letter to Project Open Hand.

C: Yeah.

T: Because that just makes a lot of sense. It could even shape what you do when you coach again. Since you really have that connection, it just seems to me that, why not? That would make sense and, otherwise, do the schedule and continue the writing. And I think you have a lot coming up in terms of pursuing the coaching stuff . . . and, uh, I want to be kept posted, please. So what do you want to do about us?

C: I'd like to come back in a month—I really need it.

## THREE MONTHS LATER

T: So, you know, what do you want?

C: What do I want? Is that the question you always ask me?

T: Sorry to disappoint you! What would you like to have happen here today?

C: Well, it's been a while since I've been here, um, and a lot has happened . . . and I've had hard times recently . . . and, uh, but on the other hand, I feel pretty good.

T: *(laughs)* How do you do that? It sounds good to me!

C: Well, I work hard at it.

T: Good, good!

C: But I wonder, you know, whether . . . I work hard at it. I think I work hard at it, maybe I'm fooling myself.

T: But if you're feeling good, what difference does it make whether you work hard or not?

C: Well, I'm never sure if it's appropriate if I'm feeling good, I'm not supposed to be feeling good, maybe I'm—see the thing is, there's a reality out there somewhere. I get my last paycheck a month from now, and I haven't figured out a way to get another paycheck, you know, the equivalent paycheck, so therefore perhaps I should be nervous about that. And I do occasionally get nervous and I have been and that's created some of my own anxiety recently.

T: Not surprisingly.

C: Sometimes I wonder should I be feeling good, you know, should I . . .

T: The answer is yes, you should!

C: *(smiles)* Yeah, yeah, I should be feeling good, but shouldn't I be worrying more? Shouldn't I be doing more? That's maybe another question, but I feel like I'm doing quite a bit.

T: They're quite different. Whether I might be doing more is a very different question from whether or not I should be worrying more. Worrying more is never appropriate, *doing* more sometimes is. Please make that distinction; it's crucial. They're not the same thing at all. One leads you somewhere, the other one impedes you.

[Therapist presents the client with a useful distinction that has implications for the future.]

C: What's possibly unreal is that I'm saying that it feels fine to me while, in reality, in a year or two I'll be miserable because I'm not coaching.

T: Okay. The reality is that you're feeling fine now and that you're dealing with your situation extremely well. What happens in the future we'll never know until we get there, and then it's the present and then we deal with it.

C: And quickly it's the past.

T: *(smiles)* So it sounds good to me. I'm delighted to hear what you're saying about feeling good.

C: *Maybe* you are, except so . . .

T: No, I *am,* and I'm quite clear that I am! *(laughs)*

C: Okay, so you are. Well, let's work on that a little bit and see if we can break that down. *(laughs)* But the fact is, my last paycheck comes in a month and . . .

T: So what are you going to do about that? What's the next step for you?

[Therapist continues to put responsibility on the client for taking action.]

C: I guess getting a job would be a good next step.

T: Sounds good. *What* are you going to *do* about that?

C: I don't know. I, uh, a couple weeks ago . . . the baseball stuff ended. All of a sudden I had nothing in front of me, you know. I had no phone calls to make to continue to network to chase something down, so I said, "Whoa!" Then I heard about this half-time position at the junior college as athletic director. It feels like this job is perfect and I'm perfect for this job, so I'm going to get all these people, like I have before, to recommend me. It feels potentially like another futile exercise . . . like it's happened a lot of times.

T: *And* you're going to do it!

C: Yeah, I'm going to do it, and I'm going to try to be positive about my . . .

T: Don't *try.* Trying does not work. *Be definite!*

C: *Trying* doesn't work?

T: Trying, think about trying: It means that you're afraid that you won't be able to do it. That's what that word means. It's a weasel word. Do not use it when you intend to have something happen.

[Therapist confronts the client with his use of words since words compel experience.]

C: Don't *try* your best, *be* your best!

T: That's it, that's it.

C: I *will* get this job.

T: "I will get that job. That is just the right one for me, and I'm going to be very positive about going for this job." Sounds good—nice place.

C: *(sighs)* It's a hard thing, kind of unbelievable. Every now and then I think about how it's going to feel when I do get a job. There's no reason to believe that I'm going to go my whole life without a job, although that's kind of what it feels like. It feels like it's all over . . .

T: Of course. So why are you smiling? *(Both laugh.)* It's just great!

C: I'm smiling because it's kind of funny that way your mind works: "Other than that I've been pretty good!" Oh, did I tell you about my journal? That's one of the methods . . . that's one of the ways I keep working at it. Every time I have a little free time I will write in my journal.

T: Excellent.

C: That's my way of keeping track of how I'm doing and all this.

T: That's great.

## THREE WEEKS LATER

T: What's our agenda today?

C: Well, I have an interview at the high school on Wednesday . . .

T: Good.

C: . . . for a full-time job teaching history.

T: Really? Great!

C: Yes, it's a step . . . it's a helpful step toward getting a job, I think. So I'm making a plan to prepare for the interview.

T: Yes, good.

C: And being here is part of it.

T: So what do you need here?

C: Uh, let's see, what do I need here? Probably some help in gaining confidence for it and a positive outlook toward it. Um, is that a reasonable request?

[Notice the client's active engagement compared to his early despondency.]

T: Sure. I mean, you can make any request here.

C: Yes, I can. Well, my thoughts regarding the interview are things like "Well, I haven't taught history and I haven't taught a curriculum class anywhere, you know, history or anything for seven years, and it's a pretty high-powered high school."

T: Um hm, but you've been teaching for the last seven years as a coach.

C: I have, right.

T: You must present yourself that way.

C: Yeah. Well, I think they bought that; that's one of the reasons that they're interviewing me. Both the principal and the vice-principal where I've been substitute teaching called for me, without my even asking.

T: How nice. Even as a substitute teacher you . . .

C: Oh, I'm a hero.

T: I'm not surprised, I've always known that! *(Client laughs diffidently.)* Really!

C: Well, they regard me as a hero. So they called.

[Mike then spends some time describing in detail how he will prepare for the interview. He uses as a model the presentation that he prepared when he was interviewed for the head coach position. That interview went extremely well.]

T: What you say sounds good to me; I'd hire you.

C: So how can I boost my confidence so *they* want to hire me?

T: Um. What I'd like to know is, when you think about it what kind of a picture do you see of yourself there?

C: As a teacher there?

T: No, in the interview.

C: Well, let's see, uh, it's a developing picture. It's in progress; it's a work in progress.

T: Well, that's what I'd like to know because I could help the work.

C: Yeah, that's what I was hoping for. Uh, couple things, I have two images to go on. One is a longtime standing image of being nervous when I went in and feeling sort of unprepared, I think. That kind of thing isn't just an interview picture of myself. However, it's changed somewhat more recently over the years. When I had the interview for the head coaching job, I knew it was going to be big, and I was nervous about being nervous. So I really prepared so that I was confident that I *was* prepared. The interview went extremely well; I was ecstatic, and the feedback afterwards was stunning. Now I think that this is the job I have to get and uh . . .

T: Well, the fact is that this is *not* the job that you *have* to get, this is just one of the jobs you would like to get. Don't forget that. *(Client sighs.)* You will not drop off the edge of the world if you do not get this job.

[Therapist helps the client realign his expectations.]

C: Feels like I might.

T: I know it, that's why I'm pointing it out to you.

C: Yeah.

T: So, what I would like you to do is a little technique called the swish. Are you ready for this?

[The reader is referred to Bandler, 1985, for details of this technique.]

C: Yeah.

T: Okay. What I want you to do is to close your eyes and make a picture of yourself nervous, the way you *have been,* the way you don't want to be on Wednesday. Have you got that one?

C: Uh huh.

T: In detail? When I say make a picture I don't mean it has to be like an etching or something but, rather, an image that has in it everything that makes you be there—the feelings, the sounds, the way you look. And I want you to be *in* that picture, looking out from your eyes. You got that one?

C: Yeah.

T: Okay, open your eyes and take a deep breath; look out the window. [This exercise is designed to get the client out of that nervous feeling state.] And now I would like you to make another picture. I would like you to use perhaps the way you were looking and acting at the end of the head coach interview, when you knew you'd done a dynamite job. And with this one, I want you to *see yourself* there, not be inside of it. You know, when you're feeling in your full power to do a good interview, okay?

C: I'm having a little trouble picturing myself.

T: Imagine that there is a mirror there to look at, so you could see yourself there. [Therapist uses feedback to revise instruction.]

C: Okay.

T: Okay, and then come back, open your eyes, and listen to my instructions before you do it. You're going to take that first picture, the one you're inside, and you're going to have it a big picture in front of you, and in the lower right-hand corner you're going to make a very small representation of the picture showing how you would like to be and it's going to be dark and small. Okay?

C: All right.

T: Now just listen to this, and then do it. I want you to make the big picture get small and dark and *at the same time* let the small picture get big and bright so that it covers up and obliterates the other picture. And then, after you've done that, blank the screen and then do it again, five times in a row. And each time that you do that swish, do it faster—and it's very important to blank the screen in between swishes.

C: Okay.

T: Great. Now *try* to see the first picture again and see what happens. *(Client laughs.)* And then tell me what happens.

C: *(chuckles)* Well, I haven't quite pictured it yet.
   [Not to be able to see the earlier nervous picture is the goal of the swish strategy.]

T: That's good, that's good!

C: I just don't seem to get it.

T: You can keep on trying if you like, but that, of course, is the purpose of this. You see, the idea is, Mike, that we get into habits of directing our brain in a certain way. Some time ago we chose a particular response, and for some reason it automated—they're often responses we don't like—and they feel like habits over which we have no control because they're so automatic. The swish invites you specifically to *redirectionalize* your brain so that when you think of one thing you immediately think of the other thing that you want. You can do it with anything. Any unwanted behavior. You just go through this process and often get the result that you did. The goal is to either erase the first picture or as you begin to get the first picture have it immediately flash to the second one. You will find that you will be feeling much more relaxed and confident in your upcoming interview.

C: There's a big difference in the two pictures.

T: I know; I heard that.

C: *(sighs)* But I know how to be the second one.

T: Yes, of course you do! And it's even more there for you now, because you had that superb experience when applying for the head coach job.

C: But it's not just that one . . .

T: *(smiles)* You don't have any other memories of competence.

C: I do, so the nervous one isn't in control.

T: You bet. Did you know that when there are things you want to give up, when you start speaking of them in the past that it enables you to give them up more quickly?

C: I didn't know that.

T: Because language compels our experience; it's all about what we tell ourselves. So the nervous picture *was* what used to be. [Therapist places the negative experience in the past.]

C: A long long time ago.

T: *(laughs, as does client)* Yes, a long long time ago. Well, of course, in some ways everything that's past *is* a long time ago. So what else do you want? You're all set now, aren't you?

C: *(pause)* I think I am. And I have a lot of things to do; there's no sense in sitting around here! *(smiles)*

T: *(laughs)* Right! Good-bye!

C: I feel that way somewhat. I was going to ask you . . . I'm glad you did—what did you call that? The switch?

T: The swish; you swish the pictures.

C: I get it.

T: You need to do it very fast and blank the screen in between. Otherwise, you set up a feedback loop; that's why that's very important there. You'd just keep seeing the two pictures going round and round. And the picture of what you want needs to be very enticing. And yours is because it's an actual memory; you didn't even have to create it. You already had it. You just want to be able to have it there all the time in place of that old one that you used to have.

C: It's good we did that. What I was going to ask when I came in was for a guided something or other, or a hypnosis thing, because I *did* want to find an image of what it would be like.

T: You got it.

C: Yeah, and the funny thing, like you said, I didn't have to create it, just recall it.

T: You just have to reconnect with it and *direct* yourself, which you've now done. And I would invite you, between now and then, occasionally look up and see that picture. Just keep on reminding yourself because as you see it, it will reinforce it. Don't try to do the other one, just do that one.

C: Oh yeah? No swishing?

T: No, you got it now. You see, if you swished it again you'd be going backwards, and you don't want to do that. You've already knocked that picture out. Don't revive it; it wouldn't serve you. Keep seeing the one you're going toward, just reminding yourself. Yes? No?

C: No, that's it, I'm just . . . time to run out of here!

T: *(laughs)* While you can still make it under your own steam!

C: *(smiles)* I'm sorry, but I have to go. I have a lot of things to do!

T: Right, you don't want to waste time lollygagging around here with me.

C: Thanks.

T: You're welcome!

## EDITOR'S QUESTIONS

Q: *You take a very active organizing role in helping to facilitate a shift in this client's mood and attitude from one of pessimism and feeling down in the dumps to one of hope and optimism for the future. Your firm directives enable him to actively take steps on his own behalf. By encouraging him to take this step or that, as you do, aren't you concerned that you will foster his dependence on you as the motivating force behind his actions?*

A: My three overall goals for all clients are increased choice, enhanced autonomy, and restored morale. With this clear focus, dependence rarely becomes an issue. I see my role as that of a catalyst who "jump-starts" the clients. This process begins with the immediate focus on what *they* want. When clients are despairing, as Mike was, they do appear dependent, and mobilizing them often takes directive activity from me. Once their motors are running, so to speak, I simply find ways to support their chosen journey. I believe this sequence is reflected in these transcripts.

Q: *Your therapy is obviously influenced by the work of Milton Erickson and the neurolinguistic programmers. I am interested in hearing about how your work evolved in this direction. How did you personally make the shift from "problems to possibilities" in your own clinical work?*

A: In 1975 when I joined the Harvard Community Health Plan (an HMO with limited mental health benefits), I was necessarily thrust into the practice of seeing clients briefly. Since I had been trained in and had practiced long-term psychodynamic therapy for some twenty years, I found this a special challenge. I began to search for therapeutic models and tools that would help me to get results in brief therapy. I was therefore delighted when I discovered neurolinguistic programming, as well as the work of Virginia Satir and Milton Erickson, for here I found the tools I needed to fulfill client requests in a time-effective manner—and an approach in which hope was engendered in both client and therapist. It then took me several years of conscious and deliberate practice to integrate these approaches into my own practice.

Q: *In the final segment of the transcript, when you've completed the "swish" process, you instruct the client to "try to see the first picture again." Earlier in the interview you chided the client for using this "weasel" word try. So the question is, why use it here?*

A: The reason that I use it here—it *was* deliberate and not accidental—is exactly the same reason that I objected to Mike's using it. The word *try* has a strong presuppositional flavor of *failure*. I objected to Mike's saying that he'll "try to be positive" because I don't want him to fail at it. When I tell him to try to see the first picture again, I want him to fail, since that is the purpose of the exercise. And while he may not consciously hear the failure presupposition, his unconscious mind does, as he can no longer see the unwanted scene. This is an example of paying attention to presuppositions and getting them to work to help the client reach a desired goal.

Q: *Your therapy appears to include a significant amount of laughter and bantering between you and the client. Obviously, in this instance, this is a person with whom you have developed a relationship over an extended period. More generally, what do you see as the benefits of humor in therapy, and how do you use humor in a way that would not be experienced as discounting the client's pain, especially when a client might present in a depressed manner?*

A: Over the past 10 years or so it has become increasingly clear to me that the more serious you are about getting results in therapy, the more humor and laughter you need to use. Psychophysiological studies in recent years demonstrate that a positive mood of hope supports both mental and physical healing. Humor and laughter both promote hope and are a direct antidote for anxiety, fear, rage, and sadness. People not only feel better when they smile and laugh but also are more receptive to change. Most humor involves some kind of reframing—seeing things in a new way—so I look for ways to offer new points of view by playing on words and posing new perspectives. I avoid discounting the client's distress by making sure that I maintain rapport even as I offer a potentially humorous comment.

## REFERENCES

Bandler, R. (1985). *Using your brain—for a change*. Moab, UT: Real People Press.

Bandler, R., & Grinder, J. (1979). *Frogs into princes*. Moab, UT: Real People Press.

Friedman, S., & Fanger, M. T. (1991). *Expanding therapeutic possibilities: Getting results in brief psychotherapy*. New York: Lexington Books/Macmillan.

Satir, V. (1986, September). Speech presented at 5-day conference, New York.

Watzlawick, P. (1978). *Language of change*. New York: Basic Books.

Wujec, T. (1988). *Pumping ions*. New York: Doubleday.

# 5

## Enhancing Views of Competence

MICHAEL DURRANT
KATE KOWALSKI

George Harrison, then a member of the Beatles, was asked at a press conference during a tour of Australia, "Mr Harrison, you Beatles have a distinctive hairstyle. What do you call it?" After some thought, Harrison replied, "I call it Fred." What do we call our model of therapy? Like Harrison, we are not sure that we wish to be categorized, but if forced to give it a name we would probably call our approach "competency-based."

There is an oft-quoted Milton Erickson story in which he recounts his experience of finding a riderless horse, which he did not recognize. Erickson rode it back to its farm, confident that the horse would know the right direction and that his own task was simply to keep the horse "on track." "And that," he says, "is the way you do psychotherapy" (Gordon & Meyers-Anderson, 1981). We often think of our therapy in much the same light; we seek to help clients use their resources, and our job is simply to keep them on track. We agree with Watzlawick (1990) that "therapy is what we say it is, i.e., what names we operate with, what explanatory principles we use, and what reality we thereby create" (p. 59). Our clients, like the horse, end up finding their own way home, our particular "theory" notwithstanding.

## UNDERLYING ASSUMPTIONS

Clearly, there are many theories or models upon which therapists can rely. Rather than argue the "truth," or otherwise, of any particular theory in seeking to say what it is that we do, we have found it most useful to concentrate on identifying the basic assumptions about people, problems, solutions, and change that inform our work. Our work together has reflected the influence of our background in the solution-focused approach of de Shazer and his colleagues (de Shazer, 1988; de Shazer et al., 1986) and in Michael White's (1986, 1989) approach and has involved aspects of the work of the Mental Research Institute in Palo Alto, California, and Erickson's pioneering therapy as well. What has been important to us in considering these influences on our work has been the extent to which they reflect similar, or complementary, underlying assumptions. We have previously outlined our main principles or assumptions regarding the treatment of the effects of sexual abuse (Durrant & Kowalski, 1990), and many of these represent the broader assumptions that underlie our work in general.

## Assumption about People's Competence

A survey by the Gallup organization found that 90% of more than 1000 Americans sampled had successfully overcome a significant health, emotional, addiction, or lifestyle problem and that professional intervention had been a factor in less than 3% of these cases (Gurin, 1990). This survey confirms what we have long believed: Most people have the ability to deal with most things most of the time. This assumption was strongly reflected in Erickson's work. "Erickson seemed to operate for the most part as if people have the possibility of changing their behavior. His therapy was usually based on the assumption that there were alternative aspects of the personality that could be brought forth and used for the person's benefit" (O'Hanlon, 1987, p. 18).

It is our contention that as therapists we have a choice about the basic stance we wish to adopt. To see people in terms of pathology or to see them in terms of competence is a matter of choice rather than of truth. We choose to see our clients as competent, while acknowledging that the patterns of behaving and thinking in which they have become caught may have hidden their competence from them.

Our assumption that people have and can build upon competence leads us to conduct our therapy in such a way as to utilize what is going right rather than to fix what is going wrong. We assume that there will be exceptions—times of success despite the problem (de Shazer, 1985, 1988)— to the problem or the view of the problem; there will be times when the problem is less of a problem or is not there, and there will be times when the client demonstrates personal competence despite the problem. We seek to ask about these exceptions as soon as possible in a session, since their identification provides already-existing solutions that might be able to be repeated or enlarged upon.

## Assumption about the Stance of the Therapist and Expertise of the Client

In our sexual abuse work and in relation to the question of whether or not it is necessary or helpful for clients to recount in detail the experience of the abuse, we have stated that our clients are the best judges of whether or not this will be helpful (Durrant & Kowalski, 1990). That is, we assume that our clients are able to be "experts" in their own treatment and, in particular, about their own futures. This assumption reflects our view that we are not dealing with pathology that needs to be "fixed"—which would require expert diagnosis and expert treatment planning—but with people who are "stuck" in patterns of belief, behavior, and interaction that they are currently not experiencing as successful.[1] Intrinsic to this view is the belief that people are capable of behaving (and thinking and feeling) differently. Therefore, rather than conduct a detailed assessment or exploration of a client's problems, we usually commence with "What do you think it would be helpful for me to know about your situation?" Our aim is that clients will feel that their expertise is being acknowledged and that they are being offered some sense of control over the therapy process.

Similarly, when a client makes a statement such as "I find it difficult to talk about this," we will often ask a question such as "So what made you decide that talking about it today would be helpful?" Such a question suggests a degree of choice and decision and so might contribute to the client's beginning to experience himself or herself as having a greater degree of personal agency.

In keeping with the theme that it is our clients who possess the expertise with which their difficulties will be solved, we often invite our clients to speculate on what the future will look like when the problem that brought them to therapy is solved. Whether this is the "miracle question" (de Shazer, 1988, 1991) or a more limited question about imagining some aspect of the future solution-state, such an invitation to speculate presupposes that our clients can envisage the future. Not only does the exploration of this future picture seem to increase the possibility of its existence, but also the questions emphasize the clients' expertise in that it is they who are defining the solution and considering its implications. Miller (1992) distinguishes between miracles and explanations in that miracles are "symptoms" of solutions while explanations are symptoms of problems. Explanations, as he points out, require highly developed therapist expertise while miracles are generated by client expertise. Scaling questions (Chapter 1; Kowalski & Kral, 1989) provide another way to build on clients' expertise by allowing them to rate their own success and anticipate what small changes will be necessary to create the desired solution.

We will sometimes explain to clients what it is we are doing and seek their opinion. Although therapy often seems like a mystery, clients need not feel that some mysterious process is being done to them. Therapy that seeks to build on strength can assume more of a cooperative climate; thus we might comment or explain to the client that our emphasis is on building on what is already working. We may ask clients to comment on whether or not

---

[1]We have "joked" in our workshops that if we are ever invited to contribute to the formulation of DSM-VIII or -IX, it will have only one diagnostic category: "stuck."

they believe something we have suggested will be helpful, believing that the process of reflecting on this may further enhance their view of their own competence, and so be an important part of their thinking about solutions.

We always invite our clients to decide if it might be helpful to have another session. Rather than say "I would like to see you again in two weeks," we say something like "Do you think it would be helpful to talk some more?" Or (if we have suggested a task): "If you decide it would be helpful to come back and tell me how you go with this, maybe two weeks would be a good time. What do you think?"

## Assumption about Experience and "Reality"

We share the constructivist assumption that people are in a constant process of making sense of themselves and their experience and that any knowledge or "reality" is a result of that process of making sense. That is, what we deal with in therapy is not "truth" but our clients' experience and their perceptions of that experience. Again, this challenges notions of norms or diagnostic criteria; every client's situation, and hence every problem, is different. Thus, we prefer not to speak, for example, of "approaches to therapy with substance abuse" or "therapy with behavior problems" since such descriptions imply a classification of the world by problem type, with the implication that different types of problems require different methods of treatment. Once we begin to think of problems as entities that may be classified and reified, we easily lose sight of the unique experiences of our clients. We assume that the important element of therapy is not that the intervention matches the problem but that the intervention fits the uniqueness of the client.

Another quote from Erickson introduces the published proceedings of an Ericksonian conference: "Each person is a unique individual. Hence, psychotherapy should be formulated to meet the uniqueness of the individual's needs, rather than tailoring the person to fit the Procrustean bed of a hypothetical theory of human behavior" (Erickson, quoted in Zeig & Gilligan, 1990).

Our preference is to talk about solutions rather than problems; however, that may not immediately fit with the experience of our clients, who often come to therapy intending or expecting to talk about problems. We do not believe that talking about the problem ("working it through") leads to change; however, we are clear that *not* talking about it sometimes leads to clients feeling unheard. Therefore, while our aim is to be alert to exceptions to the problem or to other examples of competence from the outset of therapy, we are alert to our clients' lead and to signs that they need to know that their situation has been understood and their experience validated. This is particularly likely to be the case when the problem has been long-standing, has not responded to previous therapy, or has involved some traumatic experience (such as sexual abuse, violence, or bereavement).

When clients wish to talk about the problem and an immediate exploration of exceptions or competency is premature, we seek a way of talking about the problem that renders it more solvable. In discussing the process of "inducing doubt" into the way clients see their situation (and thus making possible different ways of seeing), de Shazer (1990) suggests that his approach does so by finding exceptions while the MRI approach accomplishes this aim by reframing the problem. When clients wish to talk about the problem, reframing provides a way to do so while still challenging their problem-focused construction. Externalizing the problem (White, 1989) is a form of reframing that often offers a helpful way of talking about the problem; the technique of referring to the problem as if it were something separate from the client provides a way of discussing the problem that does not reinforce notions of internal pathology or purposiveness. However, externalizing (or any other reframing we might employ) is not an end in itself. It may be a helpful way of talking about the problem but it still aims to provide a platform for identifying exceptions and competence. Once the client seems able to begin to appreciate a discussion of exceptions, we leave behind the problem-focused, externalized description and embrace a more solution-focused discourse.

## Assumption about View of Self and the Nature of Change

The main effect of problems, we have suggested, is that they prevent people from noticing or appreciating their strengths and encourage a view of the self as a failure. Change, then, comes about through developing a view of self as competent and capable of change. Such a view of competence leads both to behaving differently and thinking and feeling differently and, importantly, makes it less likely that future difficulties will lead to the same kind of "stuckness."

The process of encouraging the development of the view of self as competent entails both challenging aspects of the old view and identifying aspects of the new. The exploration of exceptions challenges the client's old view of the self by introducing doubt as to its pervasiveness. The highlighting of continued successes, small steps at practicing new ways of behaving, and elaboration of the imagined future without the problem introduce aspects of the new view.

As clients begin to behave differently, they sometimes, begin to experience themselves differently through making sense of their new behavior (and others' reactions to it). The new view of self is built by doing (and by becoming aware of what's already been done or imagining what will be done), although this does not reduce the approach to one that simply aims for behavioral change. Often clients will begin to notice differences but will not necessarily appreciate their significance. They may, for example, attribute them to changes in other people or to circumstance. In this situation we prefer to include some specific exploration of the significance or potential new meaning of exceptions and examples of competence.

The simple question "How did you manage to do that?" or "As you continue doing that in the future, what difference do you imagine it will make?" invites clients to begin to attribute successes to their own efforts. It is not uncommon for them to be unable to answer such questions, at least initially, and this reflects the fact that they are not used to seeing themselves as having exercised personal agency. We might also respond to an example of competence or difference with a question such as "How did you decide you were ready to do that?"—another question that implies action and decision on the part of the client. Thus, the process of exploring the exceptions is one of making them meaningful.

Further, we might question the implications of these discoveries for the client's view of self. These may be questions along the lines of White's (1988) self-description questions—for example, "What do you think that says about you?"—or perhaps more explicit questions about what clients are thinking about themselves or whether they are able to appreciate certain things about themselves.

## A Map for Therapy

Our aim is that clients will build a new view of self, one based on ideas of competence rather than failure and grounded in a successful future rather than a failed past. From the ideas and assumptions noted earlier, we have derived a map for the therapy process (Figure 5.1). As with all maps, ours does not show every possible route that may be taken and is only something to help orient and guide the process. We are all too aware that it is quite possible to spend so much time looking at the map that one can run off the road! At different times different parts of the map will assume greater prominence, sometimes parts of the map will be bypassed. Often the arrows will be more complex, returning to earlier steps before proceeding.

## ANNA: A FAILURE AT EVERYTHING (EVEN THERAPY)

Anna, age 27, was referred because of constant feelings of depression and, on occasion, thoughts of suicide. She was initially seen by Kate Kowalski for five sessions. A few months after Kate left Australia, Anna saw Michael Durrant for a few further sessions.

## Session I

This excerpt begins with Anna (C) explaining to Kate (T) that she shares a house with three friends.

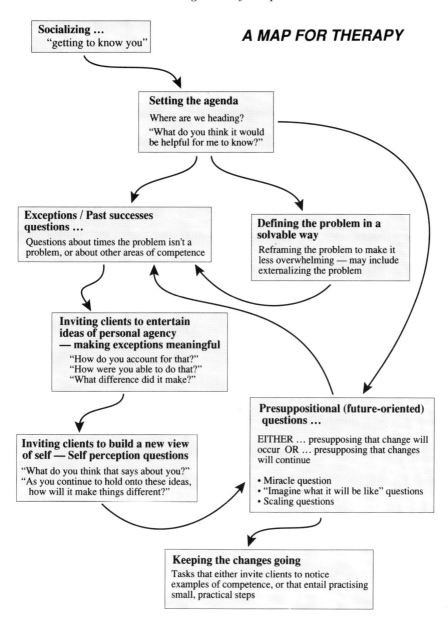

**FIGURE 5.1.** A map for therapy.

C: One of them, Sue, is my closest friend, and a lot of what I want to talk about is to do with my relationship with her. I guess it's because I've struck problems in that relationship that I wanted to see someone. Because somehow I have a feeling that that relationship is too close and I'm far too dependent. And I feel like I'm reproducing the way my mother related to me in the way I relate to Sue. And it really bothers me.

T: Okay. Have you gone for counseling before?

C: Yes, but I've never really stuck with anybody. I think I expected instant results. I didn't realize I was unhappy until I finished university. Then by the middle of the next year I suddenly realized I felt horrible all the time . . . really anxious . . . I couldn't sleep. My jaw used to ache and I had, sort of, tension in my body but particularly an aching jaw—which I don't have as much now—and a lot of other things, like an upset stomach. I had all these problems and my body felt terrible and I had no idea why. I went to the doctor but I only went once and we didn't really figure out why. But then I kept feeling so horrible, this awful anxiety, and I went to see this counselor. I think she's very understanding. I saw her every week for about five or six months. She prescribed anti-depressants after three months when I didn't seem to be progressing. I took them for four months and they didn't seem to help after the first few weeks, so I just decided to stop taking them.

T: So how do you account for the fact that you said you don't feel that same sort of way . . . your jaw doesn't ache as much.

[Anna presented as a veteran of therapy, particularly of therapy that aimed to provide "insight," but she seemed to feel that she had been a failure even at this. Already there are signs that she feels she needs to "unload," to ensure that this therapist understands how bad everything is. Mindful of the need that Anna feel her concerns are heard and validated, Kate ventures a question about an exception in an effort to encourage Anna to focus on a small example of things being better. However, when Anna uses this as a way to continue to talk about the problem, Kate decides that it is most helpful to allow her to continue. Trying to force her to focus on the exception could easily have created a struggle, with Anna left feeling unheard.]

C: I do, but not all the time. Before I saw her I think I had no understanding of why I felt bad, and she made me realize that I had a lot of anger towards my parents. My parents are divorced and their marriage was horrible and I was an only child. And she made me realize that I've never really dealt with all that stuff. And I think a lot of it's still there. And she said I was depressed and the way I was expressing it was all this tension. It was anger causing my depression. I think I learned a lot but I got really upset cause it dredged up all this stuff I hadn't talked about before. I should have written down all the things I learned, but I learned a lot about my parents' relationship and my relationship with them and how that had affected me. I think I'd just blocked it all out before. But we only just scratched the surface. She gave me lots of advice about things I could do, and a lot of it was stuff like forgiving my parents and putting all that behind me. But I don't think I really wanted to change.

T: So tell me more about what made you decide that coming for counseling now . . . that you were ready now.

C: Well, I had a talk with my minister. He said I had low self-esteem. We did this ritual where he got me to write down all these awful things about myself and we burnt them. I felt really happy but it didn't last. Then the next year I went overseas by myself for seven months.

T: Where did you go?

C: I went to Europe and I had really good experiences but I was really lonely too. While I was away I decided I need to stick with some counselor and I saw someone. But because of my job I didn't stick with her. And I found her really threatening because of what she was trying to get me to do. She used to have me sitting in chairs and pretending that that chair was my father and talk to the chair. I don't know, I think I still wasn't ready to do it all. Then I—I feel like I'm a junkie for courses and counseling and stuff—I did this course and it included a very intense weekend with all these funny body exercises to get in touch with emotions and stuff. I knew I had stuff I needed to deal with, with my parents, but I was really threatened with all those people and I was very annoyed with myself that I didn't. And they recommended meditation, but I just haven't been able to do that by myself.

[More evidence of Anna's "training" to be a therapy patient and of her tendency to attribute the lack of success of therapy to her own failure. Kate tries to redirect the focus by asking a future-oriented question that presupposes that this therapy experience will be different.]

T: Well, let me ask you this. How do you suppose you'll know that our getting together and talking has been helpful to you?

C: I don't know.

T: What kinds of signs will there be? What will you notice about yourself that will make you say, "Hey, things are going better"?

C: Well, I don't know. I think I need to talk to someone and work through all these feelings, and it's going to take more than four or five visits. I just don't know what to expect.

T: So, what kinds of things . . . when you think about how you'd like you or your life to be different . . .

C: I don't really know, I just want it to be different. That's a problem. I mean I haven't really explained to you yet what's been happening recently . . . the sorts of things I've been doing that have been frightening me.

T: Okay. What do you think it would be helpful for me to know?

[Before Anna tells the whole story, Kate wants to try to frame this process in a way that invites Anna to feel that she has some control over it, that she is the expert on what she needs to do or say.]

C: Well, I guess the way I've been treating people (starts to cry) . . . I need to see someone because . . . well, the way I've reacted to certain things really frightened me . . . because . . . I went off the deep end severely, when a couple of things happened last year. My friend told me that she was getting married, my closest friend, and I was furious. I felt really angry and really jealous and I couldn't handle it. And she was my friend. The whole time we've shared a house together neither of us has had a relationship with a man, and I have never had one. And when Sue started going out with this person, I was totally taken by surprise by my extremely jealous and angry reaction. I was just plunged into a state of depression. I just . . .

T: So it was hard to be excited and . . .

C: I just felt angry and I just don't think that's an appropriate way to react. I'd like to not keep reacting that way. But I just feel far too involved in Sue's life. I just feel excessively dependent. I just read a book about codependency and I had a horrible feeling that that's what I'm like. Like, he said that people who are dependent expect everyone else to make them happy and seem to be perpetually angry with people. I haven't been giving very much to anyone. Because I've been depressed, I haven't wanted to. I just don't feel like calling my friends. And then I feel rejected, like they don't care about me. I feel like I don't love anyone and *(very distressed)* I just feel sort of empty inside.

T: If Sue were here and I were to ask her . . . if I were to say, "Anna's saying that she is too dependent," what would she say?

C: I don't know. She knows how badly I've treated her. But I don't think she knew how churned up I felt. But a few weeks ago we had this talk and I said, "For the past year you've been going out with Ian, and I feel like you've neglected a lot of your close friends. I'm not the only one. And I'm really scared that you're going to ignore me again and I'll never see you." And for me that was quite a leap.

T: Very brave.

C: For me that's quite a big thing to do because in my family we never talk about how we feel. *(very distressed)* You just don't say anything.

T: So how did you get up the courage to say that?

C: I think I was angry with Sue but I behaved really badly. It's what usually happens. She asks me what's wrong and then we have a talk. But it's her that initiates it. So we had quite a good talk and I felt it was quite a leap forward for me. I mean, I used to lie in bed just churning. What else happened last year, oh, I . . .

[Anna has responded to another possible exception—her bravery in talking to her friend—and so Kate persists in exploring this.]

T: Can I stop you a minute and ask you some more about this talk with Sue? I'm quite interested in that. You've obviously been feeling—quite naturally—very upset about how Ian coming into Sue's life has really changed your relationship.

C: I know it's a natural reaction . . . but, I guess, I felt that I didn't manage to control my hurt feelings and it was wrong and . . . well, I've never slammed the front door and run away before in my life. But the fact we could sit down and have that talk, that's actually . . .

T: Yeah.

C: I couldn't have done that a year ago. Sue said, "You couldn't have done that a year ago, or even six months ago."

T: So Sue even appreciated that that was a big step for you. That's interesting.

[The discussion is beginning to focus on an event that implies something different about Anna, something that might challenge her view of her own failure and worthlessness. This focus seems to allow her to remember some steps she has been taking to be different, although, not surprisingly, she does not yet appreciate their significance.]

C: Yeah, I've been in a process . . . I've been trying to make myself do things that are really hard. I just have to force myself to do those hard things; otherwise, I feel like I'll never change. I'm glad I could do that, but I feel like every time there's a situation I'm going to have to force myself to do it. In the past, if I've said something bitter or sarcastic—which I don't usually do except when I'm depressed—it's really hard for me to apologize. I had a dispute with Ken the other morning and I didn't really apologize properly. I still haven't.

T: Okay, so you're still practicing.

[Anna has felt she needs some major transformation. Kate's introduction of the term *practicing* sets the stage for talking later about doing small things differently as a way of changing.]

C: Yeah. I'm doing little things. There's something else. In the middle of all this last year, and feeling depressed, there was a guy I was interested in. I finally decided to do something about it and we went out for supper and he actually brought it up, after I had been avoiding it all night, and he said, "I'm thinking about the priesthood so I can't go out with you." I think I was obsessed with him and I felt really rejected and like I had nothing to look forward to for the rest of my life. And I was feeling like killing myself because he said no. I mean, it seems really crazy now.

T: How did you get beyond that?

C: I can't remember. I know I felt so bad I seriously felt like killing myself.

T: I don't mean this in any kind of facetious way, but I'm interested in how come you decided not to.

C: I think I don't like pain.

T: What were the things that made you feel like you wanted to keep on living?

C: In the past few weeks I've felt so terrible that I wished I was dead, but I could never do it. I think maybe one percent of me feels hopeful that life might get better in the end. It's almost like a little voice inside me says, "It won't always be like this."

T: So, there's part of you that still feels hopeful that one day you'll have the kind of life that you'll like.

C: Yeah, but there's a big part . . . sometimes that part's bigger and I feel more hopeful and that leads me to try to do something. Like going to counseling. There was someone else . . . I ended up going to a psychiatrist but I only went for about seven or eight visits. I explained to him all about my parents and everything and he ended up saying, "I don't understand. There doesn't seem to be enough data in what you've told me to explain why you are the way you are. I just can't understand it." So I just gave up.

[Previous therapy has encouraged this hopelessness view that the "problem" is bigger than it appears. Seeking therapy can be seen as an attempt to do something, to take some control over things, but therapy has left Anna feeling even more hopeless.]

T: It's interesting, when you describe the counseling you've had, it sounds like . . . the tone of what you're saying is "I didn't give it enough time, I should really hang in there" and so on.

C: Yeah.

T: But at the same time it also sounds like you've made some decisions about what's felt okay to you, what's been helpful and what hasn't. You've made some decisions along the way that either certain people or certain methods were not the most helpful for you.

C: So I had a valid reason to stop?

T: Yeah.

C: But in that book [on codependency, mentioned earlier] he talks about patients who go to him for a year or two years. They might go for a year before they reach an important point, and that sort of depresses me. I think, "Gosh, will I have to go for that long?" But I think I realized that whatever it is inside me that makes me feel so worthless inside and so empty isn't going to go away just by me trying to make little changes in how I behave, because the underlying feeling inside is still there.

T: And I can understand that, but what I want to say is, don't underestimate some of the small changes you've been making. They seem small on the surface but they sound quite significant. And any kind of change that a person decides to make comes in small steps.

C: I think in the past I expected that I'd go along to this person and they'd change me, they'd resolve all my problems. And I'm just realizing that it takes small steps that I have to do myself. But I also think there must be stuff I haven't talked through or resolved because . . . I realize I have to take small steps, but I just can't see how I'm going to start liking myself by taking small steps. And, reading this book, I've been having some really weird thoughts about my mother. And I find it hard to remember things that happened when I was a child, but that seems to be a very significant time. I still feel like I need help, because I don't know enough about how to be different.

[Competing thoughts are occurring. It seems that Anna is beginning to feel that she can do something to help herself feel differently; however, the idea that someone else must solve her deep problems is pervasive. Her emerging view that she can feel differently might be able to be built upon in a way that will challenge her pessimism.]

T: Are there times . . . I mean, what you've been talking about is, sometimes you find it hard to like yourself, to feel good about yourself, to appreciate . . .

C: Most of the time

T: . . . the good things about you. When are the times when you're able to appreciate things about yourself, when you're thinking, "I guess I'm not perfect but, well, I'm not too bad."

C: Sometimes. It's not very often. I mean . . . it's hard to explain, but at the moment I feel very depressed. I can't sleep, everything feels really grey, and even if it's a bright sunny day I still don't feel like smiling. And when it's like this I start not seeing anything positive. I can't think of anything good about myself at all. No matter what positive things people say about me, I don't think they're true. I think they're sincere, but somehow it's different from how I see me.

T: Okay, but when are the other times when it's easier to . . .

C: Then there are other times . . . yeah, when I think I'm seeing things as they really are and I have a kinder assessment of myself and my value and I . . . but they seem to be very short periods where I feel intensely happy. But long periods where I feel negative all the time.

[The periods when Anna feels differently or notices different things about herself are brief but are coming into slightly greater prominence. Asking her to elaborate on them might help them become more real.]

T: And what have you noticed about those times when you find that it's easier to . . .

C: To feel more positive.

T: Yeah, to feel a bit more positive and to appreciate yourself.

C: 'Cause I haven't figured out . . . I mean, there are these periods where I feel happy and in control of my life and that my life is going somewhere and I have something to look forward to. They sort of stand out like a lighthouse, you know what I mean?

T: Yeah.

C: Like, before I went on holidays, I had several months where I felt quite happy and I was enjoying my life. And I went around being amazed and saying to my friends, "I feel happy." I couldn't really understand why. I mean . . .

T: Wait a minute. When was this? Just a few months ago?

C: Yes.

T: Oh, okay

C: I don't really understand it. I mean, I have a horrible feeling it's connected with my relationship with Sue, because when she'd broken off her engagement and I was seeing more of her was when I was feeling happy and life seemed more like the good old days.

[It is not surprising that Anna attributes the difference in her mood to something external. Nonetheless, Kate continues to try to bring this difference into greater prominence, since the presence of such differences might inject doubt into Anna's prevailing all-inclusive view of depression.]

T: So what was different at that time?

C: Yeah, it was different. I can't describe to you the incredible difference in our household when she wasn't going out with Ian. But I think my period of happiness was starting even before she broke up with him. I think I was just starting to come to terms with her and Ian. I can't remember when I started feeling happy but—maybe it was after I quit going to the psychiatrist—but I remember it was for quite a few months, in the first part of this year.

T: You were feeling a bit better.

C: Yeah. But I went on holidays and I was with these friends and I got really angry and depressed. It always seems to happen when I go on holidays. I think it's because I'm always with friends and they are all couples. I'm in my late twenties and single, and all my friends are in relationships or getting married and I feel like "What's wrong with me?"

T: Yeah, I know that can be really frustrating. I mean, I'm single and there are times it can be very freeing, times when I feel good about being single, but there are times when I feel "Hey, I'm sick of being single. How come every one else can meet people but I can't?"

C: Yeah. *(laughs)* I can only appreciate the freeing part of it in those periods when I'm intensely happy, and that's not often. Most of the time I feel rejected and alone, and I think about it all the time. I feel like a failure because I don't have a man in my life. I've just had a lot of short-term skirmishes. I don't feel I have much value and I don't like myself. And the great feeling about that period of time when I felt happy early this year was for the first time I felt okay about being unattached. I was doing lots of things in my spare time.

T: It sounds like you felt more confident.

C: I did.

T: Just generally more satisfied with your life and able to appreciate those things about yourself that . . .

C: Yes, I did. But I don't really know what brought it on. And then suddenly I've gone into this really depressed stage. And I don't want to contact my friends because I don't think they'll like me. It's like this black blind gets pulled down and everything I feel about myself is negative.

[The experience of feeling more satisfied still seems to Anna to be an aberration. In her next question about it Kate expresses her assumption that Anna's satisfied feeling can happen again.]

T: So when you imagine yourself feeling a bit better, where you're feeling less depressed, less down and out, where you're able to say, "Hey, this feels better, this is good," how do you suppose you'll be able to tell, what kinds of things will you notice that . . .

C: Well, it's really an obvious difference. It's hard to explain. The main thing I notice is that I have more energy to do things, so everything in my life that needs to get done I will get done. I'll be more . . . I won't withdraw from people. I'll be contacting my friends, going out, and doing more things. What else? Not sitting around feeling bad about being single but seeing the advantages of it. Feeling positive about my work instead of sitting at my desk staring at a piece of paper, not being able to make decisions.

[It is interesting that Anna has begun to talk in the future tense. She has adopted the phrase "it WILL be," which suggests that she is beginning to accept the possibility of a different future.]

T: So having more energy.

C: Yes, it will really be a complete reversal. What I want is to be back like I was before, which I've experienced. I get to feeling so negative that I say, "I don't remember what it was like." But that's what I want, a different emotional climate.

T: Yes, and sometimes you manage that. As we've been talking, one of the things I find myself thinking is that it sounds like feeling kind of depressed and feeling down and out has . . . has kind of gotten the best of you. It's made it difficult to . . .

C: I don't feel in control.

T: Yes, it's made it difficult to feel in control, it's made it difficult to appreciate anything about you, it's made it difficult to be with your friends the way you'd like to be. It sounds like feeling down and out has had quite an effect on you lately.

[Referring to the depression in an externalized manner draws a distinction between it and Anna . This is a way of gently challenging the client's view that *she* is the problem, and it also sets the stage for highlighting the exceptions or successes.]

C: Oh, yes.

T: And it's interesting to me that, in spite of that, you've been able to say for one thing you've been able to remember, "Wait a minute, there was a time that I actually felt better."

C: Yes. *(laughs)*

T: Because sometimes what feeling down and out can do is totally blind you from being able to remember that sort of thing. You've said that basically all you've noticed is what you don't like about yourself. And so it seems to me that you've been able to stand up to it enough that you've still been able to remember the period of time when you felt really good. And you've been able to say, "I'm not going to let this get the best of me, I'm going to push myself, I'm going to do some things." Even "I'm going to go for counseling." I think that's a sign that you haven't totally given up hope that things can be better. I'm interested in that and the fact that somehow you've had the strength to ward off the depressed feeling enough to do some of those things or maybe to think some of those things.

C: Maybe a little.

T: Yes, and not in any way to diminish how awful you've been feeling, but you've been able to do these things. It makes me think, "Hey, this woman's got some things going for herself."

C: *(brightens and laughs)*

T: "I mean, she's obviously got to be pretty strong to be able to do some of that." And I'm not sure if that's the kind of thing you ever find yourself thinking about yourself. And I also thought that going to Europe for seven months by yourself . . . I mean, that's the kind of thing that takes some guts and where you have to push yourself.

C: Yes, I met an American girl in Rome and she said she was really surprised I'd been able to do it because she thought I was such a wimp. Yes, I guess I usually underestimate whatever I've got going for me.

T: Assuming you decide it would be helpful to come back and for us to talk again, I think it would be interesting to have more information about what's been going on for you lately . . .

C: Oh, sure.

T: . . . and in particular, one of the things about the way I go about trying to be helpful to people is that I assume that there are some things going on in a person's life that basically they feel okay about that we might be able to build on. Rather than starting from scratch, if we can find some things that we might be able to build on, then it's going to make the whole process a lot easier.

C: What sorts of things do you mean?

T: Well, what I'm thinking about is . . . what I'm going to ask you to do is just pay attention to those things that go on in your life, no matter how small or how insignificant they may seem, that you would like to continue to have happen. Just take note of those things. And I think it would be helpful for us to talk about those things next time, as a way to begin to build on those times that you feel you can continue on with the kind of life you want. It may be that we need to talk about some of those other things you've been feeling. Or it may not. It may be that the talking you've done with other people has been enough. But I'm going to ask you to decide what you think it will be most helpful for us to talk about, because I could get it wrong. So I'll want you to be in charge of that. Okay?

C: Yeah, okay.

[To contradict Anna's expectations of therapy directly would be unhelpful. Rather, Kate is trying to set the scene for Anna to feel that she has some control over the process rather than feel that she is the object of someone else's expertise. Within the context of Anna being the best judge, Kate can begin to inject some doubt in Anna as to what is necessary in therapy, that is, to raise in her mind the possibility that detailed exploration may not be necessary. If therapy aims to help clients feel in control of their lives, the context of the therapeutic experience itself should reflect this. It is more important that the client feel that she has some control over the process than that the process completely "fit" the therapist's model.]

[The task (of asking Anna to pay attention to these things in her life that she would like to have continue) was essentially de Shazer's "formula first-session task" (de Shazer & Molnar, 1984). At this stage Anna was well practiced in discounting any steps she took, and it seemed more useful simply to invite her to attend to different aspects of her behavior.]

## Excerpts from Session II (Three Weeks Later)

T: I was curious . . . when I talked with you on the phone about rescheduling our time, you said that things have been going okay.

C: Yes, but not recently. I mean, last night someone said to me, "How are you going?" and I said I felt really awful again and she said, "But you were so happy last week," and . . . but, I'd forgotten.

T: So when you feel awful, it's sometimes easy to forget . . .

C: Yes. I couldn't remember that last week I was in a good mood. Because in the last few days I've felt really grey and I've thought about ways of doing away with myself. I felt really angry towards Sue. We had a confrontation on Monday night. We had a good talk. She said she was really disappointed that I wasn't giving her any support at a difficult time in her life and . . .

T: Did the talk give you any ideas about how you might like your relationship with Sue to be different?

C: I never feel like I'm the sort of person who's able to offer sympathy or empathy. I just don't know how to do it. She said she sees me withdrawing and being hostile, then she withdraws as well. That's what I've noticed. It's kind of a vicious circle: She seems more offhand with me, so I get more withdrawn and feel rejected. Then she withdraws from me too.

T: So what would it take to break that pattern?

[Framing the interaction as a "pattern" is an attempt to challenge the view that it is all Anna's fault.]

C: I don't know. I find it really hard . . . I feel like I've got to just make myself not do it, but it'll be hard work.

T: What will be hard about that?

C: I don't know. It's just easier to withdraw or feel angry. I don't want to be like this. If I'm like this with someone who's supposed to be my closest friend, well . . .

T: So when you imagine being different with Sue, what do you find yourself imagining?

[Anna can imagine herself behaving differently, although the enormity of her distress and self-criticism easily overshadows this. Kate persists in asking her to imagine how it could be different—a way to invite her to focus on a successful future without denying the current pain.]

C: Well, sometimes recently I've been able to, when I can express my feelings but do it really calmly. I think I told you last time that we'd had that talk. And I did it on Monday night again a bit. But if I could just . . . just those few times I've been able to say how I feel and not just take it out on her by being distant. I'd like to be able to assert myself at the time and not take it out at another time by having a tantrum. But it's always the same.

T: So it sounds like you and Sue have become caught up in a kind of a pattern. When you are together for a long time, you develop kind of habits for how you relate.

C: I just feel like history keeps repeating itself, and I don't want it . . .

T: And obviously your relationship with Sue is changing over these last several months. I was wondering which of the changes you're happy with, that you've been able to appreciate.

C: Well, I guess the fact that I've realized that I'm selfish and not a good friend is a change that's positive, because it means I can do something about it.

T: So you have some sense of being able to do something about it.

C: Yes. But it's very hard. But I think that's positive and also that a couple of times I've been able to express myself calmly.

T: And based on what you've said last time, that's a big step.

C: Oh, yes. But, I mean, I oscillate between feeling like there's a little bit of hope and like I'm a monster.

T: And what usually helps you to feel like there's a little bit of hope?

C: Well, last time I was here, I came away feeling positive and "Yes, I can do something." But then, after a couple of weeks, I just go back to feeling really angry and withdrawing.

T: Like the patterns take over.

C: Yes.

T: So what would it take to keep that feeling of hope, to keep it going a while longer?

C: When I feel hopeful I feel like that gives me power to take steps to be the kind of person I want to be. And when I feel really hopeless, that sort of reinforces the bad behavior. So . . . maybe that's something I need to think about.

T: Well, to feel hurt or angry if your best friend ignores you or whatever, but it sounds like the pattern sort of takes on a life of its own; it overwhelms you.

[While Kate is cautious not to place to much emphasis on proving to Anna that what she is experiencing is normal, it is important that Kate challenge even in a small way Anna's view that her reactions are evidence of failure or incompetence. By talking about the "pattern" it is possible to draw a distinction between normal reactions and a pattern that takes them out of control.]

C: Yes, but I don't know how to do something different. And I don't know how to do positive things, like show that I care. I mean, I can think of people like Ruth and Ken, who seem to know how to be positive, but I just don't know how to be different.

T: So they do the kinds of things you'd like to see yourself doing. And it seems like you are able to appreciate that.

C: Yes, I guess. And I can do those things in some friendships.

T: You can?

C: Yes, I mean, I don't think I'm a complete failure as a friend and a person; it's just with Sue. Maybe we're just too close. Or I feel like I'm too dependent. And it's all to do with the fact that I don't have any self-esteem. And I don't know how to get it.

[Again, Anna is beginning to doubt her all-inclusive view of herself as a failure. In the following dialogue, Kate asks questions that presuppose that there are times when Anna behaves differently. Rather than prefacing questions with "*If* you can be different," she asks instead "What *will* you be doing differently?" or "How do you . . .?"]

T: So when you imagine yourself being more independent of Sue, what do you imagine yourself doing? What will be some signs?

C: Well, I guess I won't develop the sorts of angry and jealous feelings I feel. I won't feel my happiness depends on what she's doing.

T: What else do you think you'll notice?

[Kate continues to ask Anna to imagine what it will be like when she can relate to Sue in the way she wants. Anna describes such things as asking Sue how she is doing rather than waiting for Sue to ask her. She also says she would like to become a better listener and practice asking more questions that would encourage Sue to talk more openly and would demonstrate Anna's interest.]

C: I was talking to a friend the other day about Sue, and she said maybe we need to make some regular time to go to a café or to the pub and just have a talk. And maybe doing that, maybe that's something I could try doing for a start.

T: So that's an idea.

C: Yeah. Maybe I'll suggest it to her. It seems silly, but maybe how things are now is silly.

[It is interesting that Anna is able to countenance the idea of "practicing," of taking small deliberate steps to behave differently. This is in contrast to her view that change will require a major, insightful transformation, and it represents a change from her view of the previous session that simply doing some small things differently will not be sufficient. Kate decides to utilize this by directly suggesting further practice, building on things Anna has already identified as helpful. Kate invites Anna to notice what she sees other friends do in their friendships that Anna sees as a sign of being a good friend, and that she would like to try herself. She then suggests Anna try one or two small things with Sue and see how it goes. The session finishes with Kate wondering what small steps Anna will decide to practice in the coming weeks.]

## Excerpts from Session III (Three Weeks Later)

C: I've been thinking about the sort of thing you do. You don't go over and over the past, but you seem to concentrate on the future and how things can be different.

T: Yeah, I mean, there's lots of different ways of thinking about people and problems. And certainly the past and what has happened has an effect on how we think about ourselves. But some people think that the past kind of determines inevitably what we will be like.

C: Up until now I've thought, "I've got to sort out everything that happened in my past and there's some hidden key and I've got to get to the bottom of what made me what I am," where you seem to be concentrating on "Well, what are you doing now?" and "What steps can you take to be different?" And I find that helpful. It feels much more liberating to realize that I can do things and concentrate on the future.

T: So it sounds like you're beginning to think a bit differently about yourself and about possibilities.

C: Yeah, I'm feeling more positive. I mean, I've still been having symptoms of being stressed and stuff, which I think is part of the whole package of not handling life properly.

T: Not the way you'd like.

C: Yes, but I'm feeling a lot happier. I was feeling horrible for a long time, but I'm not feeling horrible anymore. I feel I'm able to do something.

T: And how do you account for that? How do you make sense of it?

C: I don't know. Every time I've started seeing someone, it helps me feel positive. I walk out feeling much more optimistic. But people keep telling me that I'm changing a lot. I feel like I'm being happier for longer.

T: That must be a relief.

C: I mean, I guess I haven't spent huge periods of time being really badly depressed like some people who end up having to go to hospital. I haven't been spending as much time feeling really anxious or . . . or depressed. In the last couple of weeks I felt really bad for about a whole week, and it still bothers me that I can't always figure out why.

T: But it seems that in spite of that you've been able to have times where you've been feeling a bit better.

[Anna's comments about seeing the process of therapy differently are interesting and lead naturally to a discussion of her beginning to see herself differently. She seems better able to respond to Kate's drawing attention to continuing exceptions.]

C: Yes. I feel more in control of my life.

T: That's interesting. For a long time you've felt anxious and down and out and then what happens is, you start to do some things differently. And then maybe you feel down for a while, and it's easy to lose sight of the time you felt better.

C: I still get annoyed about not understanding. Maybe I have to not worry about that so much.

T: Maybe. So it sounds like over the past few weeks you've had some down times but you've had times that have been better.

C: Yes, I find it hard to remember the good times. I've been trying really hard with Sue. We've had some good talks, short ones. I feel like I'm trying harder and being more aware of it. And I've been feeling much happier about where I live and my house instead of just feeling really sorry for myself. And not thinking all the time about being single. I guess I've just realized that I can choose to look at the positive side of my life instead of looking at the bad things. I think I'm finding out in practice that I have a choice, which is something I knew theoretically, but I didn't know how to exercise it. I have a long way to go. I'm just seeing all these areas where I need to change things and it's up to me to do something about it.

[What is important is not only that Anna has continued practicing taking small steps forward but that she is more able to appreciate the significance of these steps. While she still shows a tendency to downplay her successes, she is beginning to see herself as having personal agency. Thus, it is likely not only that she will be better able to acknowledge those steps she takes but also that her sense of her own achievement will lead her to see herself as having some control over her own future.]

T: Do you suppose that some of the practicing you've been doing with Sue . . . I mean, you've said that since we talked last that you've really made an effort.

C: Yes, a bit. I could do a lot more. It's Sue that takes the initiative, and it's really hard for me to approach her.

T: And what do you suppose will make the difference in helping you feel more comfortable to do that?

C: Oh, practice I guess. It feels artificial to change my behavior like that. But I just have to keep doing it till it becomes natural. And I tried it with my mother too. I think we just get into a routine . . . it's always the same. Just sometimes I rebel, and I feel like "No, I know I see Mum every weekend, but I just don't want to this week." But I still feel really guilty.

T: Uh huh.

C: But last weekend came around, and I thought I'd see Mum. And I rang her up on the Friday, 'cause I always put it off and put it off, 'cause I feel scared of what she's going to say.

T: It sounds like the guilt kind of gets to you.

C: It's a guilt thing, but she's so many times in the past said things on the phone that seem designed to manipulate me . . . to make me . . . to encourage me to feel more guilty. So I didn't say anything on the phone, but I did say, "Well, I'd like it if you rang me sometimes," and she said—well she was on the defensive. So I just sort of let it slip. Then on the weekend again I found the opportunity to tell her that I felt hurt by what she says. I made a big effort to say, "I felt hurt. I feel really hurt when you say that sort of thing." I wish I'd said more.

[Anna's relationship with her mother continues to be the area in which she has the most difficulty feeling confident. It is also the matter that she has been well schooled to believe lies at the root of her problems. It is not surprising that she continues to struggle with this relationship and is not able to feel the same degree of confidence she is beginning to experience in other areas of her life. Nonetheless, she is able to identify some ways in which she has begun to try to deal with her mother differently. Kate continues to draw attention to any evidence of Anna behaving differently or dealing differently with her feelings of guilt and confusion.]

T: That was a pretty courageous thing for you to do.

C: I guess. It didn't seem . . .

T: How did you keep the guilt from getting in the way of you doing that? Of saying those things?

[A discussion ensues about how Anna has avoided succumbing to guilt. Anna states that she has started to recognize that she has rights as a person, too, and that her mother doesn't always keep in touch with her either. She says that realizing this helps her not to feel manipulated by her mother. Also, Anna is clear that she wants a new relationship with her mother and that she now sees that she can do some things to help it be different. Realizing this helps her feel stronger and in greater control.]

T: So when you and your Mum have the kind of relationship that you'd like to have, that you're satisfied with, how will it be different? What kinds of things will be happening?

C: Even earlier this year it was starting to be different. Very occasionally we might do things together. I'd like to be able to express to her when she does something that's . . . I'd like to be able to express to her, calmly . . . I'd like us to be able to talk.

T: And when was the last time that happened? When the two of you had a talk and it felt like there was a connection.

C: Well, actually, on the weekend. I mean, it isn't always as bad as I make out, because on the weekend we actually talked quite a bit . . . and that was quite good.

[After a discussion of Anna's perception of her role as a daughter and her emerging ability to keep guilt from making her think she's not a good daughter, Kate concludes the session.]

T: What I'm most struck with is the sense that I get that you believe that you can have some effect on your relationship with your Mum and that you can have some effect on your relationship with Sue. That you can have some effect on your relationships with other people. And that, in fact, you're actually taking some steps to practice that, to try that out. And I think that's a courageous sort of thing . . . and especially since, in the past you've described yourself as someone who finds it difficult to say what you think and what you feel and to be your own person. But the kinds of things that you've been thinking about and that you're actually doing are really in the direction of being your own person and letting people get to know you a bit better by you extending yourself and getting to know them.

C: Well, I have read that sort of thing in books before. But it feels more real now.

T: But I think it's one thing to read it and think, "Well that makes sense," It's another thing to actually put it into action.

C: It's the first time it feels like I'm doing something and not just reading books about it.

## Sessions IV and V

In the following two sessions Anna continued to report small steps toward changing her relationship with her Mum and Sue and seemed increasingly to appreciate their significance. Kate continued to respond to these steps, inviting Anna to integrate them into her emerging view of her own competence. Following a discussion of Kate's impending departure from Australia, Anna decided that she was ready to continue on her own.

## Session VI (Six Months Later)

Anna returned to see Michael, saying that things had gone well for some time after seeing Kate but had now gone downhill again. She thought that perhaps her therapy had been terminated prematurely because of Kate's departure. Michael asked, "What did you find helpful about seeing Kate? What did you learn about yourself that was helpful?" After some initial hesitation Anna was able to list what she had learned: "I discovered I could feel good about myself"; "I learned that I had a future"; and "I realized that I could do something about my situation rather than just sit around feeling hopeless and helpless." Nonetheless, she agreed that it had been hard to remember these things when she went through a bad period with a relationship that did not work out (although Michael noted that she seemed to have handled this relationship quite differently from those in the past. Specifically, she stated that she had not blamed herself or become depressed). In the following transcript Anna talks about feeling "false," and Michael seeks to respond to that in a way that suggests those aspects of herself that she can appreciate.

C: Friends probably would be shocked to know that I feel this bad, because I think I pretend a lot. I pretend to be better so they don't notice.

M: So how do you do that? How are you able to pretend?

C: I don't know. I just don't want them to see how horrible I am.

M: I remember one of the things you told Kate was that you felt you ruined your relationships by always going on about yourself and about how awful you felt.

C: Yes, but I don't want to do that. I don't want them to know how horrible I am.

M: So you're able to pretend.

C: Yes, I am.

M: So, being able to pretend that you're feeling good . . . where does that come from?

C: Maybe from remembering those times I do feel better. It's not a hundred percent of the time I feel bad.

M: No?

C: No, maybe ten percent of the time I can feel optimistic.

M: Really? Where do you think that optimism comes from?

C: I don't know. Maybe I'm just stubborn. I'm not prepared to give up.

Anna also talked of her disappointment in a Bible study group to which she belonged. She was disappointed that other people in the group did not seem to be prepared to be as honest as she, and she wondered if she was being unrealistic. The session concluded with Michael wondering if Anna would be able to remember more of what she had discovered about herself during her sessions with Kate.

## Final Sessions

Michael saw Anna on three more occasions over the next two or three months. While various aspects of her life were a struggle, she continued to feel better. Anna commented that she felt more realistic and was sick of being pessimistic. She acknowledged that being realistic is sometimes harder to achieve than intense happiness but that it helps keep her more stable overall. And she realized that some of her "down" times were related to the discomfort of continuing to make changes in her life.

The following comments are from Anna's final session:

C: I've been keeping a diary of how I feel, where I write down all the things that upset me and all the times I feel awful. I was going to look through it before I came here today but I couldn't be bothered reading it.

M: You couldn't be bothered reading over the times you've been feeling bad?

C: No, I think . . . well, maybe keeping a diary like that is not very helpful. I've been feeling more like I can just get on with things. I sort of feel like I don't need to come back . . . maybe in a few months just to let you know how things are.

M: Really? So you're feeling like you can just get on with things, keep going towards the future?

C: It has its ups and downs, but that's life. It doesn't mean I need to keep coming all the time.

M: But . . . I remember you saying to Kate that you knew this whole process could take years.

C: Yeah. Well, I don't think like that anymore.

## REFLECTIONS

This chapter was written 8 months after Michael last saw Anna. We discussed with Anna the fact that we wished to use her story in this chapter, and she agreed to share some of her comments about the experience of therapy.

> My visits [to the Centre] were a source of hope and affirmation at a time when I was not particularly good at seeing my life in a positive way. In contrast with some previous [therapy] encounters, these visits ended with a renewed belief that change was possible and that I could effect it. I have been through a considerable degree of change since then, and while all of it clearly cannot be attributed to our sessions, I am sure that a lot has to do with having acquired a greater sense of being responsible for my own actions and emotions through my sessions with Kate and Michael. At the time, I was often surprised by their interpretations of events—it was good to be offered alternatives to my jaundiced views! They helped me to see that the very act of coming to see someone is a big leap forward.
>
> I felt that I found objective yet understanding listeners. Occasionally Kate or Michael would relate to me an experience which was similar to mine. At the time this often surprised me, yet it showed that they had heard what I was going through and that I was not alone in my experiences of emotions like anger or grief—that I was not "abnormal."
>
> I have to admit that the style of counseling felt frustrating at times to a client who wanted to be told solutions to all her problems! With hindsight, however, it is the best possible way to help people take control of their lives, as it gives them the opportunity to start making some decisions. My sessions with Kate and Michael helped me realize that I do indeed have within me the necessary resources for change.
>
> It would be foolish to think that I have fully resolved the problems which I brought along to counseling. Most importantly, though, I feel that I am able to see things much more realistically now. To have ups and downs is human; it does not make me a failure. And I can more happily live with unanswered questions too.

## EDITOR'S QUESTIONS

Q: *Anna presents as a depressed young woman struggling with feelings of low self-esteem who has occasional thoughts about suicide. How would you have approached this therapy if Anna had had a history of suicide attempts and had talked more seriously about killing herself?*

A: The model is a way of thinking, only a tool, and is not an end in itself. As such, what is important is that it fits. When faced with a client who is more seriously suicidal, our assumptions are the same. We would still view her as someone who is competent and has the ability to experience herself as more competent but who is stuck in her current view of herself and so sees suicide as the only way out. These assumptions would still guide our work. However, that is not to say that the same techniques would be applied in the same way. What is important is that we match our assumptions and basic standpoint to our client's experience and that the steps of therapy proceed from that.

Sometimes people experiencing distress primarily need to feel heard and to have their feelings of despair validated. While we do not believe that "getting it out" in itself leads to change, we all know from our own experience that feeling heard and supported can have powerful effects—at least in the short term. In doing this, we would not wish to explore the specific problem details in too much depth (since talking about the problem can tend to make it bigger); however, we provide space for clients to talk about their own experience and feelings of stuckness, and we seek to acknowledge the reality of this experience. Once this opportunity has been provided, it is sometimes appropriate to ask (gently) about the times that the person has felt even a little less desperate or more hopeful—without seeming to discount the experience or talk a client out of suicidal thoughts.

After this chance to feel heard, the client will sometimes, be a little less desperate, and it may be appropriate to ask questions such as "Supposing that you feel a little better after this talk, how do you imagine the next day or two will be different?" Such questions may lead to a more hopeful direction to follow in further therapy, although we still remain mindful of our ethical and legal obligations.

In keeping with our desire to treat clients as competent and as having some control over the therapeutic process, we have sometimes been quite open with clients that their disclosure to us of their suicidal thoughts places us in something of a dilemma, since we have legal and professional responsibilities if we believe someone is a danger to themselves or others. Michael remembers two particular clients with whom this situation arose. The suicidal talk of one young woman was persuasive, and Michael talked gently with her about not wanting to take things out of her hands. She had chosen to come and talk, and he was impressed at how clearly she had been able to describe the agony she felt. It was clear that she felt that her life was out of her control and that killing herself was the only action left that she could make a decision about. Hence, Michael was worried that he might be forced to take her sense of control away from her by taking action that the (Australian) law required. Would she be prepared to agree not to kill herself until at least after the next session so they could get together again and try to figure out a solution that suited them both? When she agreed, Michael was able to ask (again, gently) how she thought she would be able to do this. This discussion, which continued beyond the scheduled end of the session, did not yield magic results. However, the young woman left seeming a little more hopeful.

The second case was of a man who was facing a long period in jail, had good (or, at least, understandable) reasons to kill himself, and had tried to do so before. Michael asked Kate to join the session and told the client honestly, "We can see why suicide is the option you prefer. Unfortunately, if you go out of here and kill yourself, having told us, then we could be liable. We want you to know that our concern at the moment is for our necks rather than yours. Will you agree not to kill yourself before the next session so we do not have to phone the authorities now?" This message loses something when written down. It was *not* just a fancy therapeutic intervention but an honest statement of the position we were placed in, and our position left the client with the responsibility for what happened. The ensuing discussion was emotional and prolonged. Within the (honest and realistic) frame of wanting to be sure for our own sakes that the client was not about to commit suicide, we were able to elicit from him a list of his own reasons for staying alive (at least for the moment). In this case we made clear the seriousness of the situation as we left him to consider what evidence there was that might persuade us not to notify the authorities. Ultimately, we considered his arguments persuasive, and the very fact of his discussing with us the arguments for staying alive seemed to have some effect on him.

What was important in each case was that our response fitted the particular person. Of course, both courses of action involved risks. However, if suicidal clients return (as these did), questions about how they managed to keep themselves alive may be used.

There are times when we have no choice but to notify the authorities. We try to do this in as therapeutic a manner as possible; nonetheless, we are clear that in such situations we have left the realm of therapy and have entered the realm of social control.

Q: *You see the client on an intermittent basis for example, every 3 weeks. What would indicate the need for more frequent contacts? How do you respond to people who request weekly psychotherapy? Do you actively try to make your therapy brief, or is brevity simply a by-product of your theoretical orientation?*

A: We do not believe that change occurs primarily within the therapy room. The therapy session helps new themes and ideas gain currency, and new ideas about the person begin to emerge. However, change occurs from "going out there and doing it." Hence, an interval after a session allows time for successful experiences and for intervening events that may be discussed in the next session. This interval between sessions is also important since it makes it less likely that clients will attribute changes to us rather than to themselves. However, there are no hard-and-fast rules. Sometimes we see clients after a week, sometimes after 3 weeks or longer. Usually, we ask clients what they think will be the most helpful interval.

This question seems to ignore the context that is built by therapist and client, since what the client thinks at the end of a session may be very different from his or her initial ideas. We would not seek to dissuade someone who requests weekly psychotherapy since doing so would disqualify his or her ideas and experience. However, our experience is that by the end of a session that has focused on competence and success clients respond well to suggestions that we meet again in 2 or 3 weeks if they have been helped to begin to build a different view of self. That is, they may come in thinking that we will "fix" their problems and help them "work through" their past and that weekly sessions as necessary. If they begin to see the possibility that they may solve (or are already solving) their problems, or that they can experience something different now despite the seeming enormity of their past experiences, they are more likely to feel happy about a longer interval between sessions.

While adopting a "brief therapy" perspective, we are not sure that time is the best dimension along which to categorize therapy. "Brief therapy" has a relatively limited focus, and one can implement this focus within the context of few or many sessions, closely or widely spaced. Although we both have cases that might be termed "long-term brief therapy," a focus on competence seems more often to lead to a shorter treatment period.


Q: *Although you, Kate, are persistent in maintaining a postive, future-oriented stance, you are also very respectful of the client and the client's need to talk about "the problem." Would you comment on this process? More specifically, how do you avoid the potential risks of either getting immersed in the client's problem-saturated view or, conversely, discounting the client's pain by focusing too quickly on the positive?*
A: We are always on the lookout for exceptions early in the first session. We are also alert to signs that the client thinks it is too soon to discuss exceptions. This is a constant juggling act, and whatever we do has to fit with the client. Nonetheless, we are mindful of the research that suggests that the process of observation affects the things being observed. In quantum physics it has been found that various phenomena, such as light, may be viewed as being waves or as being particles (light waves vs. photons). Scientists have discovered that they can choose to treat subatomic phenomena as waves or as particles, and the "things" then tend to behave in a way that is consistent with the stance adopted by the observer: "How can mutually exclusive wave-like and particle-like behaviors both be properties of one and the same light? They are not properties of light. They are properties of our interaction with light. Depending upon our choice of experiment, we can cause light to manifest either particle-like properties or wave-like properties" (Zukav, 1979, p. 116).

Similarly, the degree to which clients adopt a problem focus or a solution focus is a property of our interaction with them. In constructivist terms (Watzlawick, 1990), we "create a reality" with our clients and they (and we) then tend to behave in a way that fits with that. That is, we have found that a focus on competence is more likely to lead to our clients noticing and experiencing competence.

We hope that our clients feel that we respect their pain and validate their experience. We may even ask "How did you cope?" This question allows an acknowledgment of their pain but leads to an exploration of their success.

Again, the question cannot be answered in terms of technique but in terms of the overall climate that is built into our interaction with our clients.

Q: *In the interview you, Kate, share some personal information about yourself in regard to being a single person. Would you comment on the benefits of therapist self-disclosure and why, in this circumstance, you decided to tell Anna about your situation?*
A: Therapists are people too. We tend not to set out to talk about ourselves and our own dilemmas, but we have no rules that say we should not do so. Many in our field have described the therapeutic encounter as a conversation (Goolishian & Anderson, 1992). While this expression can have a variety of meanings, we take it as reflecting our aim that our approach not become one in which we operate on our clients instead of working with them. Hence, it is not important that our clients see us as experts who "have it all together." In fact, some therapists have suggested that it is important that we actively remove ourselves from the expert position and show that we feel—and suffer—as well (Lammert, 1986). Others have talked about the use of "stories" in therapy (Combs & Freedman, 1990; Wallas, 1985). Kate's comments about her own experience as a single person were not planned, and it would be hard to devise rules for such self-disclosure. Anna was talking about something that resonated with Kate's experience and it was honest to share this. Kate wanted to introduce the idea that there are different aspects to being single. She could have made a more general statement or recounted a "story" about someone else; however, it seemed to fit her current relationship with Anna to use her own experience to introduce this different perspective.

Michael has had the experience of talking about his frustrations with his own children and finding that clients thought this irrelevant or unhelpful. This is particularly likely to be the case when he recounts a time when he managed his children successfully (few though such times may be!). On the other hand, there are times when clients seem to find his sharing of a frustrating parental experience helpful. As with any story used in therapy, what is important is that the therapist's personal account fit the experience of the client. It might introduce a different perspective, but should not demonstrate success to a degree that might leave the client feeling further disempowered. We both find that we often use "stories" about other clients if they fit and seem to be helpful. Stories about ourselves are no different.

# REFERENCES

Combs, G., & Freedman, J. (1990). *Symbol, story and ceremony: Using metaphor in individual and family therapy.* New York: Norton.

de Shazer, S. (1985). *Keys to solutions in brief therapy.* New York: Norton.

de Shazer, S. (1988). *Clues: Investigating solutions in brief therapy.* New York: Norton.

de Shazer, S. (1990). What is it about brief therapy that works? In J. K. Zeig & S. G. Gilligan (Eds.), *Brief therapy: Myths, method, and metaphors* (pp. 90–99). New York: Brunner/Mazel.

de Shazer, S. (1991). *Putting difference to work.* New York: Norton.

de Shazer, S., & Molnar, A. (1984). Four useful interventions in brief family therapy. *Journal of Marital & Family Therapy, 10*(3), 297–304.

de Shazer, S., Berg, I. K., Lipchik, E., Nunnally, E., Monar, A., Gingerich, W., & Weiner-Davis, M. (1986). Brief therapy: Focused solution development. *Family Process, 25*(2), 207–222.

Durrant, M., & Kowalski, K. (1990). Overcoming the effects of sexual abuse: Developing a self-perception of competence. In M. Durrant & C. White (Eds.), *Ideas for therapy with sexual abuse* (pp. 65–110). Adelaide, Australia: Dulwich Centre Publications.

Goolishian, H. A., & Anderson, H. (1992). Strategy and intervention versus nonintervention: A matter of theory? *Journal of Marital and Family Therapy, 18*(1), 5–15.

Gordon, D., & Meyers-Anderson, M. (1981). *Phoenix: Therapeutic patterns of Milton H. Erickson.* California: Meta Publications.

Gurin, J. (1990). Remaking our lives. *American Health,* March, 50–52.

Kowalski, K., & Kral, R. (1989). The geometry of solution: Using the scaling technique. *Family Therapy Case Studies, 4*(1), 59–66.

Lammert, M. (1986). Experience as knowing: Utilizing therapist self-awareness. *Social Casework: The Journal of Contemporary Social Work,* June, 369–376.

Miller, S. (1992). The symptoms of solution. *Journal of Strategic and Systemic Therapies, 11*(1), 1–11.

O'Hanlon, W. H. (1987). *Taproots: Underlying principles of Milton H. Erickson's therapy and hypnosis.* New York: Norton.

Wallas, L. (1985). *Stories for the third ear: Using hypnotic fables in psychotherapy.* New York: Norton.

Watzlawick, P. (1990). Therapy is what you say it is. In J. K. Zeig & S. G. Gilligan (Eds.), *Brief therapy: Myths, methods and metaphors* (pp. 55–61). New York: Brunner/Mazel.

White, M. (1986). Negative explanation, restraint and double description: A template for family therapy. *Family Process, 25*(2), 169–184.

White, M. (1988). The process of questioning: A therapy of literary merit? *Dulwich Centre Newsletter,* Winter, 8–14.

White, M. (1989). The externalizing of the problem and the re-authoring of lives and relationships. *Dulwich Centre Newsletter,* Summer, 3–21.

Zeig, J. K., & Gilligan, S. G. (Eds.). (1990). *Brief therapy: Myths, methods and metaphors.* New York: Brunner/Mazel.

Zukav, G. (1979). *The dancing Wu-Li masters: An overview of the new physics.* London: Fontana Paperbacks.

# 6

## Solution-Oriented Brief Therapy with Difficult Adolescents

### MATTHEW D. SELEKMAN

The solution-oriented brief therapy approach was developed by William H. O'Hanlon and Michele Weiner-Davis (O'Hanlon, 1987; O'Hanlon & Weiner-Davis, 1989; Weiner-Davis, 1992). The model is heavily based on the therapeutic ideas of the brilliant hypnotist Milton H. Erickson (Erickson, 1954, 1964; Erickson & Rossi, 1983; Erickson, Rossi & Rossi, 1976; Rosen, 1982); the solution-focused brief therapy approach developed by Steve de Shazer and his colleagues (deShazer, 1982, 1984, 1985, 1988, 1991; de Shazer et al., 1986; Gingerich & deShazer, 1991; Gingerich, deShazer & Weiner-Davis, 1987; Lipchik, 1988; Lipchik & deShazer, 1986; Weiner-Davis, de-Shazer & Gingerich, 1987); and the brief problem-focused therapy approach of the Mental Research Institute theorists (Fisch, Weakland, & Segal, 1982; Watzlawick, Weakland, & Fisch, 1974).

Very little has been written in either the brief therapy or family therapy literature on the use of the solution-oriented brief therapy approach with difficult adolescent populations (Berg & Gallagher, 1991; Selekman, 1989, 1991, in press; Todd & Selekman, 1991). For many therapists, having to treat adolescents with such "difficult" presenting problems as eating disorders, substance abuse problems, depression, and delinquent behavior, is their worst nightmare. When I consult with therapists on their nightmarish or "stuck" adolescent cases, some of the most common comments I heard are the following: the adolescent is "resistant"; the family is "enmeshed," "disengaged," or "chaotic"; the father "refuses to come to sessions"; complex and big solutions "will be necessary to solve the problem"; the adolescent "will require long-term therapy"; and, finally, "I have no idea where I am going with this family."

In this chapter, I present my expanded version of the solution–oriented brief therapy model. For the sake of brevity, I briefly discuss seven helpful theoretical assumptions, some of the major therapeutic tasks, and my rationale for model expansion with difficult adolescent cases. This will be followed by a case example of a 16-year-old delinquent boy.

## SOLUTION-ORIENTED
## THEORETICAL ASSUMPTIONS

The following seven theoretical assumptions are highly pragmatic and offer therapists a new lens for viewing the difficult adolescent case. Each of the theoretical assumptions offers a wellness perspective on adolescent problems and brief therapy.

### Resistance Is Not a Useful Concept

The traditional psychotherapy concept of resistance has been an unhelpful idea that has handicapped therapists (de Shazer, 1984). It implies that the client does not want to change and that the therapist is separate from the clients system he or she is treating. de Shazer (1982, 1984) has argued convincingly for therapists to approach each new client case from a position of therapist-client cooperation, rather than to think in terms of resistance, power, and control. According to de Shazer (1982), "Each family shows a unique way of attempting to cooperate and the therapist's job becomes, first, to describe that particular manner to himself that the family shows and, then, to cooperate with the family's way and thus to promote change" (pp. 9–10).

Like TV's Detective Columbo, we need to listen and observe carefully for clues that help identify our client's unique cooperative response pattern. These clues include the ways family members respond to our questions and manage therapeutic tasks between sessions. For example, if a mother is highly pessimistic that her acting out daughter will change, the therapist can first try the "miracle question" (de Shazer, 1988), rather than doing "more of the same" (Watzlawick et al., 1974) and asking exception-oriented questions, and if that doesn't work, he or she can mirror the mother's pessimistic stance by asking, "How come things are not worse?" Other ways to foster therapist–client cooperation is through the use of key client language and belief material, positive relabeling of negative behaviors, normalizing, humor, compliments, and cheerleading (deShazer, 1988; O'Hanlon & Weiner-Davis, 1989).

## Change Is Inevitable

Change is a continuous process. The families we treat are in a constant state of evolutionary flux. If you expect change will occur with your adolescent clients, your expectancy for change will influence your client's behaviors. As early as possible in the first interview with a new adolescent case, I try to convey the idea to the family that change will happen and it is only a matter of when. Gingerich and his colleagues (1987) have demonstrated that there is a direct relationship between therapists engaging in "change talk" with their clients and positive treatment outcomes at follow-up. The "change talk" therapists used presuppositional language and spent the majority of their session time eliciting what was working from the clients, amplifying the exceptions, and, when necessary, having clients imagine hypothetical solutions.

## Only a Small Change Is Necessary

Erickson believed that small changes in a client system could snowball into bigger changes (Gordon & Meyers-Anderson, 1981). Typically, when parents bring their adolescents in for therapy, they have a long laundry list of behaviors they want to see changed. The therapist needs to negotiate a solvable problem. It is impossible to change breaking curfew, not following parental rules, and truancy all at once. The parents in this case scenario would need to be asked, "Which one of these difficulties would you like to change first?"; "How will you know when that problem is solved?"; and "What will a small sign of progress look like in the next week?" The treatment goals need to be small, concrete, and realistic. Once clients are encouraged to value minimal changes, they are more likely to expect to make further changes.

## Clients Have the Strengths and Resources to Change

All adolescents and their parents possess certain strengths and resources that can be utilized by therapists to co-construct solutions. Any past successes clients have had can be used as models for present and future successes. Clients are more likely to change in a therapeutic context that supports their strengths and resourcefulness than in one that focuses on problems and pathology (Beavers & Hampson, 1990). In my therapeutic work with difficult adolescents, I frequently utilize them as expert consultants and involve their concerned peers in the treatment process. For example, I might ask an adolescent client the following question to elicit her expertise: "If I were to work with a teenager just like you, what advice would you give me as a counselor to help her out?" When working with difficult adolescents, I have found that the answers to this open-ended question can help pave the way for developing cooperative working relationships with young people.

## Problems Are Unsuccessful Attempts to Resolve Difficulties

With many clinical case situations, it is the family's attempted solution that maintains the problem (Fisch et al., 1982; Watzlawick et al., 1974). Family members are stuck viewing the identified client in one particular way and engage in the same repetitive interactions with her. For example, the more super-responsible parents are in dealing with their irresponsible acting-out daughter, the more irresponsibly she will continue to behave. Besides focusing on what the parents are doing that is "more of the same," therapists need to be aware of what they may be doing in relationship to the family that is not working. In adolescent cases that have had multiple treatment experiences, it is imperative that the therapist explore with the family what they liked and disliked with former therapists to avoid making the same therapeutic mistakes.

## You Don't Need to Know a Great Deal about the Problem in Order to Solve It

With every client problem pattern, there is usually some sort of exception when the problem does not occur (de Shazer, 1985). These exceptions or nonproblem patterns of behavior and thinking can be utilized by the therapist as building blocks for co-constructing solutions with families. Weiner-Davis and her colleagues (1987) have demonstrated that clients oftentimes take important steps toward resolving their difficulties between the time of the phone call to the clinic and the first session. With waiting list cases or where there has been any lag time between the phone call to the clinic and the first session, I have found it useful to begin the interview with "So what's better?" This question conveys to clients that the therapist believes they have the strengths and resources to change and it presupposes that changes have already occurred, beliefs that can set in motion a positive self-fulfilling prophecy for them.

## Multiple Perspectives

There are many ways to look at a situation, none more "correct" than others. For every event that occurs in the world, there are at least two or more explanations of that event. Bateson (1980) referred to this form of description as "double or multiple comparison" (p. 97). There are no final explanations of reality. As a member of the new therapist–family observing system, we will base our constructions of the family's presenting problem on our own theoretical maps and personal experiences in the world (Efran & Lukens, 1988; Maturana & Varela, 1987; Varela, 1979; von Foerester, 1981). In the therapeutic arena the therapist's constructions of the family's dilemma need to be perceived as either acceptable to or come close to fitting the family's belief system. Since there is a recursive relationship between meaning and behavior, shifts in the family members' beliefs about the problem situation can alter their problem-maintaining behaviors.

## SOLUTION-ORIENTED INTERVENTIONS

De Shazer and his colleagues (de Shazer, 1985, 1988, 1991; Gingerich & de Shazer, 1991; Lipchik & de Shazer, 1986; Weiner-Davis et al., 1987) have developed several different categories of therapeutic questions and "skeleton key" interventions that can effectively disrupt problem-maintaining patterns of interaction, change outmoded family beliefs, and further amplify existing exception patterns of behavior. Since it is beyond the scope of this chapter to provide an exhaustive discussion of all of the major solution-oriented questions and therapeutic tasks, I will present only a few of the categories of questions and "skeleton key" interventions that I have found most useful in my clinical work with difficult[1] adolescents.

### Purposeful Systemic Interviewing

Solution-oriented therapists ask questions in a purposeful manner by carefully assessing the client's cooperative response patterns and matching their questions with those patterns (de Shazer, 1988, 1991; Lipchik, 1988; Lipchik & de Shazer, 1986; O'Hanlon & Weiner-Davis, 1989). For example, if the therapist's use of exception-oriented questions are generating important client exception material, then he or she should continue this line of questioning and gradually move the client toward the future with presuppositional questions (O'Hanlon & Weiner-Davis, 1989). Presuppositional questions are powerful interventive tools for eliciting the client's outcome goal, conveying the inevitability of change, and for co-creating a future reality without problems. In first interviews, I like to ask families the following presuppositional questions: "If you were to show me a videotape of how things will look in this family when the problem is solved, what will we see changed on the tape?" and "What will be different?" The "miracle question" (de Shazer, 1988, 1991), based on Erickson's (1954) "pseudo-orientation in time" intervention, produces results similar to those obtained with these presuppositional questions. The family is asked the following question: "Suppose the four of you go home tonight and while you are asleep, a miracle happens and your problem is solved, how will you be able to tell a miracle must have happened the next morning?" With each family member the therapist needs to expand the possibilities both of what the miracle-produced changes will look like and of the differencess in that member that significant others will notice.

---

[1]Throughout this chapter, I use the word *difficult* as a common label utilized by mental health professionals to describe adolescent clients displaying severe problems with substance abuse, eating disorders, depression, and delinquent behavior. Many of these adolescents and their families have experienced multiple treatment failures.

Scaling questions (de Shazer, 1985, 1991) are useful for securing a quantitative measurement of the family's problem prior to treatment and at the present time, as well as where they would like to be in one week's time. This category of questions is a valuable goal-setting tool and helps maintain a clear focus throughout the course of therapy.

## Formula First-Session Task

The "formula first-session task" (de Shazer, 1985; de Shazer et al., 1986) was originally designed by de Shazer and his associates for clients who present with vague complaints. The clients are given the following directive at the end of the first interview: "Between now and the next time we meet, I would like you to observe, so that you can describe to me the next time, what happens in your family that you want to continue to have happen" (de Shazer, 1985, p. 137). After using this task, I have rarely had a second session without at least two client-reported exceptions.

## Observation Tasks

Observation tasks (de Shazer, 1988; O'Hanlon & Weiner-Davis, 1989) are particularly useful with overinvolved and highly reactive parents. Parents may be instructed for one week's time to carefully observe their adolescent's behavior for patterns or encouraging signs of progress in order to better assist the therapist in trying to understand the behavior. The mere act of having the parents disengage and study their adolescent's behavior can produce a difference or change in that behavior. Similarly, the parents' original perceptions about their adolescent will change as well. I also use this task with families to help to amplify their present exception patterns of behavior and to help them keep track of the changes they are making.

## Do Something Different Task

The following solution-focused task is also useful with overinvolved or highly reactive parents. I explain to parents that their son or daughter has their number, that he or she knows every move they are going to make. After this short rationale for their need to be less predictable, the parents are given the following directive: "Between now and the next time we meet, I would like each of you to do something different, no matter how strange, weird, or off-the-wall what you do might seem." (de Shazer, 1985, p. 123). In response to this instruction I have had parents come up with some of the most creative off-the-wall parenting strategies I have ever seen.

## EXPANDING THE SOLUTION-ORIENTED MODEL

Like all therapy models, the basic solution-oriented brief therapy approach (O'Hanlon & Weiner-Davis, 1989) has its limitations with highly entrenched families and with adolescent cases that are riddled with interventions by multiple helpers from larger systems. There is also very little written in the brief therapy literature on the therapist's use of self and of improvisational methods used to introduce newsworthy information into the client system, to reinforce changes, and to disrupt unhelpful patterns of interaction in the therapy room.

## Brief Therapist as an Improvisational Artist

Anything and everything goes in my therapy sessions. There are no rules! I strive to create a therapeutic climate that is playful and full of surprises—from "high-fives" to outrageous humor. Each new adolescent case is approached with passion, spontaneity, and a playful use of humorous elements of the client's story. Therapist creativity can only flow smoothly when we let go of our preoccupations with adhering religiously to our therapy model rules and our need to be technically precise (Selekman, in press).

I like to compare my therapeutic style to the musical style of jazz saxophonists Charlie Parker and Ornette Coleman. Parker once said, "Music is your own experience, your thoughts, your wisdom. If you don't live it, it won't come out of your horn" (Williams, 1939, p. 77). Coleman, one of the fathers of the jazz avant-garde movement, described his style of horn playing as follows: "One day music will be a lot freer. Then the pattern for a tune will be forgotten and the tune itself will be the pattern, and won't have to be forced into conventional patterns. The creation of music is just as natural as the air we breathe. I believe music is really a free thing, and any way you can enjoy it you should" (Hentoff, 1958).

Both Parker and Coleman trusted their intuitions, were risk takers, and refused to be governed by traditional rules of musical theory. By allowing themselves to play with total freedom, they liberated listeners from being bogged down by the familiar and opened the door for rapid changes in their thinking and feeling. They essentially used themselves as "second-order" change agents (Watzlawick et al., 1974.) By utilizing the improvisational methods of Parker and Coleman, brief therapists will find themselves being more creative, having more fun, and coproducing more meaningful changes with adolescents and their families than ever before (Selekman, in press).

## Integrating Ideas from Michael White

The Australian family therapist Michael White has made many important contributions to the family therapy field (White, 1984, 1985, 1986, 1987, 1988; White & Epston, 1990). White's most innovative therapeutic idea is the "externalization of the problem" (White & Epston, 1990). Through careful use of the family member's language and beliefs about the presenting problem, the problem is redefined by the therapist into an objectified external tyrant oppressing the family, including the identified client. For example, if all family members are referring to the identified client's problem as depression, the therapist can ask the following externalizing questions: "How long has the depression been pushing all of you around?" and to the identified client: "When the depression is trying to get the best of you, what kinds of things do your parents do to help you stand up to it?" It has been my clinical experience with some highly entrenched adolescent cases that families have a strong need to talk about their long-standing oppression by the problem and typically do not respond well to solution-oriented questioning (Selekman, in press; Todd & Selekman, 1991). Externalizing the problem can be a useful therapeutic option once the brief therapist has exhausted the possibilities with the solution-oriented brief therapy approach.

Two other useful categories of therapeutic questions developed by White (1988) are "unique account" and "unique redescription" questions. These questions invite family members to ascribe new meaning to the exceptions they report occurring with their situation. When paired up with exception questions (de Shazer, 1988; O'Hanlon & Weiner-Davis, 1989), the "unique account" and "unique redescription" questions further amplify the family members' new perceptions about themselves and their relationships, thus making these exception experiences more meaningful for them. Some examples of "unique account" and "unique redescription" questions are as follows: "How did you manage to take this important step to turn things around?"; "What were you telling yourself to get ready for this big step?"; "What does this tell you about yourself that is important for you to know"?; "How has this new picture of yourself as a parent changed your relationship with your son?"

White and Epston (1990) like to celebrate families' victories over their oppressive problems by giving them parties, certificates, and trophies. This end-of-therapy ritual empowers the family to continue pioneering a new direction with their lives. In my own clinical work with difficult adolescents, I have found that end of therapy rituals like throwing parties and giving certificates can nicely complement the positive solution-oriented brief therapy approach (Selekman, in press).

## Brief Therapist as a Collaborator with Larger Systems

Very little has been written in the brief therapy literature on how to work collaboratively with involved helpers from larger systems. In many of my difficult adolescent cases, there have been multiple helpers involved who represented the juvenile justice system, the school, drug rehabilitation programs, a psychiatric hospital, and, in some cases, the child protection system. The brief therapist cannot simply intervene with the adolescent's family and assume that therapeutic changes will be noticed by the involved helpers, who are very much a part of the problem system (Selekman, in press), which consists of all those individuals involved in "identifying" a problem and trying to solve it (Goolishian & Anderson, 1981).

Whenever I am referred a case in which there are multiple helpers actively involved, I like to conduct a macrosystemic assessment (Coppersmith, 1985; Selekman & Todd, 1991) with the family to find out from them which individuals constitute the problem system mebership and need to be included in future therapy meetings. Once the key members of the problem system have been mobilized for the family–multiple helper meetings, they will have ample opportunity to notice changes and hear the problem being discussed in different ways (Anderson, Goolishian, Pulliam, & Winderman, 1986). It has been my clinical experience that the family–multiple helper meetings empower the family, and I have witnessed quite dramatic therapeutic changes in the context of these sessions (Selekman, in press).

When it is not possible to convene some of the key members of the family–multiple helper problem system for scheduled office meetings, I schedule separate appointments with these helpers in their own work contexts to hear their concerns and welcome their collaboration with me. Oftentimes, helpers greatly appreciate the fact that I take the time to meet with them on their own turf, an act that in itself can foster a cooperative working relationship. Working collaboratively with helpers from larger systems can be an enriching learning experience for brief therapists, and in many cases, the team work can make brief therapy even "briefer" (Selekman, in press).

## CASE EXAMPLE

After spending a month in the juvenile detention center, Randy, a 16-year-old learning-disabled boy, was court-ordered for 1 year of family therapy. He was placed on probation for shoplifting, stealing bicycles, possession of marijuana, and truancy. At home Randy frequently violated his mother's rules and rarely did anything around the house to help out. Randy's parents were divorced because of the father's alcoholism problem and violent behavior. Randy's mother, Mary, worked as a mechanic for a construction equipment company. Since his early years in elementary school, Randy had been placed in special school programs for learning-disabled students. He had been in outpatient treatment twice before for his behavioral difficulties.

The good news on the intake form I was presented with was discovering that one of my favorite probation officers was involved as the case manager for this case. Bill, the probation officer, had a bachelor's degree in psychology and had received a year of family therapy training. What I liked most about Bill was his real sensitivity and dedication to helping troubled adolescents turn things around. He believed strongly in family therapy for delinquents and the usefulness of close collaboration with therapists who were assigned to his cases.

## The First Interview

Present in the first family interview were Randy and his mother, Mary (Bill had called prior to the session to let me know that he was tied up in court and could not make it to our session). As with previous cases we worked on together, Bill gave me free reign to conduct therapy in any way I wished and to determine on my own the frequency of family sessions. We both agreed that some intervention was needed with the involved and concerned school personnel at Randy's high school. In the waiting room I had Randy and his mother sign release of information forms so that I could continue my collaboration with Bill and meet with key school personnel.

After establishing rapport with each family member regarding their strengths and interests, I began the interview by exploring what pretreatment changes (Weiner-Davis et al., 1987) had occurred following Randy's release from the juvenile detention center 2 weeks prior to this initial session. Since I believe strongly in the idea that all clients have the strengths and resources for change, I was confident that the family had already taken some important steps toward improving their problem situation. Earlier in the interview Randy had referred to the juvenile detention center as the "juvie." The following is a transcription of the first interview between Mary (M), Randy (R), and me (T):

T:  Since Randy got out of the juvie, what have you noticed that is better?

M:  Everything has been great! He's been going to school and following my rules. He's not smoking that marijuana stuff. It's like he's another person.

T:  Wow! How did you get him to do all of those great things!?

   [Here I am cheerleading to make these exceptions newsworthy. "How" questions are good for having family members compliment themselves on their resourcefulness].

M:  Well . . . I told him when I picked him up at the juvenile center that I'm not going to put up with his nonsense anymore and from now on he's going to live by my rules or go to live with his alcoholic father.

T:  Have you been eating your spinach lately? Let me see your biceps.

   [I get up and feel her right bicep. Randy and Mary laugh. This is an example of my improvisational therapeutic style. I had this image of Popeye the Sailor Man flash into my mind while mother was telling me about how she has gotten tougher as a parent. My humorous comments and actions serve to empower mother as a parent].

M:  *(laughs)* I don't like spinach, but I get a good workout at my job.

T:  That's one hell of a bicep! Do you curl any of the machines you work on at your job?

M:  *(laughs)* Believe me some days it really feels like I've been curling machines all day.

T:  Randy, how were you able to do all of those great things after getting out of the juvie?

R:  Well . . . I guess I really didn't like that place and I had lots of time to think about things in there.

T:  What kind of things did you think about or tell yourself in the juvie that made you decide "I'm going to turn things around when I get out of this place"?

[Here I am utilizing a "unique account" question to have Randy ascribe meaning to what paved the way for him to embark on a new direction in life after getting out of the juvie.

R:  Well . . . I thought about how I don't belong in here. It's crazy in there, man . . . all of the fights and shit, gangbangers . . . Man, I'm just glad to be out of that place, man.

T:  What kind of things did you tell yourself in the juvie that made you decide "I'm going to be a different person when I get out"?

[I decided to rephrase my earlier "unique account" question, hoping that Randy would be more specific a bout the shift in his thinking regarding the new person he wanted to become after getting out of the juvie.]

R:  Well . . . I told myself, "I can do better than ending up in places like this"; "I have to stop smoking reefer"; "I need to stop cutting school"; "I gotta listen to my mom." Things like that, man . . .

M:  Wow! It sounds like you were really doing some heavy soul-searching in the juvie.

M:  I've really noticed that he's really trying this time.

T:  How else is he showing you that he's really trying this time?

[Here, I am utilizing mother's language to further elicit exception material. I am also keeping the "change talk" going in our therapeutic conversation.]

M:  Well, he's been really helpful around the house. I haven't seen him running with those druggy type kids he used to run around with. I haven't found any strange radios or bicycles hidden in the basement, like I used to.

T:  Wow! That's great! What are you doing differently around Randy now, as opposed to before he went into the juvie?

[Besides cheerleading to further reinforce Randy's changes and mother's awareness of them, I am attempting to make a distinction between mother's old parenting style and what she is now doing differently that is working for her.]

M:  Well, I'm staying on top of him and I'm not backing down anymore. I've told him that I'm proud of him on good days, but there are still days when he's his old lazy self . . . where he . . .

T:  How did you come up with those great ideas!?

[Most therapists would be tempted to inquire about Randy's bad days when he's "his old lazy self." However, I feel that it is more helpful to the family to keep the focus on what is working. I ask a "how" question to amplify mother's resourcefulness and to return us to our "change talk" conversation.]

M: Well, I think he responds better when I don't let him slide with things. Before, he could get away with a lot of things. The praise idea comes from how I've thought for a long time that he's got low self-esteem. His alcoholic father used to always put him down.

T: What else will you have to continue to do around Randy to keep these great things happening?

[My use of the "how" question effectively returns us to "change talk" and elicits evidence of Mary's parental resourcefulness and wisdom.]

M: Keep staying on top of him, don't let him slide with anything, keep praising him for the good stuff that he does.

T: Randy, what will you have to keep doing to further improve the great new person you have became?

R: Listen to Mom. You know . . . empty the garbage, stay away from Curt and Roger . . .

M: Yeah, he's right. Those two kids are always up to no good. Wasn't Roger in the juvenile center?

R: Yeah. He was in the juvie a couple of times. He's always bragging about it.

T: At this point, I'd like to break up the session and meet with you two separately. Mary, would you like to meet alone first?

M: No . . . I really don't have anything more to talk to you about. I've said all I had to already. Why don't you two guys spend some time alone.

[When I work with adolescents, I find it useful to give both the parents and the adolescent individual space time. I use this individual session time with the adolescent to negotiate the parental goal or establish a separate goal. I also find out from the adolescent if there is a privilege he or she wishes me to negotiate with the parents. Sometimes I offer the young client the role of "expert consultant" on adolescence.]

T: Randy, how would you like to meet alone for a short time?

R: Okay. *(Mary leaves the room.)*

T: It sounds like you have done a super job! That's worth a high-five! *(I give Randy a big high-five for a job well done.)*

[My adolescent clients are often surprised by my familiarity with the popular high-five gesture. This is another example of therapeutic improvisation.]

T: The juvie didn't sound like such a hot place.

R: Yeah man . . . I hated it in there, man.

T: You know, I work with a lot of kids that are on probation or have gotten in trouble with the cops and may be heading for the juvie. I kind of would like to use you as a consultant. Do you have any ideas about what kinds of things I could tell those kids about the juvie that would be helpful for them to know?

[Here, I am using Randy as an expert consultant to further empower him in his new direction in life as a responsible young man.]

R: Well, it's not a good place to go. They've got gangbangers in there man. Some real big dudes! Kids are always fighting. Boy, I could tell you about some things I saw in there, man. I saw a kid get paralyzed in there.

T: You did? What happened?

R: Well, there was this kid. He put his hand on this black dude's shoulder in the shower . . . and, you know . . . I guess he thought he was a fag or something. You know those plastic glasses in cafeterias? Well, he broke this glass and then stuck it in that kid's spine. The kid fell on the floor and, man, you should have seen this dude's face. And he was rolling around on the floor . . . the look on his face . . .

T: Wow! That's pretty shocking. That's one horror story I can share with kids.

R: That's not all, man. I saw fights where the staff would just sit there while one kid was banging another kid's head into the wall. They wouldn't do nothing.

T: That's unbelievable!

R: I got into one fight when I was in there. Yeah, this one dude started talking about my mother—nobody talks about my mother! He took a swing at me and I knocked him down on the ground.

T: Did you give him a left hook and right cross combination?

[I am using humor here. Some therapists might have explored with Randy how long he has had difficulties with impulse control and anger management.

R: *(smiling)* Yeah right, man . . . *(laughs)* After I knocked him down, they put me in solitary for two days. On the second day this strange dude doctor came in to give me some mind tests.

T: You didn't know you had boxing talents, right?

R: My mom's boyfriend taught me.

T: Tell me about those mind tests. What were they?

R: Well, when you get into a big fight, they give you these tests to try and get into your head, you see. That strange dude doctor told me that I will probably be back in the juvie three weeks after getting out.

T: Really!? Is there anything else I could tell those kids that are heading for the juvie?

[I made a mental note regarding the psychologist's prediction that Randy would end up back in the juvie. I felt I could use this later in the interview to set up a split. I decided to further utilize Randy's services as an expert consultant.]

R: Well, there are benefits for listening to your mom.

T: Like what?

R: Well . . . if you listen to your mom, you wouldn't end up in places like this. Sometimes they give you nice things if you're good. You've got to do your homework. I never did any schoolwork before.

T: Are you doing your homework now?

R: Yeah.

T: Really! How have you been able to do that?

[I am cheerleading and asking a "how" question to reinforce this positive change.

R: Well, I'm taking school more seriously now. I know when I get out I'll need to make money and get a good job.

T: This is great! That's really responsible! That's worth another high-five! *(I give Randy a high-five.)*

R: Thanks, man.

T: Well, thank you for your helpful consultation. I've learned a lot about the juvie, and I can tell my other young clients about your experiences in there. You know, let's prove that doctor wrong. You're going to continue to kick butt after three weeks out of the juvie, and then we can laugh in his face! *(We shake hands on this.)*

R: I can laugh in his face after nine months! Then I can laugh in his face!

[Randy was slated to get off probation in 9 months. Here I am setting up a split between Randy and the pessimistic "doctor." This strategy works well with adolescents because they love proving authority figures wrong. Randy displayed a high level of reactance in wanting to prove the "strange dude doctor" wrong, which was a good sign that this intervention would work.]

T: Okay, I'm going to take a ten-minute break to meet with myself to think about all of the things you and your mother said and come up with a helpful homework assignment. *(Randy leaves the office to join his mother in the waiting area.)*

[During the break period I came up with several compliments for each family member. Since the family had identified a wealth of exceptions, my job was made easy in constructing the compliments and selecting an appropriate therapeutic task. It was clear that both Mary and Randy were keenly aware of what they were doing and what they needed to continue to do to prevent problems from happening. The most logical intervention I could make was to give the family the straightforward therapeutic task of keeping track of what they were doing between sessions that was working, a task that would best fit their unique cooperative response pattern.]

T: *(reconvening the family)* There are a number of things that I would like to compliment the two of you on. In fact, I had to condense three pages of compliments into one page. So this is the "best of" list of compliments from the three pages. First of all, Mary, I am very impressed with how committed you have been as a parent in paving the way for Randy to become a more responsible young man. I am impressed with your recognizing that by being firm with him about following your rules, not backing down, and praising him when he is good have made him more responsible and built up his self-esteem. I am also impressed with your noticing all of the responsible steps Randy has already taken since getting out of the juvie: He's going to school, he's following your rules, he's not running with Curt and Roger, and you haven't found any strange radios or bicycles in your basement.

Randy, I am very impressed with your showing up here tonight, you could have blown me off. Believe me, I get blown off a lot. I am very impressed with the responsible and mature person you have become since getting out of the juvie. It is clear to me that you did a lot of important soul-searching in there, such as: telling yourself "This is not the place for me"; "I need to go to school"; "I have to stop smoking reefer"; "I need to listen to my mother"; and that you have to stay away from Curt and Roger. I was very impressed with all of your helpful words of wisdom you shared with me about what I could tell other kids that are heading for the juvie. Maybe I should set up some speaking engagements for you in the schools. By the way, what is your consultation fee?

M: *(laughs)*

R: *(laughs)* No charge for you, man!

T: Since the two of you are doing such a great job as a family, I would like to give you a vacation from counseling as a vote of confidence. When would you like to come back here, in two or three weeks?

M: Oh, why don't we come back in two weeks.

T: While on vacation, I would like to give you a homework assignment. Between now and the next time we meet, I would like the two of you to keep track of all of the various things you will do to further improve your relationship. You can make mental notes or write all of those great things down. I will be looking forward to hearing what further progress you will have made.

M: Thanks for everything. See you in two weeks.

R: Thanks. Bye!

*(I shake hands with Randy and his mother.)*

## Treatment Summary

I saw Randy and his mother six times over a 9-month period. Sessions 2 through 6 were characterized by major individual and family changes. Randy had no further legal or drug involvement up to 1 year follow-up. In subsequent family sessions after the first one I amplified changes and highlighted differences to consolidate individual and family gains. As a vote of confidence to the family, I gave them increasingly longer time intervals between sessions. During these intervals I collaborated with key school personnel and the probation officer to address their concerns about Randy. Two family–multiple helper meetings were conducted to give concerned helpers the opportunity to notice changes in Randy's behavior. To celebrate Randy's successful termination from his probation, I threw a party for the family. I provided them with a cake and highlighted all of their major changes.

The major joy of our final session together was hearing the well-written letter Randy planned to send to the psychologist at the juvie. Randy pointed out in his letter that he remembered the psychologist's grim prediction that he would be back in the juvie and that he wanted to prove him wrong 9 months later. After Randy read this wonderful letter, his mother and I gave him a standing ovation.

## EDITOR'S QUESTIONS

Q: *It seems clear that the therapist's attitude and expectations about change have a major influence on therapeutic outcome. Would you comment on this in the context of your work with adolescents? Also, when you find yourself feeling pessimistic about the progress of a therapy, what do you do to recover your optimism?*
A: With each new adolescent case I am referred, I believe the youth and his or her family have the strengths and resources to change. I also expect that my clients will teach me how to cooperate with them. When an adolescent shows up at the first scheduled family session, I will view this youth, no matter how disturbing or chronic his or her behavior is supposed to be, as being responsible and ripe for change.

When I feel stuck with a particular adolescent case, this is a warning signal to me that I need to do something different therapeutically. I will then pursue one of the following options: (1) I will assess with the clients if our treatment goal is too monolithic; if it is, we will re-negotiate a smaller or new goal. (2) If I am working alone with the family, I will invite a colleague to observe our next session and offer us some fresh ideas about how to cooperate better. (3) I will place the family in the expert position and invite them to tell me how to treat another family just like them.

Q: *In the particular clinical situation presented, the family came in reporting significant pretherapy change. Your efforts were focused mainly on amplifying and solidifying that change. How do you approach situations where the family comes in without such change in evidence? What steps do you take to create a "customer" of the adolescent when he or she is not initially cooperative? Do you ever work solely with the parent(s) and agency people and not involve the adolescent in the therapy process?*

A: With families who present with a lot of "problem talk" and deflect my exception-oriented inquiry, I quickly move to asking the "miracle question" or pull out my trusty imaginary crystal ball and have each family member describe in great detail what a hypothetical solution will look like in the future. Not only do these questions help pave the way for solution construction with my clients, but they also produce clear treatment outcome goals.

In case situations where the adolescent is physically present in the family session but behaving like a window-shopper, I utilize one of the following three engagement strategies: (1) I acknowledge the adolescent's position of being forced to go to therapy and accept whatever individual goal the adolescent wishes to pursue. (2) I set up a split between myself and the referring person and offer to get the latter (e.g., the probation officer) off my young client's back. (3) I adopt the one-down Columbo approach as a nonthreatening strategy for inviting the window-shopping adolescent to help the confused and incompetent therapist out regarding how and why he or she was brought for therapy.

I have worked on a number of cases in which I saw in therapy only the parents and referring person or involved helping professionals. In fact, with many adolescent cases it is the parents, referring person, or involved helpers who are the real "customers" for therapy. Since these key members of the problem system are the most invested in the change process, it makes sense to problem-solve and collaborate with them. In many adolescent cases, I accomplish all of my therapeutic changes through the parents and other members of the problem system and never need the adolescent present in the sessions. When working solely with the parents and involved helpers in the therapy sessions, I only attempt to engage the adolescent directly if changes are not occurring in him or her.

Q: *In what circumstances would you explore historical issues in the family (e.g., in the case presented, the adolescent's relationship with his alcoholic father)?*

A: Since my approach to therapy is present- and future-oriented, I tend to go into the past with parents only to explore any past problem-solving strategies they utilized that worked in resolving other problematic behaviors exhibited by their son or daughter. However, I am not so rigidly wedded to my therapy model that I do not believe that there is any room for historical storytelling. There are some families who have a long story to tell about past traumatic events and negative treatment experiences, and these should not be edited by the therapist. I once worked with a family who had

had 16 previous therapy experiences, many of which had further exacerbated their problem situation. My detailed inquiry into these negative treatment experiences provided me with helpful information about what I needed to do differently with them as a therapist.

My contract with Randy and his mother was to focus on how we could keep Randy out of further legal difficulties. Since the family had already generated some creative and effective solutions prior to our initial therapy session, I saw my job as simply amplifying what was already working for them. Not once in my therapy experience with Randy and his mother did either of them voice a desire to look at Randy's negative relationship with his alcoholic father. Having Randy and his mother talk about the former's negative past relationship with his father would have been encouraging "problem talk" and could possibly have led to the family's going backward.

## REFERENCES

Anderson, H., Goolishian, H., Pulliam, G., & Winderman, L. (1986). The Galveston Family Institute: Some personal and historical perspectives. In D. Efron (Ed.), *Journeys: Expansion of the strategic-systemic therapies* (pp. 97–125). New York: Brunner/Mazel.

Bateson, G. (1980). *Mind and nature: A necessary unity.* New York: Ballantine.

Beavers, W. R., & Hampson, B. (1990). *Successful families.* New York: Norton.

Berg, I. K., & Gallagher, D. (1991). Solution-focused brief therapy with adolescent substance abusers. In T. C. Todd & M. D. Selekman (Eds.), *Family therapy approaches with adolescent substance abusers* (pp. 93–111). Needham Heights, MA: Allyn & Bacon.

Coppersmith, E. I. (1985). Families and multiple helpers: A systemic perspective. In D. Campbell & R. Draper (Eds.), *Applications of systemic family therapy: A Milan approach.* London: Grune & Stratton.

de Shazer, S. (1982). Some conceptual distinctions are more useful than others. *Family Process, 21,* 71–84.

de Shazer, S. (1984). The death of resistance. *Family Process, 23,* 79–93.

de Shazer, S. (1985). *Keys to solution in brief therapy.* New York: Norton.

de Shazer, S. (1988). *Clues: Investigating solutions in brief therapy.* New York: Norton.

de Shazer, S. (1991). *Putting difference to work.* New York: Norton.

de Shazer, S., Berg, I. K., Lipchik, E., Nunnally, E., Molnar, A., Gingerich, W., & Weiner-Davis, M. (1986). Brief therapy: Focused solution development. *Family Process, 25,* 207–222.

Efran, J., & Lukens, M. (1988). The world according to Humberto Maturana. *Family Therapy Networker,* May-June, 23–28, 72–75.

Erickson, M. H. (1954). Pseudo-orientation in time as a hypnotic procedure. *Journal of Clinical and Experimental Hypnosis, 2,* 161–283.

Erickson, M. H. (1964). The confusion technique in hypnosis. *American Journal of Clinical Hypnosis. 6,* 183–207.

Erickson, M. H., & Rossi, E. (1983). *Healing in hypnosis.* New York: Irvington.

Erickson, M. H., Rossi, E., & Rossi, I. (1976). *Hypnotic realities.* New York: Irvington.

Fisch, R., Weakland, J., & Segal, L. (1982). *The tactics of change.* San Francisco: Jossey-Ross.

Gingerich, W., & de Shazer., S. (1991). The BRIEFER project: Using expert systems as theory construction tools. *Family Process, 30,* 241–249.

Gingerich, W., de Shazer, S., & Weiner-Davis, M. (1987). Constructing change: A research view of interviewing. In E. Lipchik (Ed.), *Interviewing.* Rockville, MD: Aspen.

Goolishian, H., & Anderson, H. (1981). Including non-blood related persons in family therapy. In A. S. Gurman (Ed.), *Questions and answers in the practice of family therapy.* New York: Brunner/Mazel.

Gordon, D., & Meyer-Anderson, M. (1981). *Phoenix: Therapeutic patterns of Milton H. Erickson.* Cupertino, CA: Meta.

Hentoff, N. (1958). Liner notes for *Something Else! The music of Ornette Coleman.* Contemporary 7551.

Lipchik, E. (1988). Interviewing with a constructive ear. *Dulwich Centre Newletter,* Winter, 3–7.

Lipchik, E., & de Shazer, S. (1986). The purposeful interview. *Journal of Strategic and Systemic Therapies, 5*(1), 88–99.

Maturana, H., & Varela, F. (1987). *The tree of knowledge: The biological roots to human understanding.* Boston: New Science Library.

O'Hanlon, W. H. (1987). *Taproots: Underlying principles of Milton H. Erickson's therapy and hypnosis.* New York: Norton.

O'Hanlon, W. H., & Weiner-Davis, M. (1989). *In search of solutions: A new direction in psychotherapy.* New York: Norton.

Rosen, S. (1982). *My voice will go with you: The teaching tales of Milton H. Erickson.* New York: Norton.

Selekman, M. D. (1989). Taming chemical monsters: Cybernetic-systemic therapy with adolescent substance abusers. *Journal of Strategic and Systemic Therapies, 8*(3), 5-10.

Selekman, M. D. (1991). The solution-oriented parenting group: A treatment alternative that works. *Journal of Strategic and Systemic Therapies, 10*(1), 36-49.

Selekman, M. D. (in press). *Pathways to solutions: Brief therapy with difficult adolescents.* New York: Guilford Press.

Selekman, M. D., & Todd, T. C. (1991). Crucial issues in the treatment of adolescent substance abusers and their families. In T. C. Todd & M. D. Selekman (Eds.), *Family therapy approaches with adolescent substance abusers* (pp. 1–20). Needham Heights, MA: Allyn & Bacon.

Todd, T. C., & Selekman, M. D. (1991). Beyond structural-strategic family therapy: Integrating other brief systemic therapies. In T. C. Todd & M. D. Selekman (Eds.), *Family therapy approaches with adolescent substance abusers* (pp. 241–271). Needham Heights, MA: Allyn & Bacon.

Varela, F. (1979). *Principles of biological autonomy.* New York: North Holland.

von Foerster, H. (1981). *Observing systems.* Seaside, CA: North Holland.

Watzlawick, P., Weakland, J., & Fisch, R. (1974). *Change: Principles of problem formation and problem resolution.* New York: Norton.

Weiner-Davis, M. (1992). *Divorce busting.* New York: Simon & Schuster.

Weiner-Davis, M., de Shazer, S., & Gingerich, W. (1987). Building on pretreatment change to construct the therapeutic solution: An exploratory study. *Journal of Marital and Family Therapy, 13*(4), 359–363.

White, M. (1984). Pseudo-encopresis: From avalanche to victory, from vicious to virtuous cycles. *Family Systems Medicine, 2*(2), 150–160.

White, M. (1985). Fear-busting and monster taming: An approach to the fears of young children. *Dulwich Centre Review,* 29–33.

White, M. (1986). Negative explanation, restraint and double description: A template for family therapy. *Family Process, 25*(2), 169-184.

White, M. (1987, Spring). Family therapy and schizophrenia: Addressing the in-the-corner lifestyle. *Dulwich Centre Newsletter,* 14–21.

White, M. (1988). Anorexia nervosa: A cybernetic perspective. In J. E. Harkaway (Ed.), *Eating disorders* (pp. 117–129). Rockville, MD: Aspen.

White, M., & Epston, D. (1990). *Narrative means to therapeutic ends.* New York: Norton.

Williams, M. (1939). *Jazz panorama.* New York: Harcourt Brace Jovanovich.

# 7

# Toward a Mutual Understanding: Constructing Solutions with Families

CYNTHIA MITTELMEIER
STEVEN FRIEDMAN

*If you did nothing more when you have a family together than to make it possible for them to really look at each other, really touch each other, and listen to each other, you would have already swung the pendulum in the direction of a new start.*

—VIRGINIA SATIR

Since the meanings and understandings we have of events in our lives are tentative and negotiable (Anderson & Goolishian, 1988; Bruner, 1987), it becomes possible to co-construct new meanings in conversation. It is such a conversation that is the focus of the clinical work presented here. Our model, the "possibility paradigm" (Friedman & Fanger, 1991), integrates elements of solution-focused therapy (de Shazer, 1985, 1988, 1991; O'Hanlon & Weiner-Davis, 1989; O'Hanlon & Wilk, 1987) with other language-based collaborative systems approaches (Andersen, 1987, 1990; Anderson & Goolishian, 1988; White & Epston, 1990). The setting in which we work (a health maintenance organization, or HMO) necessitates that we maintain a sensitivity to time and to maximizing our therapeutic contacts (Friedman & Fanger, 1991). Although we deal with many complex clinical situations, we try to "stay simple" and allow our näiveté to lead us toward the client's goal. Since being naive favors optimism (Weick, 1984), we reject complex assumptions and explanatory mechanisms and make special efforts to avoid becoming encumbered by past historical accounts and "totalizing" descriptions (White, 1991). We explore the past as a way to draw on those historical experiences that may be useful in enabling movement toward a more satisfying future state.

"Language creates a psychophysiological response in us whether we are actually having the experience or whether we are just pretending to have it" (Friedman & Fanger, 1991, p. 29). By creating opportunities for clients to experience positive futures, the therapist facilitates the change process. A "wellness" model provides a map that enables us to travel along a road of hope and optimism about the inevitability of change. We immediately engage the client in projecting a future that does not include the problem. We act as facilitators or "resource catalysts" who work "unremittingly under positive auspices" (Friedman & Fanger, 1991) to generate conversations that offer the client new possibilities and options for the future. We incorporate experiential, action-based methods that enable clients to move on their own trajectory toward change. By amplifying strengths and engaging in solution-focused conversations we create opportunities for new understandings and increase options for action.

We also incorporate behind-the-mirror clinical teams as a way to offer us and our clients new ideas and new perspectives. We initially began our work using a strategic team process (e.g., Friedman & Pettus, 1985) where an anonymous expert team sends in messages to the therapist and family. We then moved to a reflecting team model (Andersen, 1987, 1990), where the team engages in a conversation while the family listens. Although the format changed, we continued to incorporate strategic ideas in our conversations (e.g., Mittelmeier & Friedman, 1991). Most recently, we have modified our reflecting team format. Rather than make pronouncements about the family process, we generate metaphors that capture the client's attention and seed ideas. We have thus moved from a process of developing consensual descriptions to one of generating multiple descriptions leading to "polyocular" perspectives. We also use the reflecting team as an audience to embody changes in the client's re-authoring process (see Brecher & Friedman, this volume).

Table 7.1 (from Friedman & Fanger, 1991) provides an overview of the principles and strategies we have found useful in our clinical work.

As can be seen in the following clinical situation, we engage the clients in an enactment of their goals (after Chasin, Roth, & Bograd, 1989; Chasin & Roth, 1990). We accept and unremittingly attend to the clients' wishes for a "better understanding." We guide and structure the therapeutic conversation in a way that allows them to successfully and rapidly reach their desired outcome.

## CLINICAL ILLUSTRATION

### The Family

Susan (age 45), a single parent, is the mother of a 16-year-old daughter, Jane, and a 10-year-old son, Steven. The therapist (C.M.) saw Susan and Jane for three sessions a year earlier. She also had one contact immediately prior to the

**TABLE 7.1. Guiding Principles and Clinical Strategies in Brief Possibility-Oriented Therapy**

| Principles | Strategies |
|---|---|
| 1. Think small. | Try simple interventions first, based on simple assumptions. |
| 2. Complicated situations do not necessarily require complicated solutions. | Focus on solutions, on what works rather than what doesn't work. |
| 3. The client's request must be taken seriously and given primary attention. | Engage the client and maintain a focus on the original request. |
| 4. Cooperation and collaboration between therapist and client create a context for change. | Insist that the client be an active partner in solution development. |
| 5. The therapist negotiates with the client in producing clearly defined steps to a specified goal. | Frame complaints in forms that are solvable. Be active, flexible, and focused. Use possibility language as a medium for creating change. |
| 6. "Brief therapy is most successful when the client is persuaded to do just one thing differently."[a] | Work to get a small change going. Create a context in which novelty or playfulness can be introduced. |
| 7. Contained within the client (family) are the seeds of solution development. | Focus on resources and strengths. Empower the client or family as change agents. Respect and support client creativity in developing solutions. |
| 8. Change is inevitable; all clients/families undergo developmental transitions and crises. | Normalize developmental transitions. Reframe difficulties in a developmental context. |
| 9. Supportive client networks increase options for change. | Involve networks of support in the treatment process. |
| 10. The therapist needs to main a sense of optimism, naîveté, and playfulness in clinical interaction. | Cultivate a sense of humor and a respect for the "benign absurdity of life."[b] |

*Note.* From *Expanding Therapeutic Possibilities* (p. 117) by S. Friedman and M. T. Fanger, 1991, New York: Lexington Books. Copyright 1991 by Macmillan, Inc. Reprinted by permission.
[a]Weick, 1984, p. 45.
[b]Whitaker, 1976, p. 164.

current consultation. This recent contact was precipitated by intense mother–daughter conflict. Susan felt that Jane was spending too much time with her boyfriend and withdrawing from activities, and she was also concerned about Jane's drop in grades. Jane viewed Susan as overly strict. The situation escalated to the point where Jane left the house on several occasions without informing Susan of her whereabouts and was now refusing to come home after school. Susan and Jane were no longer speaking to each other, and Jane's boyfriend was no longer welcome in the house.

## Consultation

The therapist, Cynthia Mittelmeier (T in the dialogue), explains the reflecting team process to Susan and Jane and introduces the consultant, Steven Friedman (C). She asks a "possibility frame" question (Friedman & Fanger, 1991). This question allows the clients to actively guide the therapeutic process and presents the hopeful view that something *will* be accomplished in the meeting.

T:  I wanted to start with what is it that you would like to have happen here today, in this meeting.

S:  The dynamics of my household are at a point where I'm not comfortable. Because of my knowing you and having confidence in you, I need some help. I'm very gracious to try anything.

T:  So what you would like to have happen here today then . . .

S:  Maybe some tools to work with. Some things beyond what I thought about or what I've tried. Maybe a different direction.

T:  How about you, Jane? What would you like to have happen here today?

J:  I want some changes to happen, but I can't think of anything specifically.

T:  Changes between you and your mom, like what?

J:  An understanding.

T:  You'd like her to understand your point of view better.

J:  Both.

T:  And that you could understand her point of view.

[The consultant orients the clients to the future, a future that does not include the problem, and requests that they give him specific and concrete examples.]

C:  What I'm wondering about is what things will look like when they are the way you'd like them to be. You know, you talk about an understanding . . . what will that look like? Give me an example of what it would look like.

S:  This is just an off-the-cuff example. I have limitations. I have to know where she's going—naturally, with who—and when she's back. If I say you have to be back at eleven that doesn't mean eleven-fifteen or eleven-thirty. She has money on her generally, and there are plenty of telephone booths. There isn't a sufficient reason not to call, to not pay any attention to her curfew, and not accept the responsibility of a consequence. That's upsetting to me. That's just a little example of the things I find difficult on a continual basis.

[The consultant uses presuppositional statements—those introduced by "when" rather than "if"—as a way to create a hopeful stance about the possibilities for change.]

C:  What can you envision things looking like at the point when things are working with you and your daughter? You're telling me about some of the obstacles you are running into, but when those obstacles are over-come, when things are at a place where you're satisfied, what would that look like?

J: Definitely a better understanding of each other.

[The consultant asks for specificity and finds out that both Susan and Jane have a shared goal: wanting more "understanding." By eliciting this information the therapists have taken the first step in co-constructing a "well-formed outcome" (i.e., a goal that is stated in positive terms; see Friedman & Fanger, 1991). They now can turn their attention to enabling this mother and daughter to reach their mutually agreed-upon goal.]

C: And who would understand who about what?

S: Oh, both ways, a better understanding of each other.

C: Okay, and how would your daughter know that you were understanding her better?

S: I would probably ask.

C: What would you ask?

S: Do you understand how important this is to me? What it might mean to me?

[Change is initiated when clients can actually experience themselves in a future without the problem. As O'Hanlon and Weiner-Davis (1989) suggest, "the mere act of constructing a vision of the solution acts as a catalyst for bringing it about" (p. 106). Here, the consultant activates the clients' resources by requesting that they demonstrate their goals for change (after Chasin et al., 1989; Chasin & Roth, 1990).]

C: *(to therapist)* You know, what I'm thinking about is if Jane and her mother can show us what that understanding would look like when it's happening in the way they would like it to happen.

S: Role play.

C: Yeah, right. To demonstrate that understanding. Now I know you are saying it doesn't exist right now. That's why you are here; you want to get there. I'm interested in seeing how you do that, the picture of how you'd like it to be.

S: Paint the picture.

C: Yeah, paint the picture.

[Jane and Susan start to talk about what example they will use, and they finally settle on one. Notice how in the following sequence Susan recognizes that the old pattern is being repeated and stops the role play.]

S: Where are you going?

J: Shopping.

S: With who?

J: Justin [the boyfriend], obviously.

S: What time will you be back?

J: I don't know what time.

S: Jane, I need to know, about what time.

J: I don't know exactly where I'm going. I can call you and let you know from where I am.

S: I might want to cook dinner for all of us. If you're not going to be home, there are other things I could and should do. What time do you think you'll be home?

J: Why don't you cook dinner? I hardly ever eat dinner anyway.

S: *(voice rising)* I'd like you to come home so we can sit down and eat dinner together.

J: We never eat dinner together.

S: Gee, since when?

J: For a long time.

S: Okay, you've drawn me into something here that's not like the perfect picture I wanted to paint.

[The consultant moves client along and avoids a potential roadblock.]

C: Why don't we simplify it a little bit? Why don't you tell Jane how you want her to play this?

J: I know exactly what she wants me to say. She wants me to say, "I'll be home by four."

C: What I'd like you to do, just for these purposes, is to try to run through that. You know what I'm saying? This is your mother's picture. I know it's not your picture.

J: *(begins to role-play again)* What time would you want me to be home then?

S: If you could be home by five, that would be superb. We're having such and such for dinner and Papa might come up and then I'll be able to do some paperwork afterwards and so and so is coming by.

J: Okay.

S: Great.

C: *(to Susan)* Did you believe her? Is she believable?

S: At this moment, yes.

C: *(to Jane)* Now, why don't you do that. What's your picture? Let's take the same scene.

T: *(to Jane)* Let's say you're going to tell her you're going shopping.

J: I'm going shopping.

S: Great, with who?

J: Justin.

S: Where do you think you are going shopping?

J: I don't know.

S: What time do you think you'll be home?

J: I'm not sure. I can call you and tell you.

S: Well, I was going to pull a turkey out of the freezer and make up a dinner. I'd like you to be home for dinner.

J: I'm not hungry.

S: Oh, but you will be.

J: At what time?

S: Oh, how about five-thirty?

J: I'll see, depending on where I am.

[The therapist and consultant persist in having the clients "paint the picture" as they (the clients) would like it to be.]

C: *(to Jane)* What would you like to hear from your mother?

J: Just "Okay, give me a call."

C: Did you hear that from her? *(Jane shakes head no)* Okay, so we've got to run through this. What are you asking her?

J: Just to say, "Okay, what time are you going to be home?"

C: Why don't you step back to where you are asking her or telling her what you were doing.

J: *(resuming the role-playing)* I'm going shopping.

S: Oh good. What time are you going to be home?

J: I don't know what time I'm going to be home because I don't know where I'm going.

S: About what time?

J: Probably around six.

S: Okay, I was going to make dinner.

J: At what time?

S: Around six or six-thirty.

J: Okay.

C: *(to Jane)* Is that your picture or your mother's picture?

S: *(to Jane)* I thought you were going to say, "I'll call."

J: *(to Susan)* Well, I knew I'd be home around six-thirty, and you said six-thirty.

S: I was waiting to say, "That would be okay." *(turns to therapist)* Fall off my chair to say that, but I was going to say that.

J: *(role-playing)* Okay, how about seven?

S: Okay, then maybe we'll have a later dinner.

C: So that's fine. *(turns to Jane)* What about your mother asking you those questions? Was that part of a picture you have? Is that part of your understanding?

T: *(to consultant)* You mean those questions about where you'll be going and what time you'll be back?

J: Yeah, that's 'cause I'm used to them.

[The consultant normalizes Susan's questioning and then compliments Susan and Jane on their successful efforts in creating increased "understanding."]

C: *(to Susan)* That's what a mother needs to do sometimes, to ask those questions. So you did that very well. You're able to do that and that was hard to do.

S: Oh, now that's basically the type of dialogue that we generally do. The meshing of answers that you got now is not traditionally what has happened.

[The therapists take the position that Susan and Jane will be capable of reaching some new understandings when space is created for new options to evolve. Rather than searching for causes of the mother–daughter *mis*understanding (a positive explanatory process), the therapists view the situation from a position of "negative explanation" (White, 1986) by asking what restraints need to be removed to allow other options to emerge.]

C: What gets in the way of having this conversation at other times?

J: A difference of opinion.

T: But this is what it would look like when some of the obstacles were removed.

S: I have a need to know. I feel it's well within my rights as Jane's mom. If I said seven, I could expect that if she was going to be late that she would call. I would be really unhappy if that didn't happen, and this has been the case. I'm no longer a negotiator. I'm becoming an enforcer. I don't feel that role is necessary.

[The consultant restates Susan's ideas about being an "enforcer," including her preference for letting go of that role.]

C: You don't want to be in that role.

S: No, not continuously and not to that extent, no. I don't feel it is necessary.

C: And that has got to be an unpleasant role for both of you. *(turns to Jane)* You don't like your mother in that role and you don't like yourself in that role. That's very unpleasant. And Jane is getting to that age when an enforcer can't enforce very much.

S: We've known each other a long time. These expectations are not new. Some things I'm not flexible about. I need to be able to make other plans for other things. . . . Everything is hinging on approximate times of who, what, when, and where.

[The consultant uses the metaphor of friction, noting that oil is required to get the gears to mesh.]

C: *(to Susan)* So that's been an expectation for you through the years and you've experienced that. *(turns to Jane)* It's just that it seems like something is happening now that you're getting older and you are making choices for yourself and there is friction now.

S: That's a nice, tender word . . . friction.

C: There's pushing; the gears are kind of rubbing against one another. So that it needs a little oil.

T: This family needs a little oil.

C: *(to therapist)* To get the gears running smoothly but I can see that they can talk to one another and be understanding and they've got a basis for that in the past to do it.

T: Which is a positive sign. I think you're right: As Jane is getting older, she's making more choices. She's wanting to do things on her own, to try out new things, and the gears are not meshing.

S: From my own particular viewpoint as her mom, at fifteen and a half oftentimes Jane feels that she's twenty-seven and can certainly do it all. I don't believe I've ever underestimated her abilities, but there are certain things you gain a confidence over gradually. "I'm not going to be home until twelve" is just not acceptable. . . . I am not comfortable with that and now I've regressed even more.

T: You're pulling the reins even tighter.

S: We're going back to square one and we will build from there.

T: *(turns to Jane)* I get the feeling you're not crazy about that, Jane.

[The therapist moves the discussion to a question she asked Susan and Jane to consider at the previous contact. This question (after de Shazer, 1985) provides an opportunity for the clients to look at what is working well in their relationship rather than what is *not* working.]

T: I wanted to follow up on our last meeting. I gave you some homework and the homework, was for you to think about some of the things that were happening that were positive in the relationship that you would like to continue to have happen. *(turns to Susan)* So what is it that is happening with Jane that you would like to have continue to have happen?

S: I guess to learn to grow together and come to terms with each other in a more understanding way. I don't feel I've come over on the wagon train. I can remember very well how difficult many many aspects of my own life were growing up. I'm still growing, the book isn't written yet.

T: So despite the friction now that you both are feeling, what's going well in the relationship? What do you want to see continue to happen in your relationship with Jane?

S: She's my daughter and she will always continue to be my daughter.

T: So your love for her is something you want to see continue to happen.

S: That's a given. That's not in jeopardy.

T: *(to Jane)* How about you? What is happening in your relationship with your mom that you would like to see continue to happen?

J: Right now, there is nothing happening. There is no relationship, no definite relationship.

C: You're not doing anything together. Shopping or something.

T: It's just the enforcer and the enforcee, right now?

[The consultant pursues the idea that there may have been times in the past when things were going well.]

C: But how about in the past? How about two years ago? Okay, what are some of your memories in the past of positive contact between you and your mother?

J: Sharing feelings.

T: You would talk to her and she would share things with you.

J: Not all the time, but when we really needed to.

C: You could get support from one another.

J: One thing that stands out in my mind was when my grandmother died. We had a really good communication of feelings.

C: When was that?

J: Five years ago.

[The consultant continues to request specific behavioral descriptions. He also asks if Jane would like to *reclaim* those moments of understanding that she experienced with her mother in the past.]

C: And what did that look like when you say communication of feelings? What were you doing?

J: Just talking.

C: That was a loss for both of you. You were close to your grandmother. So it took that kind of crisis to bring you into talking together. So you're capable of doing it. Would you like for that possibility to be available to you and your mother again?

J: Yes.

C: *(to Susan)* Do you remember that time?

S: Most definitely.

T: Do you share Jane's ideas that there was a meaningful discussion between you two?

S: I can't remember one discussion. Unlike Jane, right now there have been many discussions about Jane's grandmother and there have been other losses that we have certainly been through together and worked through. But my recollection of the past is very different than Jane's as far as closeness, as far as my being there.

[The consultant does not allow himself to get pulled into a discussion of differences but tries to home in on positive experiences.]

C: *(to Jane)* But this particular time you have a clear recollection that things were working in a way that you liked and was helpful and useful. Now was that right after your grandmother died?

J: Some right after. It wasn't one conversation. It was spread over time.

T: How did your mom let you know that she was there for you and wanted to listen to what you had to say and share feelings?

J: She didn't really let me know, it just happened.

T: So that was kind of a natural thing.

J: At the time, yeah.

[The therapist picks up on and amplifies the idea that there were several times in the past when mother and daughter achieved some understanding.]

T: *(to Susan)* When Jane was talking a minute ago, I got the impression that you were saying your feeling was that you had many more of those moments.

S: Not just moments.

T: So you think that is an underestimation.

S: Right.

*(The mood becomes heavy in the room.)*

C: I have this sense about people's sadness at this point. I'm just wondering what that's about. *(to Jane)* Can you say?

J: *(tearfully)* Not really.

C: What are you thinking about at this point?

J: Just because it feels like we were crying together and that was just a really sad time.

C: But it was also a time when you were close.

T: [The therapist is aware of other losses this family has experienced.] *(to Susan)* Were you thinking about other losses as you started to think about your mother?

S: My cousin. He was very significant to Jane. He died last year, and that was a tremendous loss for Jane and for myself . . . sure.

[The consultant uses the clients' previous experiences of shared loss to enable them to move toward their goal of mutual understanding.]

C: *(to Jane)* And how did you talk about this? Was it like what happened with your grandmother?

S: The circumstances were different. My mother had been seriously ill for a long period of time. . . . Brad's death was quick and sudden. It was a significant loss—that's an understatement. He was someone I could relate to as a friend. He always had a special place in his heart for Jane.

T: Jane, do you think that is what some of your sadness is about? Dr. Friedman was saying that instead of seeing a lot of anger, he's seeing sadness. Do you think so?

J: Yes.

[The consultant uses the memory of this special cousin and his positive relationship to them to help Susan and Jane get reconnected.]

C: What advice would he have given the two of you?

S: To me, he would certainly know, without really having to articulate, some of my own feelings about Jane. He would have told me to just rely on my faith and hang in there.

C: *(to Jane)* Would he have given you advice too? What do you think he would tell you about this?

J: *(laughing)* "You've known your mother a long time. She's a pretty hard person to deal with, but just hang in there."

C: So you both would get the same advice.

T: You both would be told to hang in there.

C: And it seems like you both are doing it.

S: His philosophy would have been for me to rely on my faith. Perhaps my faith is not as strong. I can't rely solely on just my faith. I feel I need to act and change whatever seems to be the difficulty.

[The therapist takes a future orientation, one of hope for the family.]

T: Do you think he would be optimistic that you could overcome this?

S: Of course.

T: So he would be hopeful. So he would think you could win over this problem.

S: I don't want to sound like I'm not hopeful . . . I just would like whatever tools I don't have and that I feel I need.

T: Maybe a little oil.

S: WD-40. Whatever it is—that magic key. Obviously, I haven't found it yet.

C: Maybe we should invite the team to come in now. *(The family leaves the room and goes with the therapists behind the one-way mirror. The team enters.)*

[The team is made up of Edward Bauman, PsyD, Sally Brecher, LICSW, Ethan Kisch, MD, and Jonathan Simmons, PhD]

EB: I had a thought as I was watching them. I was thinking of an analogy that might be a little bit on the silly side . . . about a pair of shoes. As one's feet are growing, sometimes the shoes start to feel a little bit too tight. This is when it can feel like one needs a new pair of shoes. Parents, having some responsibility over how one's feet might be growing, might want to try to make sure the shoes are the right size. I guess sometimes parents might worry that if shoes are too big one might trip or hurt themselves in some other way. One of the things that seems to me is happening is that there's been some growth . . . growth in Jane. At the same time, it is going to be very scary for a parent who wants to make sure that things are going to be okay and the child is doing well in their life. It can sometimes help for a parent to feel more comfortable if one can see the toes, that they are growing. I guess that checking in, making sure that she is safe and she is doing okay in her life, is sort of a way of seeing the toes. The other is to see that they are growing and they can fit a new shoe. In some ways Jane might be saying, "Here are my toes. I can fit these shoes because I'm being more responsible." That was one thought.

JS: Because you know the way you sell shoes. An infant just gets shoes. When they can't speak, they don't have a choice. Sometimes a three-year-old can say, "I want the red ones (or the blue ones)." But when you're an adult . . . Imelda Marcos can have any shoes she wants. When you're not Imelda Marcos and not a two- or three-year-old, it's hard to know how to sell the shoes. Sometimes you have to adjust your sales technique.

EK: So here the daughter wants to buy a pair of jellies and mom wants something that would be a more durable and sensible shoe . . . You know, I was interested in seeing that when Dr. Friedman asked each of them . . . what their ideal picture would be like, it didn't seem to me to be that they had to really struggle very much with that. That to change what they were doing was very minor . . . moving dinner back from five to six. I was struck by the fact that the daughter really feels comfortable for the mother to know where she is and knowing that the mom wants to take that kind of interest. It seems to me that the daughter appreciates her mother's continued care and involvement with her. So, although I understand this family felt like they were at loggerheads, it's surprising to me to see really how close together they are and how much agreement they have.

SB: It's not particularly surprising to me that they are here today talking . . . because I think that mothers and daughters at this age really begin to go through a transformation: a certain transition where the daughter is no longer the mother's little girl . . . where the mother, in turn, isn't sure how much she needs to protect, should protect, and how much she can kind of let go and allow the process to continue. I think it is a very painful time for the mother and daughter in a way. It's an exciting time because the daughter is becoming her own person. It is very clear when we heard these two women today sitting here, they both are very strong individuals and that Jane is emerging as her own person. This is very exciting, while at the same time there is a sadness about the mother losing the little girl that once was more dependent on her. There has been a shift there, and that is not an easy time for them to get through. My own feeling from my experience is that, often, trying to be open about things, trying to share more of one's inner feelings and concentrate a little less on rules and limitations, sometimes is a way of maintaining the contact or the closeness while growing up is actually going on. I think it is normal where they are and I think the mother has done an exceptionally good job in bringing Jane to this point. But it's bittersweet. I guess that's what I'm hearing . . . is that it is somewhat bittersweet.

[The team returns to their position behind the one-way mirror and the family returns to the interview room with the therapist and consultant.]

T: Okay, we wanted to follow up on what the team said that fit, and maybe some things that didn't fit.

S: I certainly appreciated looking at things in a lighthearted tone. When he had spoken about the shoes, I could relate to that analogy and, yes, this is very true in part. When the psychologist had spoken about the bittersweet of the mother–daughter relationship, yes, but Jane and I crossed roads four years ago when she first began dating. The dynamics that I feel now are different from what I was feeling in that initial type of separation in the growing process. I have been a firm believer of allowing reasonable risk for growth not only for my children but for myself. But where she might see us right now, I feel that we have crossed that road perhaps a couple of years ago. This is yet another dimension in that road.

T: So there were some things that fit and some things that didn't fit.

S: Right, sort of like the pair of shoes—some that did and some that didn't.

[The consultant comes back to the metaphor of shoes generated by the reflecting team and offers his own idea that changes and accommodations occur over time.]

C: The thing about shoes is that even if they don't fit right initially they come to fit your foot over time. There's a meshing there between the foot and the shoe.

S: That's right and good leather.

T: Jane, how about for you? What were some of the things that the team said that fit for you?

[Jane is smiling and seems to be noticeably brighter in spirit.]

J: I was thinking about the foot growing. You need to buy a new pair of shoes. It's not going to grow right; it is going to hurt if you don't get a new pair of shoes sooner or later. I disagree with her about us coming to that crossroad four years ago. I think we might have come to an intersection, but the crossroads is now.

T: What makes you say that?

J: Because I mean four years ago, it was a matter of me going to the pizza place and the movies with the boy in the fifth grade. A few years ago, I had no problem being home at six-thirty on a weekend.

[The therapist specifies that a developmental step has been taken and uses the shoe analogy to make her point.]

T: This feels like a bigger step with more pressure on the shoe now than there was before. Your're saying the shoe still fit then, even, though it was getting a little tighter. But you're saying now it's time for a new pair of shoes.

[Discussion ensues about Jane's relationship with her boyfriend, Justin, and her perception that her mother is rude to him now. The consultant looks for a way to help Susan repair this relationship as a way of getting closer to her daughter. Susan then talks about her fears that Jane is making choices that are not good for her future and that are a function of her "overinvolvement" with her boyfriend, whom Susan describes as "idolizing" Jane. The consultant normalizes Jane's intense feelings about her boyfriend and also supports Susan's hard work.]

C: *(to Susan)* It's my sense that Justin is seeing in Jane some of the positive qualities that you've been responsible for helping her achieve. *(to Jane)* I think having a boy in your life is a big pull right now . . . It's very important to you. *(Jane nods agreement.)* And *(to Susan)* you're wanting to see Jane take the right steps in her life and not step out or make choices that are going to end up hurting her.

S: I would like her to do—and I mean this wholeheartedly—I want Jane to have everything . . . I want her to have it in a way that she's going to be able to make choices that are appropriate for her and that are significant to her. I might not like them, but I'll live with them. Now is not the time for it all.

[A distinction is made between choices and changes as a way to help Susan see her daughter's behavior in a less fixed and immutable way.]

C: Yeah, but you see, I'm not seeing Jane making those major choices. She's making changes. She's trying on a new pair of shoes but I don't think she's making major choices in her life and I have a sense that you have some respect for Jane's ability not to get involved in drugs or not to get into trouble in other ways. Is that not so?

S: Right, but that is something that we talk about openly.

T: *(to consultant)* You're making a distinction between choices and changes.

C: These are the sort of experiments that teenagers try. They sometimes say, "Oh, I'm giving up sports; I'm not going to participate in this." At some point they might come back to it, they may not.

S: I see what you are saying. I do understand that and I myself have had many of the same things. But I'm not one hundred percent convinced that it is solely by Jane's choice—and not with maybe additional pressure—to have dropped out of so many activities that she had invested in for so long that, for all practical reasons, I believe they bring her lots of joy and pleasure. To wipe everything out across the board gives me reason to be very very concerned.

C: So it feels like a lot all at once.

S: That's right.

C: And not gradual.

S: Right, but also that I need to feel concerned because this is atypical of the person that I know who processes and makes decisions for herself . . .

C: So you already have the sense that Jane is not one who's easily coerced.

S: No, no.

C: I can see. *(Everyone laughs.)*

T: The team members commented that these two people are both very strong individuals, they both have their own ideas.

[The consultant brings the discussion back to "next steps." He emphasizes the idea of reclaiming what has existed before in their relationship and requests that Susan and Jane find some small ways to show their good faith in working toward a better understanding.]

C: Let's see what we can do, because we are going to have to stop. Let's see about a step the two of you can take to try to reclaim some of the positive feelings that you've had . . . one of the people was saying that you are not as far apart as it might seem. You're *(to Susan)* understanding the need for some limits and you *(to Jane)* understand that your mother has some requirements about dinner and you have some responsibility to communicate with her about when you are going to be where and how. So what would be a reasonable plan at this point? What's a slight variation . . . that's going to be more satisfying . . .

T: To go more towards that ideal picture.

C: That's right. So what is it that each of you can do, one small thing, that will move it a little closer to the picture that you have of understanding and less friction on those gears? You each get a chance to put a little oil on the gears to get them smoother.

C: *(to Jane)* What do you think is a small thing that your mother would appreciate from you? Something that would be possible for you to do.

J: I really don't know.

C: Can you offer something and see if it's something that would be appreciated? She can say whether she appreciates it.

J: Nothing.

C: Would it be okay if your mother came up with something to offer to you?

J: Yeah, if it is reasonable.

C: Do you have something reasonable that you could suggest that Jane do, but it would need to be small.

[Susan comes up with a realistic small step toward change in asking that Jane not hang up on her when they are talking on the phone.]

S: To not hang up.

C: So that means that no matter what's being discussed, the two of you hang in there. Okay, so that's a good one. And how about the other way around now? *(to Susan)* Can you think of something that Jane would appreciate?

S: Well, she was told that she was not going to be able to go out Friday night—that was a consequence for getting home later than expected. Perhaps we can renegotiate that.

C: "Perhaps" means what?

S: Well, I'm waiting to see if this is something that appeals to her.

C: *(to Jane)* Would you appreciate that?

J: Yes, considering I was planning on going anyway. . . .

[The therapists sidestep Jane's provocative comment and move the discussion back on task.]

S: See? (as if to say "Look what I put up with")

C: Okay, she would appreciate that.

T: *(to Susan)* And you would appreciate Jane not hanging up.

[The therapist and consultant end the interview and another visit is scheduled.]


## The Next Session (One Week Later)

The following is an excerpt from the initial part of the next session.

T: You had some homework and I wanted to follow up on that. You each were going to make a small change towards that ideal picture.

S: There's been no hanging up.

T: So there was no hanging up. How did Friday night work out? You were going to renegotiate with Jane.

S: Yes, she did go out Friday night. Actually it was assumed to mean that she could go . . . no further consult on that matter. I let that go . . .

T: You thought that was a smaller issue.

S: I'm going for the larger issue.

T: And the larger issue is what?

S: *(says emphatically)* A better understanding.

T: A better understanding, okay.

[The therapist, in an effort to continue on the track of creating the opportunity for increased understanding between Susan and Jane, introduces an adaptation of the "reformed past" exercise (after Chasin et al., 1989; Chasin & Roth, 1990).]

T: I wanted to do something this evening that is working towards the goal of a better understanding. Last week you painted your ideal picture, if you remember. Tonight I'm going to ask each of you to do something that's different than that. I'm going to ask you to think about a time when you did not receive understanding from somebody in the past.

S: Uh oh. *(starts to laugh)* Many things come to mind. Many things will remain unshared.

T: I want you to think about it for a minute. The idea is that the more concrete the example, the better. Okay? So, I'll be asking each of you to come up with an example of a time when you wanted somebody to understand you but you felt like they didn't. And then afterwards we are going to do something a little different [i.e., the "reformed past" exercise]. I'll explain that when we get to that point. So think back for a minute. It's a time when you really felt that you just weren't understood.

*(silence for several minutes)*

[Susan then relates an example from her past when she was a senior in high school. She told her mother she wanted to leave school, and rather than trying to understand her thinking, her mother just accepted her decision without discussion. Susan says she would have appreciated from her mother some "affirmation of my own worth." The therapist then asks Jane to play the role of her mother's mother and to enact the old scene in a new way. Jane agrees to try this.]

T: *(to Jane)* So did you hear some of the things your mom would have liked to have happen that would have told her she had gotten her mother's understanding? Let's do this one now where you are playing your grandmother and your mom is now a senior in high school.

S: *(role-playing)* I'm going to drop out of school and work full-time.

J: You're what?

S: I've been thinking about dropping out of school and working full-time.

J: How long have you been thinking about this?

S: I've given it some thought, and there's no reason I can't work full-time.

J: You're into full swing in your senior year.

S: That's really not that relevant to me.

J: I can value your *choice* because a lot of young women are going out these days and working, but don't you think you should stay in school? There's only a little time left in comparison to the other three years that you stayed in school and the other twelve years that you've been in school. Why would you give all that up?

S: I figured I could put more money in. There's really not enough money to get together for college, so why don't I just start working now?

J: Because at least you'll have your high school degree.

S: It's really not that important.

J: Well, to me it is. I'll tell you what, I'll talk about it with your father and we'll see how he feels about it. You know how I stand on it. It's ultimately up to you.

[Following this role play the therapist discusses the enactment with Jane and Susan and then asks, "What aspects in this made you feel like you received better understanding?"]

S: My Mom as characterized by Jane?

T: Yes, exactly.

S: Well she has seen the other side to it.

Although the role-playing by Susan and Jane seems very matter-of-fact, it was a very powerful interaction. Jane had an opportunity to provide understanding to her mother in a way her mother had once wished for it to happen. Susan had an opportunity to *receive* understanding from her daughter in the way Jane wanted understanding from her mother in the present. Both Jane and Susan seemed to enjoy this shifting of roles. This "reformed past" exercise was repeated with Susan in the position of offering Jane understanding she did not get in the past. The therapist then suggested some homework for Jane and Susan in order to follow up on the work of the session. She also sent them the following letter as a way to highlight the main theme of the meeting and to review the homework suggested for the next session.

*Dear Ms. Smith and Jane:*

> ". . . the growth of understanding follows an ascending spiral rather than a straight line."
>
> —JOANNE FIELD

*At times, following a session, I like to share my thoughts in writing.*

*During this last session, we focused on the goal of "a better understanding," something that the two of you seem to want. I was impressed by the openness each of you showed in reenacting scenes from previous experiences when such understanding was not forthcoming.*

*We all have had experiences in our lives when we did not receive understanding. These experiences may leave us confused, anxious, sad, and angry. Similarly, we all have felt there were times when we were understood. At these times, we may have felt listened to, taken seriously, and have experienced a deep connection with another person.*

*As I mentioned at the end of our last session, I would suggest you take 10 minutes (5 minutes each), two to three times weekly, to discuss with each other times when you have felt you have been understood and times you have felt you have not been understood in your relationships with others. At each sitting, just choose one incident to share with each other.*

*In addition, I would like each of you to think about times when you feel you have offered another person your understanding. It seems to me that offering understanding can be thought of as a special gift that one gives another. It seemed appropriate to mention this during this holiday season.*

*I am looking forward to seeing you at our next meeting.*

*Sincerely,*

*Cynthia Mittelmeier, PhD*

## Final Session (Three Weeks Later)

T: I wanted to follow up on our discussion of understanding and hear a little more about how you've been achieving understanding over the past few weeks. How do you think you have come through this in terms of your understanding of each other? How did you make it over this hurdle?

[The therapist asks about the homework and learns that Jane has broken up with her boyfriend. Some discussion focuses on this event, and then the therapist turns her attention to how Susan and Jane have been achieving understanding.]

J: Only in some situations. Like dumb things. If she's in a bad mood, I'll say, "Who pissed in your Wheaties?" She'll tell me now what happened at work.

T: So she's being more real with you or letting you into her life in a more real way.

J: Before we just didn't talk.

T: Okay, so you're getting a better understanding of her in what way?

J: If she's mad at me now I know it's for a reason—not a good reason, but a reason. I can also understand her worrying and always interfering. *(Mother groans and looks away.)*

T: How do you understand that?

J: 'Cause she's worried about me. Although I told her there was nothing to be worried about because there wasn't anything to be worried about.

T: So now you can understand her motives . . .

[Later in the interview.]

J: I think she should be in tune with trying to understand me, but I don't want her to interfere with me and say, "This is wrong." I'm going to learn by what I try.

T: So you'd like her to let you try on those new pair of shoes sometimes.

J: Yes *(laughs)*

[The therapist again raises the subject of the homework from the previous meeting. Susan reported that they never set up specified times to talk. She felt that by pursuing Jane to do this she would be considered a "dweeb." However, both Susan and Jane felt that many situations arose spontaneously where there were opportunities to share thoughts, feelings, and memories. This was fueled in part by the holiday season, which allowed for many conversations about past holiday events and spending more time together.]

[Later in the interview.]

J: And you should know that I've never been put in a position where things are out of my control.

T: I think Jane is telling you you've done a good job.

S: In a very roundabout way, yes.

T: You've given her a lot of skills.

S: They're survival skills.

T: She knows what she's doing. It seems as though you agree with that, but you feel there still needs to be some influence there: "I have to be around in case there is trouble."

J: What's going to happen in two years, Mom? I'm going to be in college. You're not going to be there saying, "I think this is sabotaging behavior."

S: There are many things that will happen for you and to you in the following two years before you cross that bridge.

J: The point is you're not going to be there.

[The ensuing discussion centers on Jane's leaving home and going off to college.]

S: In a sense it will be a tremendous change and in part a loss, but that's part of growth.

T: So you feel like you'll be prepared when the time comes.

S: I think so, after the initial "boo, hoo, hoo."

Final excerpt:

T: So how do you think the two of you are doing?

S: I think things are back on track. I feel that maybe I need to touch base with you for my own personal agenda at some point . . .

T: Sure.

S: *(to Jane)* How do you feel?

J: I feel fine.

T: Do you feel like things are better?

J: Better, yes.

T: How so?

J: I really don't know. There's not one thing, just the overall.

T: What feels different?

J: Everything feels different.

T: Is that a good feeling?

J: Yes.

S: No doubt we will walk this road many times.

T: I'm sure, but maybe you'll have a little more of a road map this time. It's important when you walk this road that you come through it and you can see some light, some sunshine at the end, and it seems like you've successfully maneuvered this, which could have gone the other way. I think you were able to do some things and work some things out together, and it kept the situation in perspective. So I'm hopeful in the future if another thing comes up like that, you'll be able to weather those other storms. As I was saying earlier, this was a tough time and a time when your relationship could have gone either way, either pulled further apart or closer together. So I think it is good that you were able to deal with this one. You deserve a lot of credit.

The therapist continued to meet with Susan on an intermittent basis, at her request. The sessions focused on Susan's interest in improving her relationship with Jane's father. Susan reported that her relationship with Jane continued to be positive and that she was successfully negotiating the variety of issues that emerge in parenting an adolescent daughter.

## EDITORIAL QUESTIONS[1]

Q: *How does the setting in which you work, a managed health care facility, impact on your therapeutic approach?*
A: Obviously, the setting in which you work impacts on your maps and methods. As psychologists who work in the mental health department of a large health maintenance organization (HMO), we are continually challenged to provide high quality mental health services in a time-effective manner (Friedman, 1990). We see our role as consultants who look for and amplify those client resources that will maximize change while decreasing the possibility of institutional dependence. When we do see people over longer periods of time (e.g., 2–3 years), it is on an *intermittent* basis (e.g., once per month). A sensitivity to time requires that we engage in a process of helping clients reach their goals with minimum cost, both financial and psychological (Budman & Gurman, 1988). As therapists working in an HMO setting, we have come to understand that our responsibility is to serve a population, as opposed to a small number of select clients (Bennett, 1988); we must consider the whole population of clients served by the health facility and allocate resources in a way that meets the needs of both the individual and the larger population. Since the volume of clients is consistently high and the demand for service great, careful allocation of resources is essential. Because we are faced with the challenge of seeing a large number of people for a relatively brief period of time, we have learned to be flexible and creative both in therapeutic approach and in management of time (Friedman, 1989a, 1989b, 1990, 1992; Friedman & Fanger, 1991). Our team at the Harvard Community Health Plan, for example, sees over 400 new families each year, or approximately 125 families per full-time staff. We have found that by taking a strength-focused approach we set the stage for a more time-effective therapy

Q: *In the clinical situation presented you use historical material (i.e., losses experienced) in a very specialized way (i.e., to help the mother and daughter move toward a more positive future together). You could have accessed*

---

[1]Special thanks to Terry Carik, MSW, Robin Hasenfeld, PhD, and Brian Meyer, PhD, for generating questions for this section.

*other historical information (e.g., regarding father's role in the family or other losses). What is your position on exploring client history in therapy?*
A: Our therapy is one of *amplification* rather than *excavation*. By pursuing history for it's own sake we run the risk of becoming lost in the myriad complexities of people's lives. Our goal in the case presented was to use history as a resource to enable this mother and daughter to achieve a more satisfying relationship. The mother and daughter were able to recall times from the past when they felt close to one another in ways they wanted to reclaim. By pursuing these positive past experiences they were able to move beyond their impasse and toward a future that included their shared goal of "a better understanding." Our interest is always in how the past can be used to help people move forward in the future. In the same way, the mother's and daughter's memory of the deceased cousin was used to help them get perspective on their own relationship. An exploration of the past without a future direction can leave both the therapist and client immersed in a problem-saturated reality that impedes solution development.

If we had found ourselves at an impasse with this family, we might have asked the mother and daughter what they each thought was getting in the way of achieving their desired goals. By so doing, the historical context would have been enlarged, perhaps leading to the generation of new perspectives enabling this mother and daughter to move toward their original goal.

Q: *You ask the mother and daughter to engage in several enactments during the course of the therapy. What are some of the clinical guideposts that you use in determining when action-oriented techniques are useful?*
A: One of our goals is for family members to experience themselves, as quickly as possible, in a new way in relation to the problem. When this occurs the family has already begun a shift from a "problem-view" to a "solution-view." Since change is more likely to take place through a multi-sensory experience, we believe that "getting them up and moving" increases the possibility that these new ways of interacting will become a reality.

We use action-oriented approaches when we find ourselves getting bogged down in the details of a repetitive interaction or when complaints are vague. By asking clients to engage in a role-play situation we create opportunities for greater clarity of the desired future state. Action-oriented techniques are also activating and involving for both client and therapist and engender an atmosphere of playfulness and hope.

## REFERENCES

Andersen, T. (1987). The reflecting team: Dialogue and meta-dialogue in clinical work. *Family Process, 26,* 415–428.
Andersen, T. (Ed.). (1990). *The reflecting team: Dialogues and dialogues about dialogues.* United Kingdom: Borgmann.

Anderson, H., & Goolishian, H. A. (1988). Human systems as linguistic systems: Preliminary and evolving ideas about the implications for clinical theory. *Family Process, 27,* 371–393.

Bennett, M. (1988). The greening of the HMO. *American Journal of Psychiatry, 145*(12), 1544–1549.

Bruner, J. (1987). Life as narrative. *Social Research, 54*(1), 11–32.

Budman, S. H., & Gurman, M. J. (1988). *The theory and practice of brief psychotherapy.* New York: Guilford Press.

Chasin, R., Roth, S., & Bograd, M. (1989). Action methods in systemic therapy: Dramatizing ideal futures and reformed pasts with couples. *Family Process, 28,* 268–274.

Chasin, R., & Roth, S. (1990). Future perfect, past perfect: A positive approach to opening couple therapy. In D. Chasin, H.Grunebaum, & M. Herzig (Eds.), *One couple, four realities: Multiple perspectives on couple therapy* (pp. 129–144). New York: Guilford Press.

de Shazer, S. (1985). *Keys to solution in brief therapy.* New York: Norton.

de Shazer, S. (1988). *Clues: Investigating solutions in brief therapy.* New York: Norton.

de Shazer, S. (1991). *Putting difference to work.* New York: Norton.

Friedman, S. (1989a). Brief systemic psychotherapy in a health maintenance organization. *Family Therapy, 16,* 133–144.

Friedman, S. (1989b). Child mental health in a HMO: A family systems approach. *HMO Practice, 3,* 52–59.

Friedman, S. (1990). Towards a model of time-effective family psychotherapy: A view from a health maintenance organization (HMO). *Journal of Family Psychotherapy, 1*(2), 1–28.

Friedman, S. (1992). Creating solutions (stories) in brief family therapy. In S. Budman, M. Hoyt, & S. Friedman (Eds.), *The first session of brief therapy* (pp. 282–305). New York: Guilford Press.

Friedman, S., & Fanger, M. T. (1991). *Expanding therapeutic possibilities: Getting results in brief psychotherapy.* New York: Lexington Books/Macmillan.

Friedman, S., & Pettus, S. (1985). Brief strategic interventions with families of adolescents. *Family Therapy, 12,* 197–210.

Mittelmeier, C., & Friedman, S. (1991). The Rashomon effect: A study in constructivist conversation. *Family Therapy, 18*(1), 17–36.

O'Hanlon, W. H., & Weiner-Davis, M. (1989). *In search of solutions: A new direction in psychotherapy.* New York: Norton.

O'Hanlon, W. H., & Wilk, J. (1987). *Shifting contexts: The generation of effective psychotherapy.* New York: Guilford Press.

Weick, K. (1984). Small wins: Redefining the scale of social problems. *American Psychologist, 39,* 40–49.

Whitaker, C. A. (1976). The hindrance of theory in clinical work. In P. Guerin (Ed.), *Family therapy: Theory and practice* (pp. 154–164). New York: Gardner.

White, M. (1986). Negative explanation, restraint and double description: A template for family therapy. *Family Process, 25,* 169–184.

White, M. (1991, October). *Re-authoring lives and relationships.* Workshop at Leonard Morse Hospital, Natick, MA.

White, M., & Epston, D. (1990). *Narrative means to therapeutic ends.* New York: Norton.

# II

## NARRATIVES OF LIBERATION

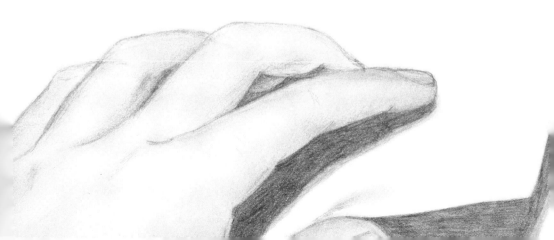

# 8

## The Monsters in My Head

### FRANK LANGELLA

I was sure he was coming to get me. First a hard step on the gravel and then a foot dragging behind. Step–drag, step–drag. I lay frozen in my bed. The long alleyway between our family house and the neighbor's was hardly three feet wide; dark, covered with black dirt, gravel and tufts of weeds and grass just barely able to survive the sunless space. The two windows of my room faced the clapboard wall of our neighbor's house, and Venetian blinds remained permanently closed against the nonview.

It was the mid-1940's. I had just seen a movie about a mummy. I don't remember the name of it. Just the image, so powerful even still, of a man wrapped in grayish cloth around his ankles, legs, body up to the top of his head. Eyes and mouth exposed, one arm drawn up against his chest, elbow close to his side, hand clawed. The other arm dangling alongside the leg that dragged. Several strips of cloth hung loosely from that arm, swaying with each step–drag, step–drag. I don't remember where he was coming from or going to in the movie. It doesn't really matter. I knew that he was coming for me.

For so many nights I heard him as a I lay alone in my bed. My heart pounded as I waited for the good foot to land. A pause, then the slow drag. I would get up from the bed, pull the blind as little as I could away from the glass; and, with my chin just a little over the window ledge, I would stare hard into the dark alley. There were no outdoor lights, so I never could see him clearly. But he was there. He stopped when he saw me. I would get back into bed and wait. He usually left. Sometimes I fell asleep, and he returned, waking me. Other nights, he spared me and moved on.

I never told anyone about him. I don't know why. Shame, I suppose. It was that he seemed to be my private terror, and as much as I was frightened of him, I was also frightened of losing him. One night, he deserted me forever, and I was not to think of him again for 40 years, until my own son, this year, at age 4, began calling out in the night: "Daddy, daddy! There's a monster in my room. Come kill him." His room, several floors above the street, looks out over a New York alleyway to a brick wall. The windows are covered with louvered shutters. I found him sitting up in bed, eyes wide, starring at the tilted louvers, pointing at his monster. "He's coming in the window, daddy. He's going to get me."

I grabbed a pillow and did a dutiful daddy fight with the monster, backing him up against the closet door, beating him toward the shutters, leaping onto the window seat and driving him back out into the night. He was a sizeless, faceless creature to me. My son told me he was blue, with big teeth.

This ritual went on for weeks. Sometimes, several times a night. I continued my battle, and, as I tucked him back under the covers, I explained that daddy would keep the monster from him always. I was bigger and stronger; as long as I was there, no monster was going to get my boy. I was wrong. No matter how hard I battled, the monster returned when my son wanted him to. I was forced to accept the fact that my macho approach to protecting him from his fears wasn't working. My dad never told me he would save me from my monsters. I don't think he knew they existed.

As I thought back to my mummy and his eventual disappearance, I realized that he had never really gone away. He was with me still. He changed shapes as rapidly as I grew up. He became a wild bear at the foot of my bed. Then, later, an amorphous flying object swooping over my head. In later years, he was my first day at kindergarten, the agony of my early attempts at the diving board. He was hurricanes and the ocean, a mysterious death next door to us, my brother's ability to outdo me in all sports. He was hypodermic needles, even early haircuts. Still later, my first date, my first night away from home, at 16, alone in a small boardinghouse as an apprentice in summer stock. The first woman to say no, the first woman to say yes. And then, he became my ambition, my fear of failure, struggles with success, marriage, husbandhood, fatherhood. There's always a foot dragging somewhere in my mind, it seems.

My son called out again. This time I went into his room, turned on the light and sat down facing him. His eyes were wild with fear, wilder than the earlier nights we had gone through this ritual. I asked him to listen, but he couldn't hear me. He kept screaming and pointing at the windows. "Kill him, kill him for me, daddy!" he cried. He grabbed the pillow and tried to get me to do my routine. I felt I needed to speak to him without the ritual's having happened first. When, at last, I could quiet him, I said with trembling voice that I was never going to kill the monster again. I explained that this was his monster. He had made him up, and only he could kill him. I told him that the monster was in his head and leapt out whenever he wanted him to. I said that he could make him go away whenever he chose, or that he could turn him into a friendly monster if he liked. He sat expressionless. He had never stared at me so hard. I said again that I would no longer perform the particular battle for him, but that I loved him and would always love him. A slow and overwhelmingly beautiful smile that I shall never forget came to his face and he said: "You mean, I can make him do anything I want?" "Yes," I said, "you're in charge of him."

I went back to bed and lay there waiting for the return of the monster. He didn't come back that night and has never again appeared in that form. Sometimes he's being driven from the living room by my son with his He-Man sword aloft, its scabbard stuck down the back of his pajamas as he cries out, "I am The Power." And sometimes he is under the covers in the big bed when the whole family plays tent. We just ask him, politely, to leave. He stays for dinner now and then. He's everything from 10 feet tall to a small tiny creature in the cup of my son's hand. He's blue, green, and sometimes he's a she.

As my son grows, I know we will be able to face his monsters together. And now, when all I was once so sure of has become a mystery to me, I'm hoping he'll be able to help me face the unknown ones yet to visit themselves upon me.

# 9

## *The Turtle with Wings*

JENNIFER C. FREEMAN
DEAN LOBOVITS

This chapter illustrates the integration of narrative and expressive arts approaches, and explores some ideas that are evolving for us through the practice of narrative therapy. The theoretical ideas that underlie this integration are introduced. Recent developments in our practices and relevant critiques of the narrative approach are discussed. A clinical example is then presented in which a series of therapeutic dilemmas are resolved through the co-creation of the therapeutic process with a family.

### INTRODUCTION TO NARRATIVE THERAPY

Our sense of self is inextricably imbedded in and defined by the social, cultural, political, and economic ecologies within which we humans live. We tell stories in our thoughts and conversations about who we and others are. These narratives not only constitute our descriptions of self and others but shape how we behave, interact, and experience life.

Initially, in therapy a person tends to relate a dominant story about his or her problems (White & Epston, 1990). The dominant story is problem-saturated; it filters problem-free experiences from a person's memories and perceptions of his or her experiences. Family members and other significant people in a person's life tend to be involved in a process of co-validation of dominant stories. As experiences that do not fit with the dominant story are filtered out, threads of hope, resourcefulness, and capability are excluded from a person's descriptions of self.

A narrative approach seeks to empower a person or family to re-author a liberating or alternative story to the dominant problem-saturated story (White & Epston, 1990). The re-authoring process involves continual invitations to persons to separate their identity from the problem, to reflect on unique outcomes, and to consider previously undistinguished choices. Unique outcomes (Goffman, 1961) are unnoticed exceptions to the dominant story that "provide a gateway to what we might consider the alternative territories of a person's life" (White, 1991, p. 30). Thus, the therapeutic conversation highlights new and rediscovered understandings and previously unnoticed choice points that are valued by clients and weaves them into a new story. Substance and depth are given to these meanings and choices in a way that facilitates the creation of this alternative and preferred story.

## EXTERNALIZING CONVERSATION

Michael White (1991) has developed the idea of an externalizing conversation.[1] An externalizing conversation consists of a dialogue that objectifies problems rather than persons. This opens space for an empowering relationship between a person and a problem. Externalizing conversations can separate a person from internalized shame and guilt and stimulate personal agency, creativity, and choice in a person's relationship with a problem. White (1991) utilizes a reflexive and externalizing grammar to separate a person from a problem. He identifies a relational space within which new ideas can evolve:

> As persons become engaged in these externalizing conversations, their private stories cease to speak to them of their identity and of the truth of their relationships . . . [and are] no longer transfixing of persons' lives. Persons experience a separation from, and an alienation in relation to, these stories. In the space established by this separation, persons are free to explore alternative and preferred knowledges of who they might be; alternative and preferred knowledges into which they might enter their lives. (p. 29)

The externalizing therapeutic conversation may wend its way through a series of problems, dilemmas, possibilities, and solutions as they arise.

## THERAPEUTIC DISCOURSE

Therapeutic discourse is conducted primarily through language. Gergen and Gergen (1991) state that language is an "expression of the relationships among persons. From this viewpoint, it is within the social interaction that language is generated, sustained, and abandoned" (p. 78). Language as a descriptive symbol system that maps the world or reflects a speaker's internal processes of cognition or intention can be contrasted with its performative function. Gergen and Gergen emphasize that language is

---

[1]Externalizing conversation is an expansion on White's original concept of externalizing the problem (White, 1989).

performative in a social context, in the sense that as we speak with others we mutually coordinate, negotiate, and shape our values and meanings, consequent choices, and behavior.

The performative power of language can pathologize a person and limit his or her choices to those permitted by the dominant story. On the other hand, language can free a person from being defined by a problem. An essential activity that is coordinated in the therapeutic discourse is the exploration of the client's or family's value system. Culturally determined stories tend to contain a normalizing value system that is taken for granted and unexamined. Through a process of reflexive questioning (Tomm, 1987) we choose to deconstruct together with a person not just the personal basis of his or her story but the dominant cultural ideologies[2] that are defining him or her in a limiting or oppressive way.

Therapy is inescapably a moral endeavor. If the therapeutic discourse accepts the dominant story without question, then the underlying core values will be accepted a priori as well. Erving Goffman (1961) aptly observed that the acceptance of the values contained within the dominant cultural story that defines a person as a mental patient not only pathologizes the person but shapes his or her "moral career," which can be defined as the behavior or lifestyle permitted within the confines of the value system in operation.

Exceptions to the problem lifestyle can be discovered and explored in a way that allows a person to shape his or her values, rather than be limited by those prescribed by the problem. Persons are invited to explore personal attributes and values that underlie unique and problem-free outcomes in the past. This can lead to new possibilities in the future. Under these conditions hopeful threads of meaning and empowerment will tend to emerge that can be woven into an alternative story.

## EXPRESSIVE ARTS THERAPY

In this chapter we are interested in extending the performative functions of spoken language into a broader range of externalizing discourse, including nonverbal means of expression, by integrating expressive arts therapy methods. For example, the particulars of a person's problematic lifestyle or a unique outcome, choice, or alternative story can be expressed visually, dramatically or kinetically. According to White (1989), externalizing conversation "frees persons to take a lighter, more effective, and less stressed approach to 'deadly serious' problems" (p. 6). We see the integration of expressive arts as especially supportive of this spirit and outcome since it employs inherently creative and playful means of expression. Expressive

---

[2]Narrative conventions are to a large extent determined within the context of the dominant culture. If therapy serves as a cultural institution to promote adaptation to those conventions, it can coerce persons to define themselves according to the explanatory systems of the dominant culture (Hare-Mustin & Marecek, 1988).

arts can also facilitate the qualities of playfulness and creativity in relationships in family or couple therapy.

Art therapy evolved with the medical model of psychotherapeutic treatment. There has been a tendency for the therapist to use artwork as a diagnostic, interpretive, or rehabilitative tool. There is an important distinction to make between an expert interpretive understanding of the symbols produced in creative activity and our current emphasis on the performative aspects. Art therapy has primarily focused on the representational aspects of client productions. Expressive arts therapy, in the context of its integration with narrative therapy, emphasizes the performative and reflexive aspects of play and creativity. An invitation to nonverbal performative conversation can be extended to persons through different expressive art forms. Expressive arts include painting, drawing, sculpture, mask and puppet making, sand tray, drama, puppet theater, storytelling, music, dance, and movement. Although applicable to individual adults, couples, and families in therapy, this approach is especially useful in joining the realms of meaning that children inhabit.

Expressive arts therapy, as it has been evolving (Rogers, 1980; London, 1989), calls for an atmosphere of mutual respect for each person's unique experience and expression, a nonjudgmental attitude with regard to artistic productions, and a facilitative intent, rather than a critical or interpretive approach to working with a person's creative expression. An example of this evolution is Natalie Rogers's (1980) "person-centered approach to expressive therapy." In describing the function of the expressive arts therapist, she writes:

> A person-centered therapist will find him/herself guiding people through movement with awareness, through art experiences which are opening, through improvisations with music and role playing, in an atmosphere which is understanding of differences, respectful of each person's world view and current problems. Such a therapist will create an atmosphere of trust and communication between people and he/she will be open to learning from the participants, allowing the group process to emerge into a co-creative endeavor. (p. 8)

## CHILD-FOCUSED FAMILY THERAPY

We see the integration of narrative and expressive arts approaches as especially relevant to the development of a child-focused family therapy. In such a family therapy children are not isolated or marginalized from the therapeutic conversation by its dependence on spoken language. Language can function to exclude children and disqualify a child's knowledge of a problem and its possible solutions. Children are sometimes seen as being solely reactive to therapeutic intervention with the adults. But children are proactive in constructing family realities. They love to play, and they learn easily this way. It is our task to include them on their own terms and join them in their own ways of expression.

Children may express their experience of abuse or other danger with "acting out" behavior that is identified by adults as problematic. Epston (1989) warns therapists treating temper tantrumming children, for example, that "it is of vital importance that the therapists scrupulously distinguish families tyrannized by [the child's] tantrumming from those families in which a young person's outbursts of anger represent a legitimate rebellion against sexual, physical, or emotional abuse" (p. 14). Expressive arts may provide a way for children to communicate this experience nonverbally.

## CHALLENGES FOR OUR PRACTICES

In this section we review some important critiques of the narrative approach to therapy that are relevant to the case presented in this chapter and identify some new ideas that have evolved in our practices.

The narrative approach encourages the therapist to be an active and creative participant in therapeutic conversation. We are grappling with the issue of how, in a respectful manner and without imposition or coercion, to invite persons who are oppressed and in pain to be curious and imaginative of new possibilities. Waldegrave (1990) has provided us with a guiding metaphor when he speaks of clients' "stories of pain and hope." He and his colleagues at the Family Centre consider these stories to be "sacred" in the therapeutic context. This approach implies a fundamental respect for these stories. It focuses on persons' preferred stories of hope and requires great care with regard to the imposition of culturally based therapeutic constructions. We find that when presented with moral choices in an atmosphere of hopefulness, clients tend overwhelmingly to prefer stories, metaphors, and symbols that are life affirming, freeing, and socially responsible. We have found Tomm's (1988) ethical posture of empowerment to be a guide to respectful practices as well. This posture is based on a facilitative intent and the practice of employing reflexive questions. According to Tomm,

> the intent behind [reflexive] questions is predominately *facilitative*. It is assumed that family members are autonomous individuals and cannot be instructed directly. . . . One major presupposition behind these questions is that the therapeutic system is co-evolutionary and what the therapist does is to trigger reflexive activity in the family's preexisting belief systems. The therapist endeavors to interact in a manner that opens space for the family to see new possibilities and to evolve more freely of their own accord. (p. 9)

## SOCIAL CONSTRUCTIONISM, REALITY, AND VALUES

The importance of respecting persons' stories of pain and hope, especially in their cultural context, is central to our practice. On the other hand, we the authors see ethical relativism as a central problem of the theory of social constructionism. We feel that ethical relativism goes hand in hand with the denial of objective reality.[3] Our theorizing confines itself primarily to epistemology and does not question whether there is an independently existing ontology (von Glasersfeld, 1991). It is the experiential reality of persons that can be constructed or deconstructed in the therapeutic conversation. Human understanding of the world may be mediated through social constructs, but that does not mean there is no world out there. An interactionist paradigm is emerging in the social sciences that sees culture not only as performing mediating functions but as an evolutionary outcome of the biologically developed capacity for choice making in humans (Freeman, 1979). This capacity for making choices is a valuable asset for people in changing their relationship to problems. Even difficult universal problems such as destructive aggression toward others can be mediated by the ability to think critically and to choose values and behavior consciously.

The social constructionist notion that our reality is constituted through language often does not deal directly with issues such as the objective reality of a person's descriptions and the power imbalances in society, in the family, and in the therapeutic relationship.

Our field has already made the grievous error of constructing theoretical conventions that fictionalized the stories of oppressed and victimized persons.[4] Basic ethical guidelines and constraints that have emerged in the field of psychotherapy are based more on reactions to the pragmatics of trial and error, including abuses of power by therapists, than on positivist theoretical assumptions. Perhaps it is time to engage in further clarification of the role of values in social constructionist theory and practice, rather than settle for a vague moral relativism. This requires grappling with the values that we inevitably bring into the room as therapists and choose to support in our clients.

It is a matter of common sense and fairness that if a psychotherapist has the power to participate in the construction of a person's experiential reality, then there is a commensurate social responsibility and accountability for the distinctions that can be made regarding the person's meanings and narratives (Krippendorff, 1991; Waldegrave, 1990). For example, Waldegrave (1991) suggests that therapists attend to the power structure in relationships by asking, Who has the most influence in determining beliefs in a relationship? and Who is most served by those beliefs? He concludes:

> The denial of objective reality in observer descriptions can lead therapists to treat the attributions of meaning given by different family members as being

---

[3]We utilize the notion of objective reality in the sense that it is espoused by Popper's (1986) theory of falsification.

[4]See, for example, Masson (1984) on Freud's suppression of his seduction theory. Closer to home for family therapists, Dell (1989) has articulated how the functions of the domain of theoretical explanation differ from the domain of experience in order to explain how cybernetic theorizing historically disqualified notions of power and inequality in relationships by characterizing them as an illusion.

of equal value. The stories of abused children and women are more likely to reflect what really happens in a household, than the reduced story a person who abuses often gives. Issues of responsibility and blame are very significant in these situations and cannot be discounted. Abusive behavior has to be opposed, and abused people relieved from blame. (p. 7)

Moral relativism can lead to confusion over our "right" to impose our values on others. This is a thorny issue that cannot be avoided. Our individual notions of what is respectful of the moral values of others should not deter us as professionals from evaluating the consequences of harmful conduct and making the choice to condemn social values that condone or support the oppression of people.

## THE IMPACT OF METAPHORS

We have been examining White and Epston's (1990) text analogy and our metaphors for the impact they have as socially constructive forces in the lives of persons with whom we work. We prefer to reflexively examine our practices and theories for the social and ecological impact of the meanings or narratives that we employ and those that we may marginalize, contradict, or place outside our ordinary awareness.

For example, members of the Berkeley Family Study Group[5] and others have critiqued narrative therapy metaphors that encourage persons to relate to problems in a fashion that denotes power over the problem. These metaphors appear to be somewhat militaristic in nature and include fighting, kicking out, undermining, winning over, or beating a problem. They may serve to support tendencies toward practices of dominance and aggressiveness in social relationships and may, through their heavy-handedness, discourage a lighter or more playful approach. However, metaphors that are heavy-handed to some could be mobilizing for others under certain circumstances. Rather than take responsibility for the use of a particular metaphor, the clinician can consider and discuss alternative metaphors with clients.

We are interested in the idea of conscious choice making in relation to problems, using White's (1991) approach of facilitating an exploration with clients of their preferred meanings and stories. As an alternative to these metaphoric power struggles, we have explored metaphors of power in relation to a problem, as in metaphors of relationship, such as those used in the following expressions: "dealing with an old friend you've grown out of," "a friend you are miscommunicating with," and "communicating with those who are imposing their ideas on you." We may discuss with clients ideas of "turning away from" or "seeking other options to" the externalized

---

[5]The Berkeley Family Study Group includes Andrea Aidells, Jennifer Freeman, Ann Jauregui, Dean Lobovits, Jane Loebel, Michelle Martin, Michael Searle, and Suzanne Pregerson.

problem. In cases where a person has the experience of the problem's being a part of themselves or declines to participate in externalizing the problem, we can borrow from Gestalt and psychosynthesis to talk about "how to have this part come into alignment with what you want for yourself" or "sort out any useful part that you want to keep, from aspects of the problem you wish to discard" or even "how to make friends with this part." A personified externalization may also be a useful concept along these lines. For example, persons may discover that when they come into better relationship with their personified "critic," it has some wisdom to offer.

We have found metaphors that articulate personal agency through protest or resistance appropriate for more oppressive problems. (D. Epston, personal communication, March 9–10, 1992). Metaphors drawn from the tradition of nonviolent resistance may be suitable to some persons, metaphors such as protesting, standing up to, liberation from, and "freeing oneself from" the oppressive requirements and definitions imposed by the problem. Severe problems that impose a life or death ultimatum on persons, such as anorexia nervosa, may warrant more aggressive protest, a power struggle, or more warlike metaphors.

Concepts drawn from lifecycle changes may be useful and can be verbalized in expressions such as "growing out of a certain phase and moving into a new one" or "embracing this transition." With children, metaphors of "readiness for a change," based on signs of maturity, may be particularly helpful. For some people, metaphors that relate to spiritual practices may be more suitable, such as "rising or climbing above," "letting go of," or "balancing in relation to" problems. In the case presented here the language evolved during the course of therapy from power-over to power-in-relation-to metaphors. The family chose to emphasize protest and spiritual metaphors.

## TRANSPARENCY

A practice that has recently evolved within the narrative approach is demonstrated in the case presentation. This practice has since been named *transparency* by David Epston (personal communication, February 22–23, 1991). Our focus on transparency involves making the choices and dilemmas of the therapist available for communication and reflection by clients. In the case presented, invitations were accepted to engage in co-creating the therapy as it unfolded, both in form and in content. This practice was particularly useful at times when the therapeutic process seemed stuck. Mutual reflection on the process of communication, on the philosophy and rationale for practices, and on both therapist's and clients' ideas for growth and change made the therapy transparent and available for revision. This encouraged respect for the wisdom of each participant, opened space for new possibilities for therapeutic movement for this family, and engaged their individual and collective creativity. Through the process

of co-creation of therapy, a unique approach emerged that allowed for the
extension of narrative therapeutic discourse into nonverbal and somatic
realms in a way that suited the therapist and family members.

## CLINICAL ILLUSTRATION OF OUR APPROACH

We describe work in which a young person and his family sought to
transform their relationship to anger and to empower their son to free his
life from the domination of temper and misery. Members of the family
were invited to reflect on their choices in relation to a series of externalized
problems and to examine the influence of dominant cultural practices on
related ideas and behaviors. They evolved alternative and preferred interactions and descriptions of their lives together.

The persons involved included Yoshi, 8; his mother, Mariko, who was
46 and of Japanese descent; and his father, Ari, 40, who was born in
Sweden. Mariko and Ari had been separated for 3 ½ years and had formed a
two-household family with Yoshi. Yoshi's time was divided equally between the two households.

Mariko called and came in initially with her son. The first issue they
discussed was the constant fighting, competitiveness, and tension between
mother and son. Mariko stated that she had lost patience and the stamina to
work things out with Yoshi, that she didn't like him anymore, and that she
was ready for him to live most of the time with his father. She agreed with
her son's estimate that her patience had shrunk from 200%, when he was
younger, to a current 1%. When fights occurred there were threats on both
sides to break off the relationship. Yoshi was suffering from night fears and
bad dreams. He also had problems at school, particularly at after-school
care, and with homework.

In the first conjoint sessions with Mariko and Yoshi, Jenny (the therapist) following the approach of Epston (1989), began the therapeutic dialogue with a basic externalization of "the fighting" between them. Mother
and son readily engaged in this externalizing conversation and explored the
impact the fighting was having on their lives and relationship. Jenny wondered if they might be interested in teaming up to free their relationship
from fighting. Mariko and Yoshi started to strategize to this effect. They
became enthusiastic about reporting unique outcomes, such as instances
when mother found ways to step back from the anger and times that Yoshi
was able to calm his temper more readily. An alternative story developed in
which the relationship gained a new identity as a peace-making team.
Within a few weeks the fighting diminished in the relationship, and mother
and son decided they were able to continue living together. The influence of
this particular problem on their relationship was reduced.

An externalizing discourse will sometimes wend its way through
several problems before an alternative story can be estblished that redefines
a person as having agency in relation to problems. For Yoshi, the alternative

story of a fight-free relationship between him and his mother was just the beginning of the changes he was to go through in developing a comprehensive new story about himself.

At this point Ari joined the therapy. The family now turned their attention to school-related problems. These included constant complaints from the after-school program teachers and Yoshi's defiance of his teachers, fighting with other children, suspensions for disruptive behavior, and struggles over homework. The child had been described in school reports as "defiant, rude, and disruptive" and as having a "bad attitude" and difficulty with "adult authority figures." (Later, his mother admitted that she had worried when he was in kindergarten that he would be a criminal in adult life.) Although there had also been long periods of adjustment at school, these problems recurred periodically and began in kindergarten, where Yoshi was asked to leave the school due to disruptive behavior. The boy's school identity was saturated with shame and anger, which were focused on his relationships with his after-school program teachers and on the detested subject of spelling. Yoshi said he hated school, especially his after-school program, and hated to do homework. Although he appeared tense and would not enter further into discussions about school, he was able to make the brief comment that he thought he was stupid and slow.[6]

During this phase of therapy the problem was externalized alternatively as "the temper" or "the misery." Jenny encouraged Yoshi to bring his success with calming temper at home into his relationship with the after-school program. Since he had lengthy periods at school that were relatively problem-free, he was also invited to reflect on those and to draw the same success into his after-school program. However, the approach that had worked before now appeared to fail. Despite his initial investment in this therapy and the promising results, Yoshi became increasingly inaccessible to therapeutic conversation. He started a slow-down protest by dragging himself into therapy growling or muttering. He said he hated both school and therapy, and no matter how much Jenny strove to dialogue about the problem or solutions to it, he remained closed down, sullen, and angry.

## Transparency and Co-Construction of Method

Jenny realized that the struggle to engage Yoshi in a verbal conversation was aiding the temper, hampering the therapeutic relationship, and defeating her creativity and empathy—perhaps as it had for Yoshi's teachers at the after-school program. She decided to be "transparent" with Yoshi about the dilemma of not being able to communicate verbally. She asked him if they

---

[6]This raised concern over possible learning disabilities, so Yoshi was referred for evaluation. The learning specialist reported that he could use some tutoring in spelling, but results showed no major disabilities that would explain his problems at school.

could find another way to communicate, perhaps nonverbal, that suited him better. This made the communication dilemma open to Yoshi's input. Consequently, both were able to free themselves up and engage in the co-construction of a more effective approach. They discovered a new method of conversing together: Jenny asked questions, to which Yoshi either nodded in agreement or shook his head and growled menacingly. Through this process they decided that she could ask him questions verbally or in writing to which he would scribble *yes* or *no* or other brief answers, and that she could ask him to express himself in other ways, including drawing or using sand tray, puppets, or movement. Since he had shared in its design, Yoshi was now empowered to participate in a therapeutic conversation that engaged him on his own terms and included his own means of expression.

## Expressive and Somatic Conversations

Problems at school were having a powerful influence on Yoshi's external and internal worlds. Shame and misery were being strongly felt, acted out, and communicated at a somatic level. Since Yoshi was so caught up in his somatic experience of them, these problems were not as available for verbal conversation as those he had experienced with his mother, and they had not yet been sufficiently expressed in therapy. The therapist had moved ahead of him by imposing the construction that he could transfer the knowledge he had gained at home from the success of calming the temper and fighting to his school situation.

Jenny attempted to move forward an externalizing conversation through an experiment with other forms of expression. Yoshi had previously brought in some of his cartoons. He showed an interest and talent in this medium. Now that a preferred method of communication was agreed upon, Yoshi was invited to draw an answer to the question "What happens to you when the temper shows up at school?" He drew the school and himself blowing up in an atomic explosion and took up the invitation to perform the drawing in gestures and noises (see Figure 9.1). In the drawing a nuclear explosion obliterates not only Yoshi himself and his school but practically the whole earth as well. He was encouraged to express also in movement how temper made his body feel. In response he showed how his legs got shaky and he collapsed on the floor. Yoshi was now able to express his "story of pain." He talked about his "bad" (angry) feelings about school and of how "embarrassment" tortured him there. He could now explore the effects of the "misery" or "temper" on his school life. Jenny proposed the idea that these problems might be influenced by "the curse of perfectionism," having observed that perfectionism was often a factor in his relationship with his schoolwork. Yoshi agreed and added, "It makes you feel like you have to do everything right and you can't stand to have any area of failure, like spelling, in your life." Later his parents reflected on their own "push for perfection" and its influence on Yoshi.

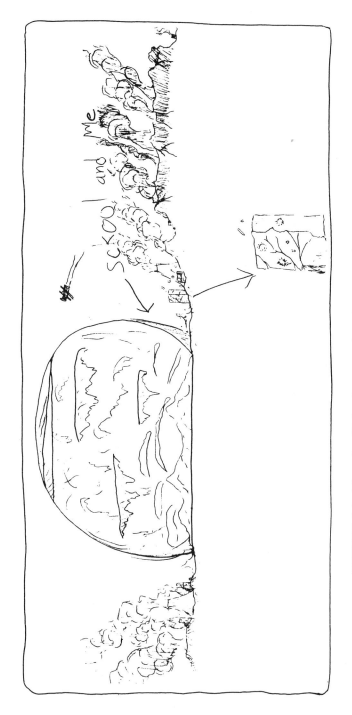

**FIGURE 9.1.** Therapist: "What happens when the temper shows up at school?"

When Yoshi's means of expression expanded, a realm of possibility was extended for him. Yoshi learned he could communicate his somatic experience of temper and misery through drawing or movement, which allowed Jenny to join him in a more emphathic way, to map the influence of the problem, and to attend to alternative meanings.[7]

Reflecting on our practices, we think we may have tended to interpret situations where a person seemed to reject our invitations to explore the influence of a problem or to consider an alternative to the dominant story as a failure of the method. We wonder now if, instead, there might have been a need to participate in alternative modes of therapeutic conversation. During the first phase of treatment the externalizing conversation constructs the description of a person's current relationship with a problem by mapping its specifications and lifestyle. These aspects of the problem need to be expressed so that they are well understood by both parties. A central concern is to find an externalizing approach that does not disconnect from or disqualify a person's efforts to communicate his or her pain and oppression as it is experienced in the body. London (1989) has described a creative process that is based on "a somatic act." He says, "If we turn our conscious attention to monitor what our body is already expressing, we will be provided with revealing information" (p. 94). Information about problems may be lodged at this somatic level even when they are barely within conscious awareness. Approaches are then needed to bring experiences that are based in the body into focus. In addition to just focusing on the feelings in the body, these may include drawing, movement, or acting the problem out with mime, sand tray, or puppets.

## Conflict in Models

In Yoshi's case, the expressive process continued for a phase of individual child therapy, wherein the child chose primarily to draw and to make a series of sand trays. Yoshi portrayed scenes of protracted struggle, with devastating and hopeless outcomes in which a weak figure was pounded time and again by dominant forces. Hopeless battles were enacted that no one was able to win or where the heroes ended up dead along with everyone else. After a while the sand-play stories began to seem repetitive and problem saturated.

Jenny was caught between theories. In her training in play therapy Jenny was taught to trust that children would naturally work out problems in their play within the supportive therapeutic environment. On the other hand, her studies in narrative therapy had encouraged her to be more active in the development of meaning. Should she let the story unfold in sand play

[7]Jenny has since experimented with having the parent be the voice of the child if the child cannot engage in this process. She has also tried producing some art herself (or a puppet play or some other expressive symbolic activity) to enable her to respond to the child nonverbally.

and trust the healing process or provide guidance for Yoshi to move through the series of "problem-saturated trays" into unique outcomes and a new story? She resolved that from the point of view of narrative theory this dilemma with nondirective play or art therapy was parallel to the question of directing spoken therapeutic conversation. Therefore, she decided to proceed with the process of reflexive questioning, whether in spoken or art form. She encouraged Yoshi to reflect on the meaning of these problem-saturated images and to question whether these meanings were inevitable or whether he might have a choice in changing them. Since he had already had a good chance to express his story of pain, could Yoshi be actively invited to consider a story of hope?

## Problem to Possibility: Choice and Empowerment

Since he was now more open and connected, perhaps Yoshi was ready to deal with the temper and misery that were still ruling him and move into a world of new possibilities. At the next conjoint session with father, Yoshi was questioned as to his hopes and readiness to change his relationship with the temper and misery. Although future possibilities were hard for him to consider, Jenny told Yoshi that there was a Temper Tamers' Club of Australia and New Zealand, consisting of kids like him that had dealt with tempers, and suggested that he consider joining it if he could complete the job of taming his own temper. Despite her discouragement about the continued domination of the temper, Jenny had an inspiration to use the Temper Tamers' Club as an audience. She thought that the idea of joining with an exotic audience of children from "Down Under" might appeal to Yoshi.

Ari was supportive, saying he thought his son could tame the temper. Yoshi was interested and curious right away and decided to consider a turnaround. He came to the following session announcing that he was sick of temper and misery ruling his life. He had decided, in his words, to choose "a life free of misery." Yoshi said he had just become aware that "the misery" meant that he got into trouble all the time and that it stopped him from being able to "play and have fun." Jenny asked him to pick one of the sand-tray miniatures to symbolize his choice for freedom. What would show his strength in creating a life free from the temper and misery? He chose a small green porcelain turtle, in sharp contrast to his previous hero figures (dinosaurs, monsters, or warriors) in the sand trays. He wouldn't say much about it at this point, and Jenny did not interpret it, sensing that it had something sacred or numinous about it.

A playful nonspoken dialogue ensued in subsequent sessions in which the turtle would mysteriously show up somewhere in the room. Yoshi might find him watching quietly from a chair or on Jenny's hand during key points in the conversation. Other times Yoshi would pick him up and handle him as he talked. The turtle functioned as a constant symbolic reminder of the unique story that was developing about Yoshi's choice to tame his temper and be misery-free. The use of a concrete symbol in the process of re-authoring a narrative in therapy removes it from the domain of representation to the domain of performative discourse. Whether chosen or self-generated in art, a symbol can be incorporated as a powerful reminder of an alternative choice or of a redescription of a person.

## Exploration of Choices

Subsequently, there were improvements for Yoshi at home and especially at school. However, several weeks after he accepted the idea of being a temper tamer, temper made a major comeback and reminded him that his primary identity was as a troublemaker. Yoshi stated the dilemma that although he wanted to be misery-free, he found himself once again liking the idea of being a "bad dude" rather than a "sissy temper tamer." In fact, he revealed that he had for some time been strongly identified with a gang of "bad boys" at school. Just that day, he said, they had thought of and carried out 115 bad things to do behind the teachers' backs! His father added the information that he was a ringleader in this gang of bad dudes. How could the identity of a "sissy temper tamer" possibly compete with this?

At this point Jenny invited Yoshi to consider the choices he might make. Jenny asked Yoshi to respond in art to the following question: "If you chose a career as a bad dude who has not tamed his temper in school, what would your future look like in five and ten years?" In this drawing (see Figures 9.2) Yoshi showed how his temper would turn him into a teenager who is "plotting to destroy the school by planting a bomb on the door and tricking the teachers into trying to be nice [to him] while [he is] hiding behind a locker laughing. Then the bomb goes off and [he says] 'Dye, dye [sic]!' " Yoshi said that if he is not wounded, he will be carted off by the police and that he couldn't think about his future in 10 years since he would "probably be dead or in jail." The depth of Yoshi's problem-saturated view of himself as a "bad dude" was a revelation to Jenny.

Yoshi was then asked to respond to "future-forward" feedback questions (Penn, 1985). The form of these questions mapped current developments that, if pursued, would lead to his preferred future. As Durrant (1989) explains it, Yoshi was encouraged to "compare two accounts of his future, and it is in [that] comparison that the possibility of a future without the temper literally becomes a reality" (p. 8). An extension of this intervention would have been to invite him to consider an alternative dilemma in expressive work by asking "Would you like to chose another picture of your future or is this the one you prefer?" or "What would that picture (or story or dramatization) look like?"

In our experience in applying the narrative approach we have found that therapy does not necessarily move forward in neat phases; the process seems less linear and more circular or reiterative. Even after important choices are made (such as Yoshi's choice for a misery-free life) and an

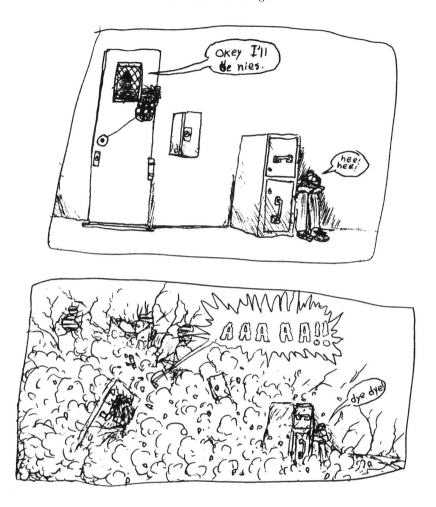

**FIGURE 9.2.** Therapist: "If you chose a career as a 'bad dude,' what would your future be like in five years [at age 13]?"

alternative story begins to develop (temper tamer), the problem may reassert itself for various reasons, which are important and need to be respected. These include an unexpressed specification of the problem ("bad dude" identity) and a need to work further with members of the defining audience for the story (Yoshi's parents) or those who serve as part of the life support system of the problem (such as the gang at school; White & Epston, 1990).

We think that this demonstrates the wisdom and autonomy of the person or persons who live with the specifications of a problem and who are affected by it on a day-to-day basis. As Andersen (1987) writes:

> Every living system is organized as an autonomous system, and only the system itself knows how and when it is ready to change its structure. . . . It is

important to respect the stuck system's resistance to that which is too unusual. The only way to know if one is on the right side of this boundary is to be sensitive for signs the system itself gives us when it closes itself to our questions. So we must let our imagination fly freely, but not too freely, in order to find questions that will be different enough but not too different from those the system usually asks itself. (pp. 416–417)

Aside from the effect of Yoshi's identity in the gang, Jenny had been wondering if there was something in his parent's ideas about therapy that was inadvertently restraining the changes he said he wanted. It seemed that perhaps the family was interested in but, for some reason, reserved about these ideas for change. Mother came in for a session with Yoshi, and while he played Jenny shared her experience that sometimes children have trouble moving forward if parents feel disconnected in some way or have questions about the therapeutic process. She wondered tentatively if this fit for Mariko and if she would like to talk about it. This is another example of the therapist being transparent about a dilemma. As the therapist offers her experience to clients as local knowledge rather than expert opinion (White & Epston, 1990), the effects of observer bias and status differences are reduced. Mariko was willing to discuss the fact that she had significant questions and doubts about therapy in general. She presented her concerns. Jenny and Mariko then engaged in a lengthy dialogue about their theories of growth and change, including their philosophical and spiritual orientations.[8] This conversation identified each person's approach to the problem. Some common ground emerged in their theories and values. A connection between them developed over the practice and philosophy of Aikido, a spiritually based martial art. Ari also had a background in Aikido and a similar philosophical orientation. Aikido-inspired metaphors provided an ongoing concordance between Mariko's, Ari's, and Jenny's unique experiences and worldviews.

Jenny invited Mariko to reflect on the therapeutic process and her own ideas for change. She also made her own approach to the therapy transparent and available for collaborative dialogue, including her philosophy and rationale for her practices. This deconstruction of expert power and knowledge opened space for co-construction of shared ideas about change and growth and for a more reflexive process. Possibilities for growth and change for the family, generated by Mariko's wisdom, might have been marginalized and disqualified had this conversation not occurred.

In subsequent sessions Mariko discussed with Jenny the morals and values in society that negatively influenced her and her son, such as the social context that supports machismo-like aggressiveness. Specific ideas

---

[8]Charles Waldegrave (1991) and his coworkers at the Family Centre eloquently articulate the importance of encouraging the broad range of human experience, including spirituality, in therapeutic conversations.

about the social validation of aggressiveness and power in young males were explored (Jenkins, 1990; White, 1991).[9] For example: How is aggressive behavior supported by cultural practices? How do these practices undermine lives and relationships? How can parents counteract the reinforcers for aggressive behavior toward others that young persons are exposed to by watching television?

Mariko reflected on the kind of moral development she wanted for her son and how she could consciously communicate her values to him. She considered her personal knowledge about how to create assertive rather than aggressive social interactions and clarified her alternative peace ideas. As she developed her own "anti-knowledges" (D. Epston, personal communication, March 9–10, 1992) to dominant cultural practices on the use of aggressiveness to solve problems, Mariko continued to experiment with interactions that invited peaceful solutions instead of temper "burst-outs" and noticed when Yoshi was doing likewise.

Simultaneously, the therapeutic conversation with the dyad of Ari and Yoshi focused on articulating Ari's respect for his son so that Yoshi could see himself as competent and growing in his father's eyes. This seemed to be an essential element for Yoshi to solidify the alternative image of himself as a capable, misery-free person.

Things now improved for Yoshi at home and at the after-school program to such an extent that we decided he might want to apply to the Australian/New Zealand Temper Tamers' Club and get ready to graduate from therapy.

## Performances of Meaning: The Validation and Circulation of Alternative Stories

In the "text analogy" (White & Epston, 1990) persons need an audience in order to consensually validate alternative stories about themselves. We have found this concept difficult to integrate because of the dominance of therapeutic ideologies such as the importance of maintaining strict boundaries between clients and between the "therapeutic container" and significant persons in a client's life. The practice of recruiting audiences for the performance of meanings about new stories has challenged us to reach beyond the therapy relationship to others who have influence in a person's life.

There are several types of audience available. A defining audience consists of those in a person's life who interact with and influence his or her unfolding story. We have found that it is most helpful in the process of re-authoring clients' stories for these people to be identified and included as

---

[9]Michael White (1991) enumerates four invitations to men engaged in abusive behavior: to take responsibility, to make amends, "to challenge attitudes that justify such behavior and the conditions and techniques of power that make abuse possible," and to "be engaged in the identification and the performance of alternative knowledges of men's ways of being" (p. 39).

an audience for change. The alternative story about Yoshi as a temper tamer was strengthened as his parents, teachers, and others observed his influence in the life of the problem.

Ari had been working hard to help Yoshi with his problems at the after-school child care program. This included having frequent conversations with the teachers when he picked up his son at the end of the day. It so happened that while Jenny was considering writing a letter to the after-school teachers to include them as an audience for Yoshi's changing story, one of the teachers spontaneously became an audience for the boy's positive developments and simultaneously began to regard Ari as a parent to be emulated. He wrote the following appreciative note, which was brought in to therapy by Ari and Yoshi (making Jenny an audience for this audience):

> Dear Ari,
>    I wanted to take some time out to tell you that I really, really appreciate you and your support of the staff here at childcare. Yoshi's attitude and behavior seems to be a lot calmer lately and most importantly he seems to be trying. He's only been here one or two days a week, but mostly I'm referring to the few weeks before the break. I know it's not an easy task raising a son, and as a man I can really appreciate the time and energy you give your child. I'll remember you and Yoshi when I have children of my own.
>
> Thanks,
>
> Kevin

In addition to members of the defining audience, other people or groups that the client could connect with as peers can be included as an audience. Jenny asked Yoshi to interview for the *Temper Tamer's Handbook: How to Cool Off and Be Cool.* She had previously started this informal handbook to circulate the knowledge of children on the subject of temper taming. The handbook provides children with an opportunity to share temper-taming techniques and perform meanings for an audience of their peers. Yoshi wrote about how he had decided to have a misery-free life so that he could get on with playing with his friends and having a good time in after-school care rather than always being in trouble and miserable because of the temper.

Another group that was an audience for Yoshi's alternative story was the Temper Tamers' Club of Australia and New Zealand. Its president, David Epston of the Family Therapy Centre in Auckland, New Zealand, was recruited by Jenny at this point as an "exotic audience" for the performance of meanings about Yoshi's temper-taming ability. Jenny and he co-authored the following letter of application for candidacy in the club. This initiated a sequence of letters and drawings from each participant in the therapy. The following is a letter from David and Jenny inviting Yoshi to join the Temper Tamers' Club:

*Dear Yoshi,*

*Jenny told me that you might be a candidate for the Temper Tamers' Club of Australia and New Zealand. If you were to be successful, I guess you could set up a branch office in Berkeley and be our American agent. The next board meeting is in a month's time. So far, from what Jenny told me, you are looking good.*

*However, I need to ask you for some further information. I have some questions for you and your mother and father to answer in order to back up that what Jenny and you say happened has really happened.*

*1. Is it true that your temper didn't want you to come to therapy and work with your family to get rid of it in the first place and that you refused to go along with your temper?*

*2. Is it true that you freed yourself from its grip and are now more able to talk for yourself and to turn around some things in your life that were bugging you? Was this hard? Are you finding it easier the more you do it?*

*3. I was excited to hear that you and your mom came up with some interesting peace ideas to stop the temper and fighting that were coming between you. Could you let the people in Australia and New Zealand know what your favorite ideas were and which worked out the best?*

*4. Do you think your temper is in favor of your decision to choose happiness instead of misery in your life? Do you think the temper now knows clearly that you will not put up with it giving you or anyone else a hard time?*

*5. What benefits have you seen in your home and school life now that you have struggled and freed yourself from temper and misery and can enjoy a life more for yourself (and less for temper) and a life of your own choosing?*

*6. Mariko, what benefits have you noticed at home since you teamed up with Yoshi to liberate your relationship from the temper and fighting?*

*7. Mariko and Ari, what changes have you noticed in how Yoshi is being seen in the eyes of other people since he made these changes: in your eyes, in Jenny's eyes, the eyes of his teachers, classmates and friends? How do you think his own view of himself (in terms of self-respect, liking, etc.) has changed?*

*I am looking forward very much to hearing from you through Jenny. Once I have, I will give this information to the board and inform you about their decision. From what I have heard so far, I am confident on your behalf.*

*Yours sincerely,*

*David Epston*

Here, members of the family are invited to plot a history, in the landscapes of action and consciousness (White, 1991), of their story of liberation from the temper, misery, and fighting. The questions encourage them to detail Yoshi's and Mariko's and Ari's relative influence in the life of these problems and to build a series of unique outcomes that render the dominant story obsolete (White & Epston, 1990).

Question 1 begins by plotting Yoshi's first steps to tame his temper (landscape of action). Question 7 asks for information on how others view his changes and then asks about Yoshi's thoughts, feelings, and motivations within the alternative story (landscape of consciousness). Questions asked from these perspectives invite persons to reflect on and perform meanings about their preferred choices, values, abilities, and agency in relation to problems. The following is the letter of response from Mariko:

Dear David Epston,

1. When we first started bringing Yoshi to Jenny's he would verbally and almost physically refuse to go, saying he hated it, it was stupid, he refused to go, etc., and literally walked in painfully slow, inch-at-a-time steps to the door. Originally, I brought Yoshi. It got to be so much of a drag that we switched to Ari bringing Yoshi. If Yoshi resisted it was half-heartedly, then not at all, so we switched back to me for a while. At this stage he once said he actually enjoyed it and asked if I got to see a therapist.

2. I believe one never truly frees oneself from the grip or tendency to react a certain way under pressure: i.e., to get off balance. However, getting back on balance comes more quickly, until others may not even notice, as in Aikido. Yoshi has come a long way to go a short way, so to speak. He still occasionally has outbursts or burst-outs as he calls them! But they are never of the intensity and ugliness they were before. And when he does burst out, he calms himself down within often 5 minutes or so, can apologize with integrity, and "let it go." Sometimes it will even be before the parent! He has less burst-outs, it seems, with his friends too, less playtimes that end with "I hate Jeff," etc.

3. Peace Ideas: One was for me to try to differentiate under pressure between when I was the one who was angry and when Yoshi was angry initially. If it was me, I would try to say I needed a short break, say 10 or even 20 minutes, as the situation allowed. Then we would come back to the issue and "chill out," as they say! If it was Yoshi coming off the wall, I tried to maintain my own good mood and not be infected negatively by his: "Please remain calm; it's no use both of us being hysterical at the same time." The trick was to remain neutral under fire if the other was bouncing off the wall, yet not patronize nor turn off.

4. This question is a tricky one to answer for me. I don't think the temper clearly knows Yoshi will not put up with it getting out of hand, but it is not the predominant force between the two of them any more. I don't have a clear sense of the response to this one, but Yoshi's father may.

5. Benefits: Home: Upon reflection, we rarely have strong disagreements and arguments anymore. I recall sitting down once near the middle of the therapy and negotiating about Yoshi going somewhere I wanted and he didn't in exchange for me taking him somewhere he wanted, after an initial strong reaction from Yoshi.

After School Care: Father deals more with this aspect now as he has Yoshi there 3 days and I only one for a short time. There have been less and less complaints/reports about his behavior, defiance, disrupting, but I'll let Ari tell you more.

6. <u>Benefits for Mariko:</u> I <u>like</u> my little son again!! That's a <u>major</u> benefit.
I had got to the point where I said, "Mother love notwithstanding, I
couldn't care less if he stays with me when he's like this!" Damaged little
psyche or no, that's where our fighting had led me.

7. <u>Others/Own View:</u> Some happenings come to mind:

   a. His teacher volunteers at her daughter's private school as a parent in
      the classroom. She was doing a dinosaur presentation and asked
      Yoshi and 2 friend/classmates to be the resident student experts and
      accompany her to this class. It just happened to be the same school
      Yoshi attended in kindergarten from which he was essentially ex-
      pelled for uncontrollable temper. He loved it! The presentation, that
      is.

   b. Yoshi was verifying a fact with me in front of his friend, who he
      thought had said something opposite. His friend said, "No, I didn't
      say that"; Yoshi said, "I thought you did. It's okay to make a mis-
      take; I make mistakes." When his friend continued to say he hadn't
      made the erroneous statement, Yoshi did not insist he had.

   c. He talks less and less about his initial inability to get something
      right as "I'm so stupid."

   d. Other parents have said things like "I've seen Yoshi like that, but I
      haven't seen him fly off the handle or get ornery or moody or de-
      fiant lately."

   e. I notice that I am impressed frequently with him—I can't say ex-
      actly what—but I recall saying "I'm impressed" somewhat regularly
      now. One is his spelling, which was a hugely difficult area when
      we first came to Jenny. But also in other aspects of his behavior.

In response to Question 2, Mariko states that she believes that "one
never truly frees oneself from the grip or tendency to react a certain way
under pressure." This implies that one needs to have an ongoing relationship with a problem, instead of being able to vanquish it. We appreciate
Mariko's contribution of a power-in-relation-to-a-problem metaphor in the
context of an ongoing relationship with it. She distinguishes between the
idea of freeing oneself from the grip of a problem and the idea of getting
back on balance quickly from one's tendency to react a certain way. Mariko
articulates the nuances of Yoshi's new relationship with his temper wherein
her son can "let it go" and regain balance quickly.

In response to Question 3, Mariko contributes several "peace ideas"
based again on the idea of maintaining balance under pressure. What
worked for her was neither patronizing Yoshi nor turning him off but
remaining neutral under the fire of anger. Mariko's ideas have since continued to develop and to be useful to her and her family. They were referenced
in future conversations in the therapy and woven into the new family
narrative. In a follow-up interview Mariko wrote up a sequence of peace
ideas she had been practicing: "Take a moment to step back (count to ten);
ask myself: 'What is my part in this episode? What am I doing to escalate?';
neutralize; de-escalate; ask for space to be angry or disgruntled for five
minutes; and let others know I will be okay but need to let off steam first."

The following is the letter of response from Ari:

1. *Yoshi's temper did not want him to come to therapy for a long time and in fact had the upper hand in the struggle. Eventually, Yoshi did refuse to go along with his temper and got control of his life.*
2. *Yes, he has been able to turn some things around in his life. I see him having a happier, more equal relationship with his friends, where he doesn't have to be in charge of the playing as much as before. Also, he has, for the most part, done well in after-school care.*
4. *I don't think that Yoshi would necessarily be able to say that his temper knows that he will not put up with it. I have some problems with the wording or language in the question. I assume this is from therapy and that the direction is to externalize "temper" as something to fight. How does that relate to responsibility, and does it not encourage Yoshi to split off aspects of personality rather than unifying them?*
5. *I see Yoshi being willing to reconcile much faster than he was before, sometimes even before I'm ready. Also, see #2.*
7. *He seems to be more at ease with himself, not as insecure as he was before. This is more of a feeling than a fact at this point. He still doesn't want to get involved in classes, teams, groups of any kind. I do believe he has more self-respect and self-esteem. All in all, we—Yoshi and I—have more fun together. [Ari marked questions 3 and 6 "N.A."]*

Ari's response to Question 4 parallels the critique of metaphors and responsibility discussed in the introduction to this chapter. Ari directly questions the fighting metaphor and asks whether this metaphor encourages personal responsibility. After Jenny read Ari's response, she discussed this issue with him. He said that he thought it was important to "unify aspects of personality" and was concerned that externalizing a problem might mean "splitting off aspects of personality." He also emphasized a moral relationship with the problem rather than denial or power over it. Ari's question invited Jenny to consider whether externalizing temper as something to fight encouraged Yoshi to separate himself from his relationship to the problem and responsibility for its consequences. She brought this up again with Ari and discussed with him a distinction similar to that made by White (1989) in addressing this issue:

> While the practices associated with the externalizing of problems . . . enable persons to separate themselves and their relationships from such problems, these practices do not separate persons from responsibility for the extent to which they participate in the survival of the problem. In fact, as these practices assist persons to become aware of and to describe their relationship with the problem, they enable persons to assume a responsibility for the problem that they could not do so [sic] beforehand. (pp. 21–22)

Ari's concern about personal responsibility provided us with a caution to distinguish the process of constructing solutions to problems from any absolution of a person for the consequences of his or her behavioral problems.

Yoshi responded to David Epston's letter by taking up Jenny's suggestion that he illustrate his success in temper taming and establishing a misery-free life. He created a series of cartoons and a story, which Jenny wrote down for him (see Figures 9.3–9.5). Yoshi's story, "The Turtle and the Temper," follows:

*The Turtle is Me. He uses his wings. He chooses to feel a certain way, and the Temper passes him by and can't catch him. He stays free. The wings don't exist except in his mind . . . he can use them. The Temper used to spin around and catch Yoshi up in it. It would suck him in and let him out and teach him how to be bad [Figure 9.3]. The Temper had gotten so big it destroyed its creator (the black wolf), who used to run it. The Turtle concentrates on his power, but he can't feel it anymore because he's just so concentrated. At first you have to concentrate, because the Temper wants to be your master, and you have to want to be free, not a slave, and to have your own life. The Temper used to be so powerful it had me under its control all the time. The Temper used to suck up everything and sucked up even the first sun [Figure 9.4]. It would demolish everything and sucked up even the last little bit of dirt! The last little piece of dirt was being sucked up by the Temper [Figure 9.4.]. Then the Turtle appeared, saying that he was feeling stronger [Figure 9.5]. The White Wolf, his ally or creator, also appears, saying bye to the Temper. The Turtle decides it's time to face the Temper, saying, "I must face him." He flies off and has an encounter. It's intense but he says, "That wasn't bad." So now he's really ready to face the Temper himself, who shows up with a many-snake-headed face. Turtle is amazed and says, "Wow!" as the snakes try to get him under their power. But he gathers his strength and blasts them away. Most of them blow away but there is one left, and when Turtle faces it he just smiles and the snake is zoomed off into space past the moon, where it ends up on another planet.*

*THE END*

Jenny then provided a commentary on Yoshi's story, which was shared with the family, sent to David Epston, and presented along with Yoshi's drawings in a show of children's art made in therapy at Jenny's office. Yoshi's drawings and story have also, with the family's permission, been circulated among other children and families who are dealing with similar issues. These presentations served to widen the audience and affirm Yoshi's pride in his story of freeing himself from temper. What follows is Jenny's story about Yoshi's story:

*This series of drawings [Figures 9.3–9.5] was made by way of response to a series of questions designed to elicit the story of Yoshi's success in dealing with his temper. It emerges as a kind of hero's journey of magnifi-*

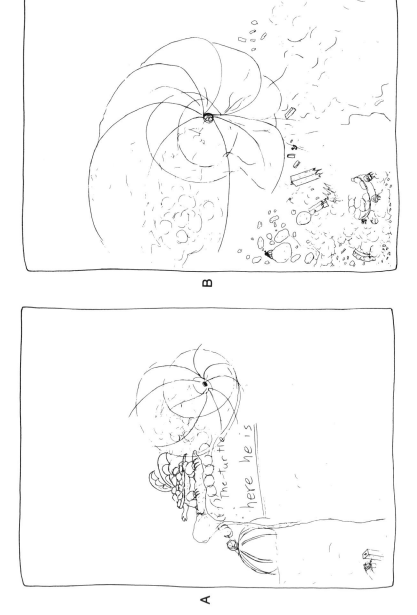

**FIGURE 9.3.** *A:* "The turtle chooses to feel a certain way, and the temper passes him by." *B:* "The temper used to spin around and catch him up in it and teach him how to be bad."

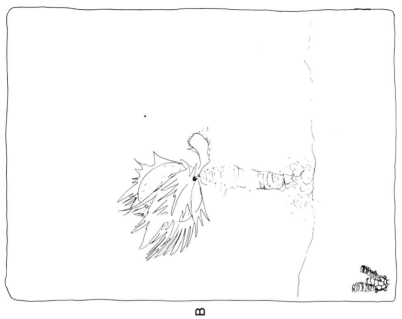

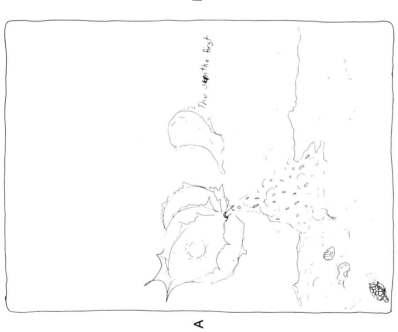

**FIGURE 9.4.** *A:* "The temper used to suck up everything in its power." *B:* "Even the first sun."

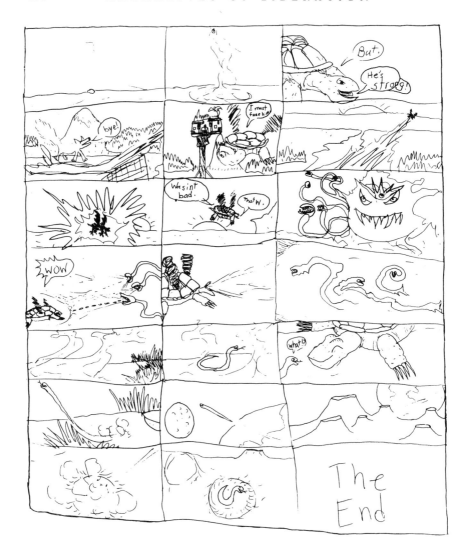

**FIGURE 9.5.** "The turtle decides it's time to face the temper, saying, 'I must face him.' "

cent proportions. The turtle had been discovered as a symbol for Yoshi's ability to choose not to go along with the temper at the point at which he had made his decision for a misery-free life. When the turtle emerged as the hero in the temper tamer's story, it was transformed with wings. The turtle without wings seems faintly reminiscent of Yoshi's earlier image of himself, of being slow and dumb and feeling powerless at school. How delightful that such a small, slow, and insignificant figure as a tiny turtle could magically outwit and blow away a huge storm of a temper!

*Now the turtle developed new and surprising abilities, much as Yoshi had in stopping the temper. The turtle sprouted wings and turned his smallness into an advantage. He could maneuver and fly out of the way of this dangerous temper; perhaps this was a necessary first step. Then he could turn around and face it. As if he were combining Yoshi's mother's Aikido philosophy with his father's philosophy of responsibility, the turtle then met the temper with a light touch and room to move. As Yoshi's mother might have said from Aikido philosophy, meeting a force with force of equal weight would have ended in an explosion. After standing up to the temper, the turtle ends up actually blowing it away with a great breath and a smile, sending it out to the stratosphere. I think this reflects the power of playfulness in dealing with difficult problems such as temper. A creative, lighthearted approach is a relief for therapist and client alike.*

Jenny then sent a package consisting of Mariko's and Ari's letters, Yoshi's drawings and story, and her commentary to David Epston. David wrote back accepting Yoshi as the first U.S. member of the Temper Tamers' Club:

*Dear Yoshi, Ari, and Mariko,*
*1991 has been an extremely good year for Temper Taming here in New Zealand. Mark, aged 8; Andrew, aged 9; and Julian, aged 9, have all made rapid comebacks from the misery their tempers had put them in. So I read with great interest, Yoshi, your brave story and drawings showing how you stopped getting "sucked in" by your temper, and your commentaries, Mariko and Ari. From what I both saw and read, I am more than satisfied that you, Yoshi, have tamed your temper and are free to live the kind of life you want to live. Yoshi, have you found, like Julian, that you are feeling more happiness inside of you? Mariko, like Andrew's mother, who for the first time ever heard her son whistling with happiness on his way home from school, have you observed Yoshi taking more delight in himself? Have you found yourself delighting in him more than you were able to in his old temper-enslaved days?*
*Mariko and Ari, the most convincing evidence for candidature is, of course, the confirmation by those who were formerly complainants. So I read with great interest your comments, Mariko (Others/Own View), and yours, Ari (see Q. 7). Yoshi, I was particularly impressed by your dinosaur presentation and the way your returned to the site of your expulsion and showed your ex-teacher the kind of person you truly are. And I was amazed that you could admit your mistake to your friend and moreover say that mistake making is OK. You could even accept that your friend wasn't as mature as you are. And Yoshi, you have been able to get other parents to appreciate your Temper Taming. Both your parents only too happily note that although your temper wasn't much fun, you certainly are and that now they can get to know more of you. This tells me that you are pretty much free of your temper.*
*Yoshi, can you imagine what your life would have been like if you had allowed your temper to lead it? Mariko and Ari, can you imagine what*

*your relationships with him would have been like if he had allowed his temper to shape them?*

*So, Yoshi, even though I know your brave story only through Jenny, yourself, and your mum and dad, there is nothing but evidence for your Temper Taming. For this reason, the Temper Tamers' Club of Australasia (New Zealand and Australia) grants you full membership. Your member-ship number is 131, and I am proud to say that you are the first citizen of the United States to be either nominated or accepted. So we are proud to have you in our club.*

*This membership entitles you to give advice and counsel to any young person about your age who seems in danger of having their life made mis-erable by their temper. It also means that you can represent the Temper Tamers' Club in giving speeches to your classmates at school if they are curious about how you overcame your temper.*

*Yoshi, I need to warn you that as you become more proud of yourself, it is very likely that your temper might get mad at you and try to make a comeback in your life. On such occasions, you could draw your temper's attention to your Membership Certificate. Our members have found that their temper just gets lost when it finds out that you are a qualified temper tamer.*

*Good luck in your future! If you have the free time, I would be glad to hear from you so I can keep up with your development as a free person.*

*Yours against temper-controlled lives,*

*David Epston*
*President (Elect)*

This letter serves as a "counter document" (White & Epston, 1990). It documents the re-authored story of Yoshi's relative influence in the life of the problem, then welcomes him to a new status in an alternative communi-ty. The letter concludes by describing his new responsibilities and privi-leges. Thus, Yoshi is empowered to intervene with his confirmed expertise in any recurrence of temper's attempt to exert influence in his or another person's life. Yoshi was later awarded a Temper Tamer's Certificate. When David Epston writes that "the most convincing evidence for candidature is, of course, the confirmation by those who were formerly complainants," he places the evaluation of a change in behavior in local hands. A letter such as this can be circulated to a wider audience, in order to reinforce its perform-ative power.

At the final family therapy session a celebration was held. Family members were asked by Jenny if they would like to draw their "experience of the misery-free life that has settled in." Yoshi drew the turtle visiting the Temper's former lair (Figure 9.6). It is now boarded up and a snail may be seen on one of the signs, which says STAE OUT (the other says KEEP OUT). Inside, covered with cobwebs, are the old weapons that the Temper left behind. The little turtle can be seen basking in the sun on a plant on the structure off to the right-hand side. Dad drew the turtle resting peacefully

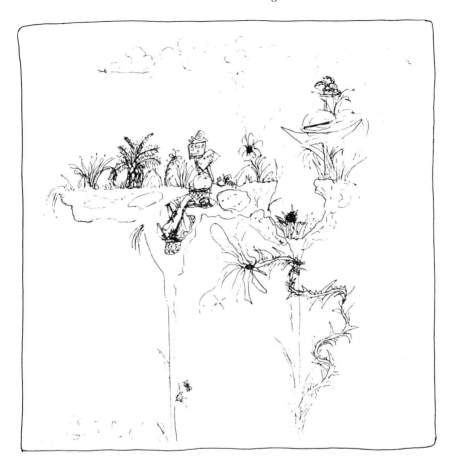

**FIGURE 9.6.** Turtle visits the temper's former lair.

on a rock (Figure 9.7). and commented on how much he was enjoying this new life. This provided a lovely confirmation, beyond words, of the turtle's new position in the family's alternative story.

## Follow-Up

Mariko called to check in 6 months later, after there was a hiccup of temper's getting the upper hand on Yoshi at the video store. In between the call and the therapy session that was scheduled, a family meeting was held without the therapist. The family was able to resolve the issues raised by the incident. Aterward, Mariko and Yoshi decided to come in for a visit anyway. Jenny was caught up on recent developments, functioning as an interested audience for the continuing performance of the alternative story. Both mother and son had generally been keeping their clarity in working

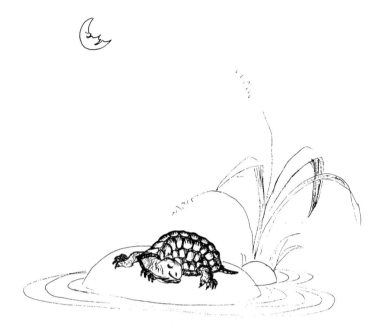

**FIGURE 9.7.** Ari's drawing of the turtle in his "misery-free" life.

with anger and maintaining relative harmony between themselves. Their ideas for peace had continued to unfold. When asked about his experience of these changes in relation to anger, Yoshi commented "I'm happy and colorful, and not dull like I am when I'm mad. I have a lot of energy." He was feeling proud about being on the honor roll in spelling, having just scored 100% on a test.

A follow-up interview was held with all three members of the family a year after therapy ended. They each agreed that they were enjoying their relationships and that life in their households had been peaceful. Ari commented that Mariko now talked, in contrast with her remarks during the previous alienation caused by the fighting, of wanting to have more time with Yoshi. Ari was enjoying more physical closeness, such as hugging, with Yoshi. Mariko and Yoshi were taking Aikido classes together, and he was learning some Japanese. Aikido practice and philosophy seemed to have developed further as a fruitful source of common experience and metaphors for adaptation and change for the whole family.

There were, of course, still plenty of opportunities for minor altercations in daily life, but the temper rarely made it onto the scene. Both parents commented that they had not used the temper-taming metaphor much as they still did not feel comfortable with it. Mariko maintained that "there is a difference between taming something by force and working with it." They continued to experiment with peace ideas such as "balance," "taking a moment to think," "giving space to the other person to be mad when they need it," "apologizing when you did something," and "forgiving."

Several ideas had become part of the story of family life. For herself, Mariko had found it especially important to put into practice the idea of "stepping back." When an angry mood was impending, she found herself able to take a moment to step back and reflect on her choices. Taking the space to decide how she wanted to feel and act had allowed for a separation from anger, and a sense of agency and choice. Yoshi too had been practicing this method with success. He and his mother regularly used their idea for Yoshi to identify with the special abilities of his new cat, Zen Kitty, who displayed particular equanimity and poise. It seemed to Jenny that Zen Kitty was now a playful element in the family's quest for balance in relationship to oneself, others, and the world.

School life was proceeding smoothly for Yoshi. He related a recent event at school that highlighted his development in the use of assertiveness without temper. When he was taunted by another child to fight, he had simply faced him, saying, "I don't want you to do that," and walked away. Jenny and his parents were delighted and impressed with his poise and self-confidence. He playacted for them his role in the scenario, showing himself delivering his message with firmness and a calm smile. This reminded Mariko of his series of drawings about facing the temper, where at the end the turtle had simply smiled at the last bit of temper, sending it flying off into space.

The family reviewed the therapy with Jenny, discussing many of the issues raised earlier in this chapter, such as values, types of metaphors, transparency, and co-construction of the therapy. Mariko, Ari, Yoshi, and Jenny each talked about what worked for them in the narrative process and which ideas had endured. Some of these ideas were subsequently incorporated into the writing of this chapter. The continued willingness of each person to reflect on personal philosophic preferences and practices at length in the interview confirmed the hopes of the therapist for engaging in a reflexive, mutually respectful, and co-creative endeavor.

## EDITOR'S QUESTIONS

Q: *You refer to the idea of therapist "transparency" and describe several examples in your paper. I would appreciate it if you would further discuss the importance of this process in therapy and how it differs from the more traditional notion of therapist self-disclosure. What does it mean to be "transparent"?*

A: Traditional concepts of self-disclosure, in the authors' view, involve revealing personal information in the hope of either increasing the client's identification with the therapist or providing some kind of model for the client on how to live his or her life. The purpose of transparency is to deconstruct that aspect of the therapeutic hierarchy that is based on unrevealed expert ideas about what is best for the client. If the therapy is approached as a co-creative endeavor, transparency is a methodological guideline that allows for the therapeutic process to be shared between therapist and clients. Thus, the therapist can bring his or her therapeutic and personal knowledge into the discourse in such a way that the client has an equal voice and choices in setting the course for the therapy that he or she desires.

Our idea of transparency arises from a reflexive practice of discussing more openly with clients the therapeutic practices and ideas of the therapist. Disclosure by the therapist of personal information may be one aspect of this, especially in the context of being explicit about what personally informs one's ideas. White (1991) describes several components of this practice. One consists of getting feedback and evaluation of the therapy itself, another of encouraging clients to interview the therapist about his or her "thoughts about the actual process of the therapy across the interview" (p. 38). At this point the therapist may disclose personal experiences, imaginings, or intentions, which may allow for discriminations by clients as to whether the therapist's ideas are relevant to them. For example, in the follow-up interview, we invited the family, after reading this chapter, to reflect on Jenny's practices and discuss her ideas during therapy.

Previously, we were used to keeping private most of our theory, formulations, and therapeutic decision-making processes. Now we are more inclined to engage clients in discussion and feedback about the process of the therapy and our thinking about it, especially on questions and dilemmas and therapeutic pathways that we are considering. This invites persons to co-create their therapy and seems to be especially useful at stuck or choice points in the therapy, as it was in the case presented.

Q: *I am very interested in your comments about the therapist's use of "power in relation to" metaphors in contrast to "power over" metaphors. Since our language represents our view of the world, this distinction is an important one. Would you elaborate further on the usefulness of this distinction in your clinical work?*
A: In discussing both gender and multicultural perspectives on narrative work, several people have commented that they feel oppressed by the aggressiveness of power-over metaphors and do not wish to adopt the value system of forcefully defeating problems, with its social/political implications.

In our experience an analysis of questions based on this distinction has been useful to women clinicians who were previously uncomfortable implementing narrative questions. These ideas are somewhat influenced by Jean Baker Miller's (1988) writing on the self-in-relation theory. The concept of "power in relation to" metaphors has opened the possibility of focusing on different forms of relatedness between persons and their problems. Such metaphors may encourage coexistence and relatedness within the family. For example, in recent work with a family dealing with temper the family decided that instead of just helping their 4-year-old to tame temper they would like to engage in a "peace-family project" as well. Instead of defeating the problem, they deconstructed the influence of multi-generational patterns of aggressiveness in family relationships and focused on finding ways to promote harmony between them.

Mariko's preferred relationship with the problem came from the Aikido idea of balance in relation to anger, as opposed to the initial oppositional "fighting against" metaphor we proposed. We have recently discovered that these ideas duplicate observations reported by Tomm, Suzuki, and Suzuki (1990). Their paper elaborates on the response of Japanese therapists to a presentation on narrative therapy in Tokyo. Tomm recounts that "at the conclusion of the workshop, a couple of participants . . . came to me to point out that the basic Japanese orientation was one of compromise and coexistence with problems, not one of confrontation and struggle against them." Mariko expressed her idea of dealing with problems in these words:

> Aikido says to maintain your integrity at all times while taking care of your opponent. There is a very practical purpose [in this]—in deflecting an attack and turning it around. If done maliciously, the opponent will be more determined to get back at you rather than feel that he doesn't want to attack anymore. He is not to be conquered or defeated. The Japanese say never to back someone into a corner or he will feel shamed and resentful.

Tomm, Suzuki, and Suzuki distinguish "inner" from "outer" externalizations, which are analogous to our "power in relation to" versus "power over" metaphors. They state that "an outer externalization supports a pattern of languaging in which the problem is talked about as if it eventually could be defeated, escaped, and left behind. Conversations about conflict, power and control tend to prevail. An inner externalization fosters languaging in which the problem is talked about as if some kind of ongoing coexistence may be necessary" (p. 105). They further describe the possibilities offered by a "personified entity within the person" as an example of an inner externalization that can reduce the restraints of shame and guilt while leaving "full responsibility with the person regarding the manner in which he or she interacts with the externalized problem" (p. 105). We are interested in further implementation of this idea with the hope that the benefits of externalization may then be gained without promoting a "power over" value system or discouraging responsibility.

Q: *In the illustration presented, David Epston is recruited as a long-distance audience for change. The parents also serve in this capacity. How important is it that such an audience exist? Is involving an outsider critical to the success of the process or can family members and the therapist serve equally well in that role?*

A: Although our training reinforces our reluctance to recruit audiences, we have found an audience outside of the immediate family to be very helpful for an alternative story to take root. However, we have observed that the audience needed does vary. In some cases it appears sufficient that the new story be performed in front of the therapist and one or two key relations; in others the involvement of outside audiences is important.

David Epston and the Temper Tamers' Club serve as an example of an outside audience for change. New Zealand was an exotic and interesting place for Yoshi, and this made the invitation to become a temper tamer more intriguing for him. This is not, however, what we see to be the most critical aspect of David Epston's involvement in the therapy. Rather, it is that David brought with him a wider audience, a community of temper tamers and their parents, and their knowledge into Yoshi's therapy. Yoshi is not the only young person—nor is his family the only family—to deal with the undermining and destructive effects of inappropriately aggressive behavior, behavior that is often reinforced and valued for males in our culture.

White and Epston (1990) have pioneered the development of communities of audiences who share knowledge and bear witness to successes with problems such as anorexia, asthma, tantrums, and night fears. It is a relief to clients to gain knowledge of other people who are struggling with similar problems, understanding their social context, and dealing with them successfully. The community also has the power to appreciate alternative stories in the making and to offer locally based knowledge and techniques for changing dominant, problem-saturated stories that equate a person with a problem. We are still experimenting with creating an audience for children and their families by utilizing practices such as inviting David Epston to share his knowledge of the efforts of other temper tamers and their families, invitations to the Temper Tamers' Club, and circulation of the *How to Cool Off and Be Cool* handbook.

A second type of outsider audience is someone who is not in the treatment unit but who is known and contiguous to the family system, for example, Yoshi's after-school teacher Kevin, whose letter to Ari is reproduced in this chapter. These persons are members of the "defining audience;" that is, they interact with the client's unfolding story. They may be recruited by the therapist as extended treatment system members who can help to develop a new consensus for a person's empowerment in relation to a problem. The engagement of an extended audience for the performance of the alternative story is analogous to the way in which audiences outside of the immediate family are required for rites of passage in important life transitions such as adolescence (e.g., confirmation, Bar-Mitzvah, or Bat-Mitzvah) or marriage.

Q: *I don't have a sense of the time frame involved in your work with this family. How long did the therapy process last and how many meetings were held? Do you actively try to make your therapy brief? In general, do you conceptualize your approach as time-effective?*

A: The therapy took place over a period of approximately 9 months. This was one of the first cases where Jenny strove to integrate the narrative approach with other aspects of her background (family therapy, object-relations-based play therapy, and expressive arts approaches). The therapy moved through several "stuck" phases, which slowed things down. In fact, one of the reasons that we decided to present this case was that it demonstrates some of the common dilemmas and challenges that we and others have faced in the implementation of this approach, including theoretical model confusion and the lack of rapid, "miraculous" results.

We are striving to make our therapies generally brief and time-effective. The narrative approach is very useful in this effort. Jenny is finding that some of the tempers that come in with children these days are resolving within several months, and sometimes within just a few sessions. However, we find there is definitely a place for longer-term work, such as in cases of trauma recovery. People have different needs and interests in therapy. We include the issues of length of time and approach in the therapeutic conversation to find a match between clients' needs and the possibilities available to them, rather than making assumptions as to their best interests.

Q: *I am intrigued with your use of drawing with Yoshi as a way to join with him at his level rather than relying on spoken language. Would you comment on other forms of nonverbal expression with children that might be useful in providing a medium for externalizing discourses (e.g., movement and dance)?*

A: The media that Jenny has experimented with in this context include painting; puppet theater; creation of a minidrama or role play; sculpture; mask making; sand play; and movement. The creative process can also be continued across media, borrowing from Natalie Rogers' (1980) approach, the "creative connection." For example, a drawing may be then danced or a sand-tray theme enacted in dramatic play. Jenny thinks that stories develop from experiences that were registered through more than one sensory system. Therefore, employing the visual, kinesthetic, and auditory senses together may help to stimulate and integrate change.

For example, a 9-year-old girl who was struggling with math was questioned about the negative social messages girls get about this subject. She decided to invite a friend into therapy who was struggling with the same restraints. They formed the Anti Anti-Math Club, and both did a series of drawings about freeing themselves from these limiting messages. For example, one said she wanted to be a scientist, and realizing that these ideas would get in the way, she drew herself in the future, functioning in her chosen career. Jenny asked them to show in movement how it felt to go through the world "as a girl that didn't believe in herself" and then how it felt to move as one "who could shrug off these limits and be herself." Next they chose to do a puppet play in which some girl puppets protested to some boy and authority figure puppets who were putting them down because they were smart and could do math. The girls had a lot of fun in this process, and their interest in math and confidence in themselves improved. This could even be observed in the way they held their bodies.

Clients can be asked if they would like to represent the problem in some visual medium, such as a mask. A mask can then be worn and moved from within its persona or used as the basis for a dramatic story. For example, one child made a mask of the fear that was keeping her up at night. By making it concrete, she seemed to face this fear. She relaxed further while playing with the mask, thus transforming the fear's grip on her. Some art therapists I know have been working with the idea of "personification" of a problem or of part of a person (such as the critic in one's self) through art media with a very similar aim to externalization.

Stories of hope and solutions can also be artistically represented. One child and Jenny each created a small finger puppet with big ears called a "listening mouse." They played with them from time to time to reprise a story about listening skills that were developing in the family. A relationship with the problem can be depicted in sand play using symbols, in a play using puppets, or in movement. For example, the therapist might say, "Yesterday you described a period when you felt free of the fear. How could that freedom be expressed in movement?" Many possibilities can be explored like this. A symbol in any medium, including a pattern of movement or a song, can become a touchstone for the preferred outcome for the client—as the turtle was for Yoshi and his family. Success stories can also be celebrated through various art media, drama, or dance.

## ACKNOWLEDGMENTS

The authors are listed alphabetically; both contributed equally. We would like to acknowledge the editorial assistance and support of Andrea Aidells, David Epston, Jane Loebel, Rick Maisel, Margaret Rossoff, and Michael Searle, as well as of the family described in the case presentation.

## REFERENCES

Andersen, T. (1987). The reflecting team: Dialogue and meta-dialogue in clinical work. *Family Process, 26*(4), 415–428.

Dell, P. (1989). Violence and the systemic view: The problem of power. *Family Process, 28*(1), 1–14.

Durrant, M. (1989). Temper taming: An approach to children's temper problems—revisited. *Dulwich Centre Newsletter,* Autumn, 1–11.

Epston, D. (1989). Temper tantrum parties: Saving face, losing face, or going off your face! *Dulwich Centre Newsletter,* Autumn, 12–26.

Freeman, D. (1979, January 24). *The anthropology of choice.* Presidential address of the Anthropology, Archaeology and Linguistics Sections of the 49th Congress of the Australian and New Zealand Association for the Advancement of Science in Auckland, New Zealand.

Gergen, K. J., & Gergen, M. M. (1991). Toward reflexive methodologies. In F. Steier (Ed.), *Research and reflexivity* (pp. 76–95). London: Sage.

Goffman, E. (1961). *Asylums.* Garden City, NY: Anchor Books.

Hare-Mustin, R. T., & Marecek, J. (1988). The meaning of difference: Gender theory, postmodernism and psychology. *American Psychologist, 43*(6), 455–464.

Jenkins, A. (1990). *Invitations to responsibility: The therapeutic engagement of men who are violent and abusive.* Adelaide, Australia: Dulwich Centre.

Krippendorff, K. (1991). Reconstructing (some) communication research methods. In F. Steier (Ed.), *Research and reflexivity* (pp. 96–114). London: Sage.

London, P. (1989). *No more secondhand art: Awakening the artist within.* Boston: Shambala.

Masson, J. M. (1984). *The assault on truth: Freud's suppression of the seduction theory.* New York: Farrar, Straus & Giroux.

Miller, J. B. (1988). *Connections, disconnections and violations.* Work in Progress. Wellesley, MA: Stone Center.

Penn, P. (1985). Feed forward: Future questions, future maps. *Family Process, 24,* 299–310.

Popper, K. R. (1986). *Objective knowledge: An evolutionary approach.* Oxford, U.K.: Clarendon Press.

Rogers, N. (1980). *The creative connection: A person-centered approach to expressive therapy.* Santa Rosa, CA: Person Centered Expressive Therapy Institute.

Tomm, K. (1987). Interventive interviewing: Part I. Reflexive questioning as a means to enable self-healing. *Family Process, 26,* 167–183.

Tomm, K. (1988). Interventive interviewing: Part III. Intending to ask linear, circular, strategic, or reflexive questions? *Family Process, 27*(1), 1–15.

Tomm, K., Suzuki, K., & Suzuki, K. (1990). The Ka-No-Mushi: An inner externalization that enables compromise? *Australian and New Zealand Journal of Family Therapy, 11*(2), 104–107.

von Glasersfeld, E. (1991). Knowing without metaphysics: Aspects of the radical constructivist position. In F. Steier (Ed.), *Research and reflexivity* (pp. 12–29). London: Sage.

Waldegrave, C. (1990). Just therapy. *Dulwich Centre Newsletter, 1,* 6–46.

Waldegrave, C. (1991). *Weaving threads of meaning and distinguishing preferable patterns.* Lower Hutt, New Zealand: Author's reprint.

White, M. (1989). The externalizing of the problem and the re-authoring of lives and relationships. In M. White (Ed.), *Selected papers* (pp. 5–28). Adelaide, Australia: Dulwich Centre Publications.

White M. (1991). Deconstruction and therapy. *Dulwich Centre Newsletter, 3,* 21–40.

White, M., & Epston, D. (1990). *Narrative means to therapeutic ends.* New York: Norton.

# 10

## A Narrative Approach to Families with Adolescents

VICTORIA C. DICKERSON
JEFFREY L. ZIMMERMAN

When families come for therapy, most often the parents are the narrators of stories about their youngster. These stories are problem-saturated. Youngsters seem to have very little to say about their own story. In fact, youngsters usually have barely an outline to a story for themselves (Dickerson & Zimmerman, 1992). The younger the adolescents or the more they have been subjugated by another's problem story for them, the less apt they are to have any story for themselves. Stories, or narratives, are critical, since they become the mechanism by which persons give meaning to their experiences.

Like Bruner (1990) and White (White & Epston, 1990), the authors believe that narratives structure lives. In families with adolescents a transition must take place in which the parents' story about their child becomes less influential than the adolescent's developing story about himself or herself. However, if parents have created a story that leaves little room for their youngster's choices for themselves (Bruner calls these narratives "overspecialized"), then the young person might look elsewhere to develop her or his own narrative. On the other hand, the young person might adopt the story fully but feel little ownership and thus respond with little enthusiasm. In either case, the parents must then account for why their daughter or son is not doing the "right thing." Stories then begin to evolve to justify actions, both those of the teenager and those of the parents. For example, when parents go to extreme lengths, even treating their children in ways the parents themselves do not like, they say that their intention is to help their children reach certain goals. Likewise, when young people act out, they justify it in terms of learning to make choices and take charge of their own lives. The evolving narratives are supported by small stories from the past that bolster the story of the narrator (the parent or the child) about the other. In the clinical example discussed here, the parents say of their son, "He always looks suspicious," whereas he might say of them, "They never let me do things." Often, then, these narratives contain problem-laden assumptions about the other.

## WHITE'S IDEAS

The work of Michael White (1991; White & Epston, 1990) has been extremely helpful in guiding the interventions we use to bring forth these problem stories and to begin the process of developing new stories. In this chapter we will briefly outline some of these ideas and then illustrate the theory and interventions with a clinical example.

After finding out something about each member of the family (as persons separate from the problem) during the first family therapy session, we ask each to tell her or his story without interruption from the others. Once all are listened to, a description of the problem that fits everyone's experience is constructed. Thus, the therapist and clients co-construct an externalized problem (description) that affects all members and is supported by certain externalized habits that affect each particular member. Further effects of the problem are elicited through questions, as the therapist notices the influence of the problem on the lives and relationships of the family members. From a narrative perspective this process of externalization allows a separation between the story each person has constructed to justify his or her actions and the persons involved in that story. This begins a process of deconstruction. Questions can then be asked to further deconstruct the story (i.e., to bring forth the mitigating circumstances and the cultural specifications that have gone into the process of storying or meaning making.)

When deconstruction ocurs, there is both separation from the story and alienation, especially if the persons consider their own preferences about what "should" be occurring. In the space created, there is an opportunity to begin to notice what Michael White calls "unique outcomes": events, actions, and thoughts that do not fit into the problem story. These unique outcomes serve as entry points to alternative narratives. Once these doors are opened through a process of questioning, an alternative narrative can be developed. Bruner suggests that narratives have dual landscapes: The landscape of action focuses on what actions in what sequence are taken to certain goals; the landscape of consciousness is focused more on the goals and intentions of the members. By helping the family notice that these alternative kinds of actions, taken over time, correspond more closely with the goals and intentions and values they hold than the ones that supported the problem story, they will begin to interpret or make meaning or create stories that are quite different.

## THERAPY WITH ADOLESCENTS

As suggested in the previous section, the work of therapy is twofold. The first step is to deconstruct the problem story. This usually involves externalizing the problem, as specified by the parents and agreed to by the adolescent. This problem is supported by a reciprocal pattern of interaction. Another possibility is to directly externalize the reciprocal pattern, of which the adolescent's contribution to the problem is only one end. The therapist then looks at the effects of the problem or the problem pattern on the family. Often the personal stories (given past experience) or societal discourse about adolescence that informs the behavior patterns needs to be brought forth and deconstructed, with the intention of eliciting the preferred ideas and practices of the family. The second step, "restorying," involves bringing forth and making meaning of unique outcomes, again attending to preferred ways of being. This work is mostly done with the whole family present. Sometimes parents and youngster are seen separately, if the conflict is too great, to allow each member to present his or her own version of the problem story.

Restorying, in the case of young adolescents, is a process of helping them develop their own story for themselves. This process centers on what ideas and goals young persons might have for themselves, again attending to their preferences (Dickerson & Zimmerman, 1992). The work may seem incomplete if youngsters are not ready to develop much of a story for themselves. Sometimes, simply separation from the problem story and opening space for a new story to develop is sufficient.

In the following clinical example, the therapeutic process involved (1) externalizing and deconstructing the problem story, and (2) working with the young person and the custodial parents to construct a preferred story. The therapist externalized both the problem, as specified by the parents, and the problem pattern, which was brought forth by the third session. Restorying began by the second session and was done with both parents and stepparents, with the young person and his parents, and with the young person by himself. (Italics indicate a problem that has been externalized.)

## CLINICAL EXAMPLE

This is a story about a 12-year-old young man, David, and his two families. One family consists of his dad, Mark; his stepmom, Connie; and his stepbrother, 14-year-old Calvin. The other family includes Mark's mom, Patty, and his stepdad, Larry. This example involves a problem story of *stealing habits* and *argumentativeness* on David's part and of *lack of trust* and *suspiciousness* on the parents' part and a re-authoring process that took place over a 4-month period.

The family initiated therapy when the mother called explaining that her son had been in the habit of stealing things from his family. The boy lived with his father, stepmother, and stepbrother, spending alternate weekends with his mom and her husband. The stealing had been occurring off and on over the last 3 years, but a recent occurrence, plus their frustration about what to do, had prompted her to initiate the call.

## Session I

As is our usual approach, everyone in the family, including both sets of parents and both boys, was invited to come to the initial session. The first few minutes of the session were spent getting to know each person individually. Mark, the dad, was a postman, a job he had held for 18 years; for fun he liked camping and reading. The stepmom, Connie, had a mail-order business that she operated out of their home; she also enjoyed reading. She and Mark had known each other for 10 years but had married only within the last 2 years. Patty, the mom, was a financial manager for a large grocery store chain; she enjoyed hiking and loved going to the movies with her husband, Larry, who was an attorney. They had been married for less than a year. Connie's 14-year-old son, Calvin, was a freshman in high school and collected comics. David, who would be 13 in 2 months, was in junior high school; he was a whiz at video games and liked making model airplanes.

[This is an important step in understanding the family members as persons separate from the problem and as experts in their own lives. Some of their competencies, preferences, and important relationships are also established. Then the descriptions of the problem by those involved are examined in an attempt to appreciate their understanding of the problem.]

Each family member was asked to describe what they saw as the problem. Patty, David's mom, began by saying that the problem was that David was *taking things;* she couldn't explain why it was happening, but it seemed to occur when they least expected it. For example, just before his last birthday, he had stolen a camera. This led to lack of trust and to people having to lock things up. Connie, the stepmom, agreed that the *stealing* was what was most troublesome to her; by having to lock everything up, she felt forced to have to live in a way that "just didn't feel right" (she called it "dungeoning"). The *stealing* also led to a great deal of resentment, frustration, and anger on her part. She saw herself as most affected by the problem. Larry added another dimension by saying that he experienced a lot of *argumentativeness* and that David, who seemed to have difficulty accepting that adults might know more, tried to find his way around the rules. Mark, David's dad, stressed that things had to be locked up, that the *stealing* had led to a *lack of trust* and to the development of *suspiciousness*. He also indicated that he saw *argumentativeness* as a problem. Calvin, Connie's son, said that he knew his stepbrother was taking things but that he and David got along and he preferred to keep their relationship separate from the problems.

David agreed that he had fallen into *stealing habits* and that sometimes *argumentativeness* had led to his saying things he didn't want to say. He thought it was because he didn't take the time to think. He didn't much like the restrictions, which were consequences his parents imposed on him, but he tried to make the best of them. Mostly, he didn't like the effect of anger on his parents and stepparents and the ensuing lectures. Everyone agreed that David was a bright young man, that there had been no problems with these habits outside the family, and that they were generally very pleased that he and his stepbrother got along so well. The major effect of the meeting, which both families commented on in subsequent meetings, was that everyone had a chance to come together, state their concerns, and show their caring for David. David was the last one to speak in that first meeting, and he seemed genuinely touched by what he heard. Although everyone was troubled by the problem, the process of externalizing and looking for unique outcomes allowed the parents to speak of David as separate from the problem and allowed David to speak of the problem as something he wanted to overcome. Two subsequent meetings were scheduled, one with each family.

[As is often the case in stepfamilies, behaviors that are considered difficulties by the natural parents take on a problem status when stepparents enter the scene. Because the stepparents' responses to the behavior may be different (influenced by their own experience) from the natural parents' responses, the stories that evolve to justify their responses may involve different intentions attributed to the youngster's (and their own) behavior. The youngster's responses may also be different for the same reason; different intentions assumed on the part of the stepparents for the child's behavior lead to different interpretations and a different story justifying the responses they are making. The reader may note that this explanation differs from the one that would suggest a causal or functional relationship between the system change and the symptom (e.g., stealing as a way of providing connectedness or attempting to recapture stolen love). Externalizing both David's stealing habits and his argumentativeness allowed a discussion of the effects of the problem on the others in the family. Effects included lack of trust, anger, resentment, and suspeciousness. These effects led to habits of locking things up, setting restrictions, and looking for behavior that would indicate sneakiness and argumentativeness. A reciprocal pattern of suspiciousness on the part of the parents and sneakiness on the part of the son was constructed in a later session.]

## Session II

The next session with David, which occurred 10 days later, included Mark, Connie, and Calvin, the family David lived with on a regular basis. There had been no recurrence of the stealing habits. (The family was asked if they would allow the session to be videotaped. Because they were afraid they would be hampered by the process, they declined. In later sessions they allowed audio taping, and these sessions have been transcribed. David talked a bit more about himself, saying that he liked reading science fiction and wanted to be a marine biologist. He said he hadn't much thought about "taking things." Mark agreed that David had been pretty much doing what he was supposed to be doing. He had some fears that with a birthday soon coming up (in less than 2 months) David might revert to old bad habits. He said it seemed like a pattern: "There's always trouble before birthdays and special occasions." Connie reiterated her feelings of anger and frustration when the bad habits occurred. In this session the parents talked also about the *argumentativeness*, or what Mark called a "know it all" attitude. They did say that it only occurred about 20% of the time. The therapist and family looked at how David had, in fact, improved over the past year or so and considered that the *argumentativeness* was perhaps just the bad side of a scientific, questioning attitude. Ways that Mark and Connie saw that David had improved were that he could share, be more sensitive, keep friends, and know how to be in the world. Calvin again indicated that he enjoyed David and that it was more just an inconvenience when the problems occurred. The session ended with David saying that "not thinking" was what seemed to get him into trouble; he seemed interested in "thinking" more in order to "get the trust back."

[What seemed notable in this session was the recitation of specific examples of how David had improved over the last year. These were instances that had not been noticed earlier owing to the problem story the parents originally presented. Bringing them forth had the effect of making a distinction between the problem story and other, more preferred activities, so that all could see David's interest in having influence over the problem. Seeing his intentions as different affected the parents' interpretation, and they began the process of developing a new story.]

## Session III

The third session, which was 2 weeks after the initial session and was videotaped, was with David, his mom, and stepdad. David's time spent with them was mostly limited to every other weekend and some holidays. A similar direction was taken in this session in that unique outcomes were searched for and some time was spent with David in helping him identify that he might have ideas and plans for himself. This seems important in families of adolescents, although with younger (12- and 13-year-old) teenagers, the work is slower. The session followed a back-and-forth process between complaints by parents (mostly stepdad), attempts by the therapist to bring forth unique outcomes, and a beginning process of restorying. A transcript of portions of the session follows.

The session began with a review of the meeting with David's other family. After checking with David that it was okay to review the last session, the therapist began:

T: We talked some about the *stealing habits,* but that those habits hadn't occurred since the time before. And it hasn't occurred since then either?

D: Yeah.

T: Well, you must be pretty pleased about that.

D: Yeah, well another week.

T: Well, another week, another day, even—it's good. And then we talked a bit about the *argumentativeness* as a problem. But what Mark pointed out, which I thought was really interesting, is that he saw some changes in David over the last couple of years in ways that he was able to do some things he couldn't do a couple of years ago, in ways that he was sensitive, he seems to be able to make friends and keep them, and he knows how to be in the world. You remember your dad saying that? *(David nods.)* He's sharing things. So what he said about that is that gave him confidence that he could beat these habits, too.

  You talked, David, about how *not thinking* got you to do compulsive things *(nods),* and about how you were going to try to think about that, to catch it, to think more about what was lying ahead, to think about consequences. So, did I summarize it okay? *(David nods again.)*

T: So . . . since David spends his time between two families, why don't one of you catch me up on how things are in this family?

[Larry began by spending some time talking about his relationship with David, some of his worries, and his attempts over the years to share things with him and learn about him. He also discussed how he and David clashed around chores and how he was tenacious in requesting that David do things.]

L: But a situation where all of a sudden chores need to be done, it can start; he can go from the wonderful kid that everybody sees, that everybody in my office sees, when he's helping us, to the Mr. Hyde, just like that.

T: And it tends to come up around your requesting something from him?

L: Yes, but since a lot of life is requesting things of people, you can see how often that can happen, you know.

D: I've gotten better about that, though.

T: You think you're getting better about that, huh?

L: He is; he's getting better about that.

T: Oh, all right! Do you have some examples of that, recent ones?

D: Yeah.

P: Yeah, now when we ask him to do his regular chores around the house—can't ask him anything extra, but the regular stuff—making sure his bed is made, doing the vacuuming, the yard work he is supposed to do, he will do that without a fuss because he knows he has to do it. I mean, there's no question.

T: So, it's just sort of an expectation that he does.

P: Right.

D: *(to Mom)* You hardly have any expectations. Everything's just "go."

T: So, David, when your mom says regular things like making the bed, doing the vacuuming, mowing the lawn—those aren't expectations?

D: Those are.

T: So you do them:

D: Yeah, it also goes along with cleaning the bathrooms.

P: Yes, that's right, you have to keep your bathroom clean.

D: There's nothing else, I don't think.

L: Whatever else we may ask you to do.

T: So, David, I have a question for you. How did it happen that you got so that you just did those things without having to be bugged to do them?

D: Because they started getting more regular.

T: Oh . . . so what do you like about that?

D: They're regular.

T: So regular things just become a part of your plan of life? Tell me how old you are again?

D: *(puzzled look on face)* Twelve.

T: Because I keep thinking you're older.

L: Coming up rapidly on thirteen.

T: Okay, maybe that's what it is. Because you know the reason I asked you that, the reason I got confused there for a minute is, I don't know very many regular twelve- . . . even almost-thirteen-year-old boys who do their regular stuff sort of as a part of their plan. They always see it, not as their plan, but as their parents' plan for them.

D: More of it is their plan for me.

T: Well, you just told me, yeah, maybe so, but you've incorporated it into your life.

D: Yeah, I've done it—it's part of my life—but it's their plan for me. It's not my plan. If it was my plan for myself, I would be doing something different.

T: I understand that, but let me ask you this. No, that's probably too hard a question to ask.

D: Ask it.

T: Well . . . well, okay, I'll ask it. If you were living on your own . . . the reason I don't think I should ask this is that living on your own is a long way away.

D: Well, they've asked me this question before. *(Mom laughs; so does David.) (to Mom)* Haven't you?

T: What am I going to ask? Tell me what I'm going to ask.

D: You're going to ask me, if I were living on my own, what would I do with myself?

T: No, that's not what I'm going to ask. What I was going to ask is "If you were living on your own, would part of your plan for yourself include doing some chores?"

D: A little bit.

T: A little bit.

D: Not much.

T: Well, why would it?

D: Not as much as them.

T: Probably not. But why would it include doing some chores?

D: To keep my house clean if I was living on my own.

T: So that is somewhat important to you?

D: Yeah, I mean, I would keep it not like their kind of clean.

T: You might have somewhat different standards for yourself, but you'd have standards.

D: Yeah, I'd keep my house clean, I'd vacuum it, but I wouldn't do everything as much as they do.

T: All right. That's what I mean. That's why I said to you that I could see you've incorporated these plans into your life. Even though you might not have the same ones, you could see they were important to you in terms of living in this family.

[The therapist's intent, in this example, was to work with David in an attempt to develop an outline of a story he might like to have for himself, separate from his parents' story for him. The therapist's questions can be seen as landscape-of-consciousness questions, since they attempt to bring forth preferences, goals, intentions, and values. White (1991) points out that these questions help develop commitments in life and, with adolescents, the beginning of their own story. From a narrative perspective, David's noticing his own intentions will affect his interpretation of his parents' demands and lead to different actions.

What followed was a discussion initiated by Larry about how both he and Patty became independent early in their lives and how they expected something similar from David. These personal experiences were accounted for in the stories that influenced their response to David and led to the kinds of demands they were making. The therapist then returned to some questions around the problem.]

T: What are you thinking about? When you folks first came in here you were concerned about the *stealing habits,* and now we've had a period of time that they haven't occurred. Are you encouraged, are you a bit wary? What's your state of mind here?

P: I'm very encouraged. I felt that there was a lot of hope that came out of our first session together, just laying everything on the table. It was almost as if no one had anything to be afraid of anymore because it was all there; we all knew about it. Everyone had told David the way they felt about it. So, the worst had happened. So when David went back to school, it was like a sense of relief, like I lived through that one, it couldn't be any worse than that.

[The therapist commented on the hope and caring they showed and on the fact that they were "all on the same side, trying to fight the problem."]

T: What have you seen David do to get some charge of his life and keep that problem at bay? What have you seen him do in this period of time?

P: We've been together but in different ways than we're normally together. We went skiing and we had a lovely day. We just had a very nice day. We skied together the whole day, and David . . . it was a different David. It was not the David that was so frustrated and then would frustrate me because he'd get so angry and just not want to try anymore. He fell down a lot, but he got up every single time and never said a word about it. And, in fact, it was just the opposite . . . as I came by and said, "Are you okay?" he said, "I'm fine, go ahead."

T: What did you see . . . what do you think it was, Patty, that maybe David doesn't even see? What was it about him that he didn't even let the frustration get in there?

P: He was feeling good about himself; he was happy and confident and feeling good about himself.

T: And how did that happen? What did he do, or what happened in his family, that he was so confident?

P: I don't know specifically, but he was. It was a different attitude.

[This example shows work in which the therapist is prompting the parents (mostly mom) to notice those times when David conquered the problems and to begin to pay attention to how the victories may have occurred. In addition to these landscape-of-action questions, land-scape-of-consciousness questions brought forth a new description of David, with "new" characteristics to fit into the emerging new story.

The remainder of the session was spent continuing to help the parents and David notice more of how David does for himself and thinks for himself and takes charge of his own life. No subsequent appointment was made at that time. The next appointment was scheduled with David, his dad, and stepmom.]

## Session IV

The next appointment with David; his dad, Mark; and his stepmom, Connie, occurred 2 weeks after the last session with them and centered mostly around dad's problem with David and *argumentativeness*. David said the problem was most apt to come up when his dad didn't listen. Connie saw how both were vulnerable to *argumentativeness,* but she was also able to see how they had gotten better over time and were beginning to negotiate. And things seemed to have settled somewhat around the *stealing habits.* Connie asked if she and Mark could come in alone next time. Since the problem with the youngster seemed to have lessened to some extent, this request was responded to, and an appointment was made. In determining which family members should be seen, we believe the question that should be addressed is "what would support the most effective re-authoring context?"

## Session V

In their next session, Mark and Connie expressed their concerns, a reciprocal pattern was externalized, Connie's notion of "mind-set" was attended to, and the parents were invited to begin to attend to more preferred behavior and to what steps each member of the family had been taking to reach their goals.

C: I guess to start off with . . . what I'm still concerned with—and I don't think it's being pessimistic, I think we've accomplished a lot, all of us talking with you and talking together—I'm still concerned that something more needs to be done, that you . . . I keep thinking in my head . . . that you need to talk to David. We can sit here and talk about things and clear the air—and that's all well and good—but what I'm afraid of is those simple core issues with him. That value system that confuses him between right and wrong and "I want this; therefore I'll take it" and "It's better to sneak than to ask" is still there and . . . I'm worried. I want something accomplished with that, and I'm wondering, should something more intensive one-on-one be done with him, or is it just enough that he hears what we all have to say?

T: That's a good question. Let me ask you two questions. I guess the basic one is "has there been any recurrence of the taking things . . . of the *stealing habits?"*

C: Just one little thing. Like . . . one morning I got up, came out of my bedroom, and started down the hall, and David was coming from the kitchen and down the hallway and saw me and he does one of these things . . . tucks his arm and zips into his room . . . and it looks like he has a flashlight . . .

T: Looks suspicious . . .

C: And I just went . . . it always looks suspicious . . . he always looks suspicious . . .

M:  Yeah, when he's doing something, it looks suspicious; it's obvious.

[Connie related the incident where David had sneaked a piece of beef jerky for breakfast, which, although she saw it as minor, was an indication of a basic value system of "I want it; therefore I'll take it" or "Better to sneak than to ask."]

T:  That was really my second question. What would you call that value system that he's holding, that you think isn't good for him, that reflects that "I want it; therefore I'll take it"?

C:  That it's better to sneak around the edges and just take something than to ask permission.

T:  Sort of a sneaky . . . *a sneakiness?*

C:  It's sneaky. It's just sneaky. It's like Mark said. When I walk into a room and don't expect David to be in there, I assume he's up to something. I never walk into a room and think, "Oh, hi, David." It's like, "What's he doing?" And that's just the past behavior.

T:  Yes, that's the really important point. It's your experience of him over time, where this *taking things* . . . it's been a habit . . . and the *sneakiness* has been more prevalent.

C:  He's really done good! I'd say . . .

M:  I should think that I'm actually losing that part of the . . . I didn't really get that upset over the beef jerky thing.

T:  Mark, say a little bit more on how you are losing the feeling that . . . feeling of *suspiciousness.*

M:  I've had that *suspiciousness.* It's beginning to fade away. His behavior seems to be less suspicious. He doesn't do these kind of things. This was one incident in four or five weeks now. I'm kind of proud of that, that he's come down from that.

T:  You said that too, Connie, that he's been really good lately.

C:  Yeah, and with his birthday coming up on the eighteenth, he not only hasn't even mentioned his birthday . . .

[Two things were occurring in this segment of the session: First, the therapist was attending to the reciprocal pattern of *suspiciousness* and *sneakiness,* and second, attention was drawn to the parents' comments about how they were more encouraged and less upset, that is, about how they were losing the *suspiciousness.* What starts out as an interpretation of David's intentions and values is thus deconstructed. Perhaps *suspiciousness* invites *sneakiness* (and vice versa), and David's intentions and values are more similar to the parents' than they notice.]

C:  You have to be careful, and sometimes it's hard to be careful and not to mind-set his . . . to say, "You always do this," and they want to prove their parents right.

T:  Tell me more about that, Connie. That sounds really interesting to me. "Be careful not to mind-set his . . ."

C: Yeah, you have to be careful with your children that you don't input what you are afraid of them doing. You know, "You better not do this again." It's the negative point.

T: Does it go both ways? Could you mind-set kids to do more what you want them to do?

C: Yeah.

T: Have you ever had an experience like that with David or with your son, mine-setting him in a direction that's more what you want?

[Connie spent some time telling a story about how she was able to help her son get over some anxiety about switching high schools. She also mentioned how stepparents have to work out their differences in parenting. She talked about how well her son and David got along and how pleased she and Mark were about that.]

T: Let me get back to this. You were able to positive mind-set Calvin, based on your own knowledge of how important it is for kids to feel security, that both of you have that because of your own experience. Talk about . . . that with David. It sounds like you've already done a little of that with him, beginning to think, more in terms of what his strengths are, not looking . . . I mean, the *suspiciousness* still hangs out there for you but you're able to . . . it's fading away. You're not noticing as much. I can see, in the past sometimes the *suspiciousness* would mind-set him in a negative way and then he would do suspicious things.

C: We never got to the point where we could praise him on anything. It was real hard. You knew you should, but it was constantly something; so it was real hard to get to that point.

T: So now that he's acting a bit better, what do you see yourself doing that's sort of prompting that?

M: Helping him along? He's basically doing it on his own but . . . maybe it's just no negative feelings back, because he's not doing these things. We're not hovering around him or eyeballing him a lot, trying to find something.

T: *Suspiciousness* isn't getting you to be over him all the time.

M: A lot of the times we were just worried about what he would do next. He was home alone. Everything was unlocked just recently.

T: *(surprised)* Oh, is that right?

[The stepmom introduced the notion of "mind-setting," an idea that the therapist then used to prompt their interaction with David in a more preferred direction. After noticing evidence of David operating with his own preferred (and, in the parents' eyes, more positive) story, the parents were ready to invite him to develop his own story rather than invite him to accept theirs. By responding in this manner the parents are acting in more preferred ways themselves.

After a discussion about how the parents were watching for signs of how David might be taking charge of his own life, the therapist asked what David might be showing at 13 that he was not doing at 10 and what he was doing at 10 that he couldn't do at 7. The parents commented on his remembering things, his making and keeping friends, his being on time, and being responsible for school activities. They were less able to see improvement in the 3 years between ages 7 and 10, indicating that it was a "tough period" in which there were "temper tantrums, which he doesn't have anymore." The therapist drew attention to this last statement, asking if it was an improvement; the parents assured her it was. The therapist then summarized the change over time.]

C:  We'ver never gotten to this point before. We couldn't get to a point where we could praise him about something.

T:  So this is progress?

C:  This is the best point we've been at in the last few years as far as "Okay, there's not been an incident, there's not been something where you're not feeling drawn to that," but yet we can look at the positive and actually point out and feel good about giving . . .

[The parents then talked about David's interest in role-playing games and mountain biking and how both activities involved organized groups outside his family.]

T:  You're telling me about how inventive and creative and energetic this guy is. Tell me something. You made this statement, Connie: "This is the best point we've been at." What steps do you think each of you took to get to this point?

C:  Patience, stick-with-it-ness,

M:  A lot of talking with him.

T:  So, you said you talked more, there's been more patience. What other . . .

M:  We seem to be trying harder, at least trying.

T:  What steps do you think he's taking, that are allowing him to put more effort into this?

M:  I see him putting his dishes away; he's trying to clean up after cooking.

C:  He's trying to be more helpful. He's sticking to his own room and his own stuff and sharing that with Calvin. We'll walk down the hall, and both of them will be doing this game on the computer or computer stuff together.

T:  So in terms of your initial concern when you came in here today, of wondering about the value system . . . if you wanted to help him develop a value system that would be more forthright and forthcoming, with honesty and integrity rather than *sneakiness,* what have we talked about today—one of the things is mind-set—that might help you do that? It sounds like in the past, because of behavior, you know, that it developed some *suspiciousness* in both of you, and that *suspiciousness* got you to look at him in a suspicious way, which often got him to respond with suspicious activities, because of his being so impressionable and from that negative mind-set. I know that there is more to it than this, but I also know you've told me that over time that this young man has progressed a little, taken a little bit more charge of his life. So I'm looking at things that you two must have done to help him do that.

[The therapist was attempting to help the parents notice the steps they and David had taken toward conquering the problem and re-authoring. Developing a history to the new story, for both the child and the parents, helps support a landscape of action over time. Persons live by their histories, by what they perceive as events unfolding in time. If these events are connected to their preferences, then they can feel their lives moving forward in preferred ways (White, 1991).]

C: Maybe we didn't lay up the ground rules. He seems to be real—you know what I saw pinned over his bed? He wrote notes to himself that said "David, did you . . . ?" and there were little squares that said "brush your teeth, clean your room, do your homework, tell your parents you love them."

M: I missed this one! You didn't tell me that. I'll have to go check this out.

C: It's right by where his little head goes down . . . so this is something that . . .

M: Unless he's trying to fake us out!

T: No, it doesn't sound like he's trying to fake you out. It sounds pretty straightforward.

C: I was in there putting clothes away and thought, "This is cute!" Brush your teeth, clean your room, tell your parents that you love them. So he's really trying.

T: That's delightful. Yes, he is trying . . . much more grown-up . . .

[The parents surprised themselves, and the therapist, with this incident that suddenly came into memory. Our experience is that once outlines for new stories are in place, other incidents do "pop out."

Concerns came up again in this session, which provided a context for talking about backsliding, remembering that progress happens over time and often in fits and starts, and reviewing the notion of positive mind-setting.]

C: It's like we are almost at a point where if things continue on like they are now that he's really trying and things have gotten better.

M: We can remember the positive.

C: We can build on that momentum. It will snowball.

T: That's a good word. It will snowball.

[By the end of the session it seemed that the old story outline had begun to crumble and that the parents, rather than the therapist, were making the "new story" comments.]

## Session VI

The first part of the sixth session, a week later, was with David alone. The time was spent, in part, trying again to help David to story his life and to notice what he was doing to turn his life in a more preferred direction.

T:  What does this mean, that your mom *and* dad are both interested in having a party for you? Does this mean that there has been a kind of a turnaround in your life?

D:  Yeah.

T:  Tell me about that, David. What's the turnaround?

D:  I don't know. It's just been better lately, I guess. I don't know . . .

T:  So the turnaround has to do with that there's been less . . . there haven't been any recurrence of those *stealing habits,* right?

D:  No, no stealing.

T:  And then what about what your dad said last time, that there's been very little recurrence of the *argumentativeness?*

D:  Well, I did get kind of argumentative with my dad, but that's hard not to do.

T:  So tell me about that. How is this happening?

D:  I don't know.

T:  No idea?

D:  No.

T:  Well, I'm going to remind you about the first day I met you. It was January fourteenth. Okay. So it's not even two months since I met you. Not even two months and there has been no recurrence of these problems.

D:  Yeah.

T:  So how did you do this, David?

D:  I don't know.

T:  Doesn't this sound pretty amazing to you?

D:  I just haven't had it.

T:  Just haven't had it? So does that mean if the *stealing habits* or *argumenta-tive habits* started to sneak up on you, would you be able to fight them off?

D:  I don't know.

T:  What do you think?

D:  I don't know.

T:  Would you be interested in fighting them off?

D: Yeah.

T: You would? See, I would have guessed that. Why would you be interested in fighting them off? How would it be helpful to do that?

D: Pretty helpful. You know, I don't like feeling it in the first place, but sometimes it's just going to happen.

T: Yeah, it's funny how trouble gets into somebody's life; it just sort of happens. But you're not much interested in continuing these bad habits, are you?

D: Yeah.

T: So you'd be interested in fighting them off?

D: Yeah.

T: But you don't know for sure how come they haven't made a reappearance? Right?

D: No.

T: Would anybody else have a idea of how come there haven't been a recurrence of those habits?

D: I don't know, maybe . . .

T: If somebody would have an idea about that, who would most apt to be aware of that?

D: Probably Connie and my dad.

T: Why would you say them?

D: 'Cause they're around me a lot.

T: You think one or the other? Connie or your dad? Which one most?

D: I don't know . . . mainly Connie . . .

T: Okay. Would your mom or Larry notice it too?

D: Maybe. I'm not around them as much, so I don't know.

T: There hasn't been any recurrence with them either, right?

D: Nope.

T: Is this a puzzle to you?

D: I really don't know.

T: Is this something that you sort of suspected would happen anyway? That these habits were bad habits that you really wanted to put behind you?

D: Yeah.

T: So in some ways this really isn't a surprise to you.

D: Mm hm.

[Attempts were made to continue to develop both a landscape of action (what, how) and a landscape of consciousness (why) in the new narrative. As can be seen, it was difficult for David to notice how he was able to conquer the problem and go in a preferred direction.]

T: What is it about you as a person that you weren't much interested in these bad habits anyway?

D: I don't know, I just don't want them because they got me in trouble. And later . . .

T: So you could see that if Connie is pleased with this turnaround, how did that affect you? Since she is more pleased?

D: Well, she lets me use a lot of her office stuff. And sometimes I get home and there's a key out in the back and there's unlocked stuff.

T: So if you were to say the one thing that's become better for you in your life since some of these habits are not making an appearance, what would you say is the one thing that has gotten better? Would it be your relationship with Connie? Or would it be getting to use some things? . . .

D: Freedom.

T: Freedom for what?

D: To do what I couldn't do before.

T: Can you give me an example of one thing?

D: Well, I mean, they are just letting me do a lot more and they are trusting me a little bit more.

T: Is that something that you are glad about?

D: Mm hm.

[The therapist's questions led to some responses that seem to fit a story that a 13-year-old could construct. The remainder of the session was spent with David, Mark, and Connie, and in many ways was an opportunity to review the themes that were discussed in the previous session with the parents only.]

T: So what do you see happening now that David is developing a sense of empathy.

C: It's mainly attitude. It's nothing I could give you a real example of; it's just I know it's beginning to be there.

T: Would it be like an example of you more willing to let him use your things because you sense some respect for your things?

C: I think the respect was there.

M: I think it was something different. I think he's a little more humble and he doesn't expect it to be his to use even though it's not his. I don't think he has expectations any more that just because he's David that he's going to do whatever he wants with anybody's stuff. I think it's that feeling. I think he respects people's property a little bit more now.

[The therapist's intent was to allow David to experience his parents as an audience to the new behavior. A key development was a discussion of empathy and respect, topics brought forth to help David develop a new experience of himself. We have found this to be quite useful in the re-authoring process.]

T:  What are some of the things about you as a person that you can keep on doing it? Do you remember what some of those qualities were?

D:  I'm . . .

M:  You drawing a blank?

D:  Yeah.

M:  I think he's got persistence.

T:  That would help him keep on doing it, wouldn't it?

M:  Yeah, if he aims that need in that direction, I think he can accomplish things.

[The approach taken here was to bring forth some qualities David might have as a person that could help him go in a more preferred direction, further supporting a landscape of consciousness in the new narrative.]

T:  Let me ask you this question. Lots of times when problems have been in somebody's life for a while and then there is a turnaround, sometimes the problem casts a shadow back on your life again. And that's something you're a little bit worried about, that even after good things happen, like birthdays and birthday parties, et cetera . . .

C:  There's just too many years of hard stuff to have good stuff . . . "Okay, it's all fine now."

T:  It might be realistic for you to watch out for that shadow and not be too surprised if it were to happen, but to think of it as a shadow.

M:  Hopefully.

T:  In fact, shadows are interesting because they pass over. So that might be important for you to remember, that if that happens if doesn't mean that it's a total relapse back into the old behavior.

M:  It's really good to see him realize that he's slipping back to an old pattern. When he starts realizing that then maybe he could . . . I don't know if he'll verbalize it until he's older, but he'll say, "Ah well, I'm getting argumentative. I understand what you're saying. Yeah, I see your point of view." And then we can come to grips with . . . maybe the shadows are just shadows, and it's not going to be full-blown sunrise again.

[The therapist's intent was to prompt the parents not only to continue to notice changes in the past but to anticipate them and look for them in the future. Future looking-back questions support the parents' effort to notice the steps they all are taking in a preferred direction. The therapist was also preparing the family for the inevitable setback. This family had not experienced any relapses into old bad habits in the 3 months in which they had been coming for therapy. They were anticipating something around David's birthday, which was to occur in a week, but were hopeful that nothing "bad" would happen. By talking about shadows, the therapist was preparing the family for any event so that the momentum of going in a preferred direction would not be lost.]

## Session VII

The seventh session, 5 weeks later, included Mark, Connie, and David and was purposely scheduled to occur one month after David's 13th birthday. When Connie called to confirm the appointment, she indicated that they had a story to tell about some events around the birthday. There had been no recurrence of the *stealing habits* or the *sneakiness,* and the parents had been paying attention to "mind-setting" in a more positive way. Nevertheless, the therapist was not surprised to hear that a problem had made a reappearance. Although David said that the birthday had gone to his liking, his dad said that there had been a problem. Before his birthday David had received a poor performance report from school, a notice that required the parents' signatures, but he had not shown the notice to his parents. Mark and Connie learned about it only after they received a second notice *after* the birthday. Both parents said they could understand why David had not shown the first notice to them; he had "held back on it, so he could enjoy the birthday." However, they were disappointed. Mark felt that David didn't realize that they would have been easier on him if he had shown them the notice instead of hiding it. Connie said that "old habits die hard" and that as much as they were "trying not to mind-set [the old habits]", she was afraid they had in fact done so.

As can be seen from the words they used, the parents did not see the behavior as a complete reversal of direction but as a setback; it was a disappointment but one they could understand. They also were clearer about their participation in the problem and seemed able to separate David from the "problem habit." What was most astonishing, however, was David's response.

T:  *(to David)* Are you most concerned about the poor performance in school or are you most concerned about having fallen back into that old habit of *sneakiness?* I guess keeping the notice back was sort of a *sneakiness* habit.

D:  Yeah, it was kind of *sneaky,* but I don't think it was anything like a *sneakiness* habit. You know, it was just like . . . I didn't do it, like, because it was . . . 'cause I just felt I had to do it. It was like I did it because I thought about it, kind of, and it came out like, "Well, they probably won't let me have a party."

T:  So, it wasn't because . . . although it looks like *sneakiness* . . .

D:  It looks like *old sneakiness* . . .

T:  It looked like the *old sneakiness,* but it wasn't, because you *thought* about it?

D: Yeah. *(nods)*

T: It wasn't that *non-thinking.* You were worried that you'd be punished in a way you didn't want to be, so it was more of a decision, even though you can see now it wasn't a good decision?

D: Yeah. *(nods more vigorously)*

T: That's an interesting difference. So would you say you're not as worried about that as you are about the school performance?

D: Yeah.

T: So, if this were to happen again . . . let's say that something happened that worried you . . . do you think that you'd be more apt to tell someone next time?

D: Yeah.

[So even though the old bad habit had made an appearance, David didn't see it as the old habit. He could make a distinction between a *sneakiness* that caught up with him and got him to act in deceitful ways and a *decision* that he thought about and made in his own best interests. What he learned was that it turned out to be a decision that was not in his best interests. Much of the rest of the session was spent discussing with the parents how they might help David and discussing with David how he might learn to act on his father's promise that he would "be understanding if he came forward with the truth."

It is our experience that when clients make a distinction between the problem story's influence and their own ideas and preferences, a new story is evolving, one in which the client is narrating on her or his own.]

## Follow-Up

Two more appointments followed: one 2 weeks later with the stepmom alone, at her request, and the other a month after that with Connie, Mark and David. The latter appointment occurred after the end of the school year. Each session was indicative of the new story that was beginning to take hold. Connie was beginning to see her participation in constructing David's story; she talked about the lack of connection she had felt with David over the years and how she had not had much contact with him before she and Mark were married. This lack of connection seemed to make it more difficult for her to help David develop his own story for himself and had made her focus more on his bad habits, the *stealing* and the *sneakiness.* The direction of the session with Connie was toward developing her interest in becoming more connected with David and in validating his ideas for himself.

The last session with this family focused on the new story that was now being circulated about David. He had turned his grades around so that he, his parents, and stepparents were pleased about his school progress. His dad and stepmom talked about his summer plans, his interests in a role-playing club, his mountain biking, and the vacations that were planned. David talked more specifically about his efforts in school and his plans for the summer in a way that showed clearly his awareness of agency in his own life. In other words, he was neither responding negatively to his dad and stepmom's story about him nor simply trying to please them; he was standing up for his own ideas and goals for himself. The problem story, the narrative that included the stealing habits, argumentativeness, and sneakiness, was barely alluded to, and then only to distinguish it from the newer, more preferred story of a young man who was making decisions for himself, decisions his dad and stepmom mostly saw as good ones.

## EDITOR'S QUESTIONS

Q: *In the clinical situation presented, you ask David's father and stepmother to come in without David in the fifth session and you choose to not involve David's mother and stepfather in the later sessions, even though it was the mother who originally contacted you for therapy. What guidelines do you use to decide who you will see in therapy so that you can "support the most effective re-authoring context?" Also, how do you decide how often to schedule sessions?*

A: In families with adolescents it is important to make a distinction between the story parents have for their youngsters and the story young persons have for themselves. Often the dominant story is so powerful that it is subjugating the youngster and inviting him or her to respond with defiance. In these cases it seems more helpful to see the parents and the adolescent separately. Usually, we try to see the whole family for the first session; in this case that meant including both stepfamilies and both youngsters. After the problem story has been understood and externalized in a way that captures the experience of all concerned, then decisions are sometimes made to see some members of the family without others. Sometimes the decision is the therapist's, as when the context is too powerfully affected by the dominant story. At other times the clients may request a separate session. In this case, seeing the parents separately allowed the therapist to separate dad and stepmom a little from the problem story, thus providing some space in subsequent sessions for David to develop his own story. A similar process occurred when the stepmom asked to come in by herself. Since the therapy had by then progressed to the point where it was clear that David could have a story for himself, the stepmom could see her own inadvertent cooperation with the problem story. Had these moves been made earlier in therapy, at the instigation of the therapist rather than the family, they might have been too precipitate. We have found that it is best at first to respond to the family members' stories and then let other stories of influence make themselves known in the process of therapy.

Since the mom and stepdad were less involved in the problem story, they were not included in the therapy after the first two sessions. The mother had placed the call because she had been asked to find a therapist. All four parents came in the first time because they were all concerned. When it became clear, however, that the stepmom was the one who was most affected by the problem story, the focus turned toward the family where the problem story had the most influence.

We tend to schedule sessions at more frequent intervals at the beginning of therapy. Even so, we rarely meet more frequently than every 2 weeks; however, our sessions are scheduled for an hour and a half. This allows enough time in the session to focus on the problem of influence, and the time between sessions is long enough for people to collect information from their experience. Time between sessions is for noticing "new story" events, attitudes, behaviors, and beliefs and for building a trend for living a new story. In some ways people tend to access their own resources more readily when therapy sessions are infrequent, and thus movement is facilitated rather than hindered by the longer interval. In more urgent situations, other means of communicating such as phone calls and letters, can keep the contact high around a new story.


Q: *I am intrigued by your comment that "once outlines for new stories are in place, other incidents do 'pop out.' " Would you expand on this idea?*
A: Michael White, referencing the work of Gaston Bachelard in Wood (1991), suggests that narrative structures memory. In other words, what we remember are incidents that fit into the narratives that are currently structuring our lives. Bruner (1990) also suggests that the process of constructing narratives about ourselves involves reaching backward to find small stories from the past that we pull together and use to account for or justify the present. So when we say other incidents "pop out," we are referring to this awareness in the present of small stories from the past that fit the new story.

In a restorying process the outline for the new story must come from experience in order to be evocative. The images the new story brings will facilitate a backward-in-time process whereby experiences that fit into the new story will be highlighted. In this manner the new story will be constitutive of the person, just as the old one was. When new stories are evocative, they have a past that can be resurrected in this way.


Q: *There are clear similarities between the narrative approach you use and solution-focused methods (e.g., finding and amplifying areas of experience that contradict the problem-dominated story). Is it simply a matter of labels (e.g., "unique outcomes" vs. "exceptions"), or are there some real differences in these models? Also, how did you personally come to adopt a narrative perspective in your work?*
A: We believe that although both narrative and solution-focused models represent a trend away from deficit models and toward appreciating the

possibilities that exist for the person, there exist substantive differences between them. In a discussion of this by de Shazer (1993) and a response by White (1993), some of these differences are highlighted, although we dis-agree with de Shazer's assessment of the narrative model. One of the differences often discussed is the distinction between the labels *exception* and *unique outcome*. The first label, according to de Shazer, refers to events that are repeatable and that can then become the new rule. Unique outcomes, in the narrative approach, are less important in and of themselves; their value lies in the fact that they represent entry points into an alternative narrative. Unique outcomes in the form of behaviors that occur at very low frequen-cies seem to have little meaning to persons. Unique outcomes in the form of a different attitude toward oneself, another, or the problem become a wider door into alternative narratives. We also see the juxtaposition of the alterna-tive story to the problem story as useful in therapy. Thus, some attention is paid to the problem story in narrative therapy; this is *not* the case in de Shazer's work. Finally, we refer to White (1993) for a discussion of the role of history in narrative therapy.

The answer to the second part of the question bears further on the differences in the models. We were both initially influenced by strategic therapy models and then by Milan-oriented therapy. White's work, which has subsequently been referred to as narrative therapy, was appealing on several counts. First, narrative therapy combined a directional approach against the problem (like strategic work) with a mutually co-evolving systems orientation (like Milan work), thus highlighting what we saw as the best of both. We believe solution-focused work to be more strategic, in that the therapist is in a hierarchical position and usually decides how things should go. We no longer prefer to operate this way; we see narrative work as being collaborative in ways that fit our personal values about working with people against problems. Second, White's work, in particular, is inclined to be political in the sense that it challenges dominant knowledges that are subjugating. We feel strongly about this component of the work; the larger social context does not seem to be addressed in solution-focused approaches. Therefore, the narrative approach matches the beliefs and values that fit into the landscape of consciousness in our own preferred stories.

## REFERENCES

Bruner, J. (1986). *Actual minds, possible worlds.* Cambridge: Harvard University Press.

Bruner, J. (1990). *Acts of meaning.* Cambridge: Harvard University Press.

De Shazer, S. (1993). De Shazer & White: Vive la difference. In S. Gilligan & R. Price (Eds.), *Therapeutic conversations* (pp. 112–120). New York: Norton.

Dickerson, V., & Zimmerman, J. (1992). Families with adolescents: Escaping problem lifestyles. *Family Process, 31,* 341–353.

White, M. (1991). Deconstruction and therapy. *Dulwich Centre Newsletter,* 3, 21–40.

White, M. (1993). The histories of the present. In S. Gilligan & R. Price (Eds.), *Therapeutic conversations* (pp. 121–132). New York: Norton.

White, M., & Epston, D. (1990). *Narrative means to therapeutic ends.* New York: Norton.

Wood, A. (1991). Outside expert knowledge: An interview with Michael White. *Australian and New Zealand Journal of Family Therapy, 12*(4), 207–214.

# 11

## Escape from the Furies: A Journey from Self-Pity to Self-Love

### STEVEN FRIEDMAN

*When a person finds her own voice, she takes charge of her own story.*
—ALAN PARRY, 1991

There is a plant that grows in the western United States called *ceanothus*. This plant lies dormant for many years, waiting for the right conditions (i.e., intense heat as in a forest fire) to free its growth. Similarly, given the right conditions, the people with whom we work have the necessary resources and potential to create new futures for themselves. How do we as therapists provide the contextual conditions to facilitate the blossoming of new stories and the generation of revised narratives that are liberating and empowering?

Many of us were trained to be what Michael Durrant (Kowalski & Durrant, 1991) calls "psychological detectives," that is, therapists who search out pathology. Rather than "pathology detectors," Durrant suggests we think of ourselves as "competence detectors," therapists who seek out and amplify the client's competencies and resources. Many of the people we see are immersed in a problem-saturated picture of their lives. How do we, as therapists, set the stage for clients to detect elements of themselves and their behavior that contradict this problem-saturated view? As we all know, a problem can grow in size and importance and begin to dominate our conversations with ourselves. As we think more and more about the problem, we find ourselves further and further immersed in a spiraling cycle of negative self-talk that "waterlogs" our thinking and leaves us feeling hopeless and overwhelmed.

With these ideas in mind, it is possible to conceive of therapy as a "journey of liberation," a voyage of discovery of new possibilities and new perspectives. What would envisioning therapy as such a journey offer us and our clients? And how could we most effectively prepare for this voyage? My guess is that we need to travel light and avoid carrying excess baggage in the form of assumptions that draw us into the whirlpool of hypothesis generation and structural analysis. By freeing ourselves of these assumptions, we increase our readiness to listen to the client's story and to generate with the client new meanings and new understandings that will lead out of a problem-saturated world and into a world in which competence and a sense of personal agency become the more dominant discourse.

White and Epston (1990) talk about "supporting persons from behind" (p. 148). Rather than imposing meanings on the client's story the therapist engages the person in a conversational process that allows the client to re-author his or her own story. The "from behind" approach puts the therapist in a position of setting the stage or context for change. By leaving space for clients to utilize their resources in generating new meanings about past events and putting current events and happenings in a new framework, the therapist facilitates the process of change.

If the therapeutic process is envisioned as a journey in which clients move out of a problem-saturated world and into a world in which they can reclaim their autonomy and sense of personal agency, what is required of the therapist? What seems required is a shift in the therapist's position from a "practicing down" attitude (Hoffman, 1991) to one of renewed respect for the client's voice and self-authoring capacities, a shift from the position of an imposing director of the action to a participant–observer (Anderson, 1991; Anderson & Goolishian, 1988) or participant–facilitator (Real, 1990) of the therapeutic conversation.

This new approach is highlighted in the clinical material in this chapter, which reflects not only a client's journey of liberation from an imposing past but a therapist's journey as well. Originally trained as a strategic therapist (Friedman, 1989a, 1989b; Friedman & Pettus, 1985), I have found myself on a journey of exploration of new forms and new pathways. Just as the client discussed here generated a new view of her life, so also did I move toward a new perspective about my clinical work. This journey required that the client and I both generate new maps for understanding.

The principles that have guided me on this voyage of discovery are an integration of several elements, including what my colleague Margot Fanger and I call "possibility therapy" (Friedman & Fanger, 1991), the solution-focused methods (e.g., de Shazer, 1985, 1988, 1991), and the work of White and Epston (1990) using the narrative metaphor. These ideas are evolving ones as my perspective expands and changes. I hope that the utility of these ideas will be reflected in the following presentation of clinical material.

My initial approach with the family to be described included normalizing their predicament and maintaining my attention on the parents' initial concerns (i.e., the son's behavior).

The family consisted of the parents, Matthew and Barbara Reynolds, and their four children: Sarah, age 17; John, age 14; Rachel, age 10; Ted, age 7. The original referral contained only the following description of John: "hard to handle lately . . . big mood swings; won't talk or listen; he says nothing is bothering him." That is the extent of the information I received prior to my first meeting with the family, which included only John and his parents. As I listened to the mother I came to understand that she was struggling with forces from the past that left her feeling constrained and oppressed and were getting in the way of her being the person (and parent) that she hoped to be. As I listened to her story I engaged her in an externalizing conversation and then provided an opportunity for her to re-author her story in ways that could liberate her from these oppressive and limiting forces.

## THE INITIAL SESSION

I made social conversation, and learned the names and ages of the children from the parents. I learned that the family lives in a working-class neighborhood of an industrial city and I also learn that the father (Matthew, M in the dialogue) was to be laid off from his job of 12 years (in another month) and was currently looking for work. I learned that the mother (Barbara, B in the dialogue) was working full-time as a nursing assistant in a nursing home on the 3:00 to 11:00 P.M. shift. The oldest child, Sarah, was a senior in high school and was busy with many outside activities. John (J) had responsibility for babysitting his two younger siblings; the parents commented that John resented being in such a responsible role. I asked my standard opening question as a way to get the family focused on their hopes and wishes for therapy and to let them know that I see the process as one in which *they* will provide direction.

T: Tell me what you were hoping to accomplish coming here. Whose idea was it?

M: I guess it was my idea . . . I think, due to the fact that I'm working full-time and Barbara is working full-time and John has to do all these things—we don't get enough time together. I can't talk to him. When I ask a question—"What's on your mind?" "nothing." That's what I get out of him. I ask him to do this [a household chore] and he starts yelling . . . he blows up. I would like to carry on a normal conversation, for him to let me know what's on his mind and we can discuss things.

It really bothers me that he can't. I think he keeps things inside and it's just festering. He goes around slamming doors. It's a bad influence on the younger two. It's kind of rubbing off and I want to stop it right now.

[I then ask the "miracle question" (de Shazer, 1988): "What if a miracle happened during the night while you were sleeping, and the problems you are concerned about all disappeared. When you woke up in the morning how could you tell that this miracle had happened?" Barbara starts crying, saying, "I always thought that when I had my children everything would be perfect . . . I just feel . . . of all of them John is the quietest. He keeps everything in—which I can respect because that's the way he is—but there's no touching, like with the other three." We discuss Barbara's perception that John isn't like the other children, who are more affectionate and verbally expressive of their feelings. Barbara then presents her picture of herself as coming from a "dysfunctional family" and by so doing expands the focus from John's sense of himself to her own self-perceptions.]

B:  I've been in therapy before, by myself, several years ago. I think I came from a dysfunctional home. I learned that through therapy. It's a cycle and I want to break it. (crying again) I feel guilty about being at work when the children come home from school . . . I do . . .

T:  (returning to the miracle question) Give me a picture of what things will look like after this miracle happens? What would you be seeing that would be happening?

B:  Us, happy at our meal times. You know, communication, less fighting among the kids.

T:  What would people be doing instead of the fighting?

M:  Talking to one another, caring for each other. More time to do things. Really get to know each other, so to speak.

T:  (to John) What difference would you see [the morning after the miracle]? Can you give me any ideas about that?

J:  (shakes head no) I don't know.

B:  I always wanted to be the perfect mother . . . I don't know. . . (cries) Maybe when he gets angry at us and he says things to us, which I don't think he really means . . . because I know I say things when I'm not feeling good about myself that come from my childhood. I have to remind myself that I can't do to my kids what my family did to me. (cries)

M:  She takes the tiniest little things sometimes and blows up and has a temper tantrum. I think John gets most of his temper from Barbara's side of the family. The tiniest little things will set Barbara off sometimes.

[Barbara then describes how she compares her children with other children and wonders if her parenting is okay.]

T: You keep wishing you were a better parent. *(to Matthew)* Your wife is a tough judge of herself. She keeps giving herself messages . . .

B: I do. . .

T: They're old messages from the past.

B: I loved my father and he had problems. And I thought when he died it would be over and it's not.

T: Part of it is carrying those messages on, those old scripts that you keep telling yourself.

[The conversation shifts back to John. I tell John I think he is a sensitive guy in his own way: "You show it in what you do."]

T: I'm going to excuse myself for a moment and do some thinking. I'll be right back.

[I leave the room and go into an empty office and sit down with my pad and pencil to jot down some thoughts, which I will use as feedback to the family before the session ends. My goal is to leave the family with some new perspective or view about their situation (Budman, Friedman, & Hoyt, 1992; Friedman & Fanger, 1991). I normalize the current reactivity as a response to recent stressors in the family and represent John's perceived negativity as self-protection.]

T: I think at this point it seems the family's under some stress. *(to Matthew)* Clearly, your job situation is an important piece of that. And, clearly, when stresses are up chances are that people are more reactive to one another. Everyone is just more sensitive. And as irritability levels go up there are more chances for friction.

B: It's been good lately since we called you. Hasn't it, Matthew? Even with John.

M: Yes.

[The parents' comments that improvement has happened already since making the initial call is not uncommon (Weiner-Davis, de Shazer, & Gingerich, 1987) and I could have capitalized on this had I asked about changes earlier in the interview.]

T: I think, in some ways John, you may feel some special pressure as the oldest boy, and you've got some special responsibilities. I think when someone is feeling pressure in that way, you feel like saying no, setting some limits.

[I emphasize the areas where I know (from remarks made earlier in the session) Matthew and John have a connection—baseball, fishing, and carpentry. I frame John as caring but in a different way from his siblings. I also comment on the old scripts that Barbara is vulnerable to and work at externalizing these messages as a force outside of Barbara over which she can begin to gain control.]

T: *(to John)* And I think you have your own special way of caring about your family, and *(to parents)* I would suggest that you notice when you see John showing that he cares in his own way. And it won't be as easy [to notice] as with your other children. *(to Barbara)* I think when things don't go the way you had hoped, those old scripts get triggered for you. They get running and you start thinking you're not doing a good enough job. I'd like you to think about what you do when you resist that urge to let those old scripts dominate your life. There are times when you don't let the old history get in the way, okay, when you're in charge. What do you do so that you're in charge of your life, not the old scripts? Because you need to be in control of your, life not that old history.

B: Uh huh. I have to take responsibility. Right now the only place I feel good is my job.

T: The more in control you are going to get, the more in control things are going to feel in the family. Do you want to set another time? *(to John)* Are you willing to come back?

J: Yeah.

[The parents agree and I ask them to decide about the value of having the whole family come to the next session.]

T: Would it be valuable to have the others come in as well?

B: It wouldn't hurt, I don't think. It might be good.

## BETWEEN THE FIRST TWO SESSIONS

An appointment 3 weeks hence was set for the whole family. A few days after the initial session I sent the parents the following letter as a way to reinforce and amplify what was discussed in our meeting:

*Dear Mr. and Mrs. Reynolds,*

*I wanted to write to you after our recent meeting to share some thoughts I had. I can see how seriously each of you takes your parenting responsibilities. I rarely see parents so committed to improving their relationships with their children and making family life more satisfying. I have the impression that the two of you don't give yourselves enough credit for the jobs you do well in regard to parenting. It is easy to overlook the good things we do and notice only those things that blow up in our faces.*

*I was especially impressed with John and the way he can sensitively show his caring by the things he does. While your other children are more expressive using words, John is especially adept at showing his caring in his actions. As I mentioned at the meeting, I would encourage you to notice and keep track of when John is showing his caring by doing. In addition, I would suggest that each of you make up a list of the positive qualities that exist in each of your children (those characteristics that make them special). Feel free to share this list with your children.*

*I am concerned about the old scripts that you, Mrs. Reynolds, have let get the upper hand in impacting on your perceived competence as a parent. You mentioned that 25% of the time you didn't let the old history push you around. Do you see some ways that you can increase that percentage to 35% ? What do you need to do to get the upper hand on the old history and keep it from getting in the way of your being the competent and capable parent that you are ? Each time you don't let the old scripts effect your current life you push it further into the past. Each time you let the real you come through, the you that is not triggered by old history, the stronger you will get.*

*I was impressed to hear that John is good with his hands. It sounds like he has a special gift in this regard. I'm hopeful that you, Mr. Reynolds, will have some opportunities to work with John on some carpentry projects in the future as a way to build a stronger relationship with your oldest son. Although life has its frustrations, I would suggest that you consider what you do when you resist the urge to let frustration get the better of you. I would be interested in hearing what you come up with.*

*I look forward to seeing you.*

*Sincerely,*

*Steven Friedman, PhD*

## THE SECOND SESSION

The next session took place 3 weeks after the first, and the whole family was present (S stands for Sarah). The parents came in ready to tell me about recent positive events: Barbara requested a change in her work schedule to allow her to be home after school, and Matthew found a new job. Notice how I encourage this talk about change and how the focus has now dramatically shifted away from John to Barbara's self-perceptions.

T: What other changes have happened since we met last? What other things have you noticed that have changed?

B: I'm trying to be more in control. I'm trying to really concentrate on it. The day after our meeting the last time I had to work the next night and I asked John if he could baby-sit and he got upset. And I don't blame him. He had youth group, and I said to myself, "I'm not going to force him, I'm not going to get upset about this."

T: Yes.

B: I called Matthew at work and explained. We had to work out something and we compromised. He took the younger ones with him.

T: You worked out something different . . .

B: Yes.

T: How did you manage that?

B: It was early in the morning and I said to myself, "I'm not going to get mad at him. He has a right not to want to baby-sit. We compromised and it worked out okay. But at other times I just get triggered.

T: *(to children)* Do you know what your mother means by "triggered"?

B: Sarah [the 17-year-old daughter] understands.

T: *(to Sarah)* We were talking last time about things from your mother's past that come up and get in the way. How can you tell when some of the old past stuff is getting in the way?

S: She's usually angry.

[I begin asking questions in an effort to externalize the "old scripts" that are oppressing Barbara.]

T: How does that affect you when you see that old history come up for her . . . when the old history takes control?

S: I don't take things she says seriously when she's acting like that.

T: So you can separate out that something else is going on here, outside the situation.

S: Yeah.

B: They'll go off in their rooms. We had company a couple of weeks ago and I woke up in the morning and I felt overwhelmed and I have to have everything perfect. I woke up in the morning and I said to Matthew, "I'm going to really try hard today to have a good day" *(cries)* and he helps me.

T: What would a good day look like?

B: Everything just perfect. I can remember my father telling me I'll never be like my mother.

T: Your mother kept the house in perfect order?

B: Yes. Everything was just perfect, everything. And I can hear those messages and I want to overcome them. I just don't know.

[Following up on my letter, I begin to look at the ways the "old scripts" influence and impact on Barbara's life. These externalizing conversations are an attempt to deconstruct Barbara's constraining narrative and to objectify the "old scripts" as a powerful force that influences her life. I ask Barbara questions about how this force impacts on her life across several domains and find that she is least vulnerable to their influence in the work setting. This information serves to challenge her "totalizing" descriptions of herself and to open up new options for change.]

T: These old messages are powerful. They have a powerful effect on people's lives. They stay with you. I have the sense that you're struggling to get past them and get control of them.

B: I want to be able to say to myself, "I know I'm not perfect."

T: It's hard to let go of the messages that say you're not doing enough, not doing good enough.

B: Matthew helps me. He helps me a lot. I don't mean to be like that.

T: When this old history comes up, how does it effect your relationship with the kids?

B: I feel like I'm an outsider from them . . . not as close as I could've been. *(cries)*

T: So the old scripts have a way of getting in the way of being closer. The old messages have a way of separating you from your children . . . so that you're not as close as you'd like to be. How about relationships outside the house?

B: I work with the elderly in a nursing home, and I'm not like I am at home. I basically have a lot of patience at work.

T: Somehow you've been able to keep your work from being effected.

B: Yes, it hasn't.

[Later in the session]

T: You gave an example at the beginning where you didn't let the old messages win out, so it sounds like there are times you can get the upper hand, although it takes some effort to do it.

[I then ask for other experiences where Barbara has gotten the upper hand on the old messages, and she gives other examples of walking away from situations with John and relying on her husband's support to respond in a different and calmer way. I then shift back to follow up on our original focus on John.]

T: Did you notice when John was showing his caring by doing?

[Barbara gives me two examples in which she noticed how John showed concern for his family.]

T: *(to Barbara)* I'm wondering how you can pat yourself on the back.

B: Deep within me I know I'm a good person.

T: The old messages rear up and wreak havoc. You've shown you can get the upper hand at work and on some occasions at home.

B: I can, I can.

[I state my idea of the goal for therapy and Barbara agrees.]

T: The idea is to get control and not let those messages push you around to an emotional place. It's a push. And at times you do. And that's what the goal is—to have more and more control over your own life. I think we need to keep talking about this. You've got a beautiful family here, which means that you and your husband have done a good job being parents. And it's a tough job. You've shown that you can get the upper hand on the old messages.

## BETWEEN THE SECOND AND THIRD SESSIONS

The next appointment was scheduled to take place in a month. About a week after the second session I sent Barbara a letter. In this letter I continued the process of "externalizing" and objectifying the oppressive forces and I give them a name—the Furies.

Dear Mrs. Reynolds,

I wanted to follow up with some thoughts I had after our last meeting. I enjoyed meeting your children and experienced their playfulness and their closeness . . . I was impressed by your report of how you avoided cooperating with the "old scripts" in dealing with John and by the ways you are able to keep the "old stories" from intruding into your work life. It seems, from our discussions, that your husband has been a great source of support to you in your quest to be unburdened by the old scripts. You are fortunate to have him by your side.

I was thinking of a name for the old scripts and one that came to mind was the Furies. The Furies are forces (described in Greek mythology) that represent feelings of guilt. They are part of the irrational world we sometimes carry with us. The Furies are the false, guilt-inducing voices that have been intruding on your life. It seems to me that at times the Furies wreak havoc on your relationships with your children and prevent your home life from being more satisfying. In that way the Furies are a very powerful force. Somehow, the Furies have gotten the idea that they have a permanent home with you. The goal will be to avoid cooperating with the Furies and, by so doing, to allow your own voice of inner peace and calm to be heard.

I wonder if you could make a list of the ways that the Furies try to direct your life. In this way it may be possible to plan a challenge to the Furies' domination. By giving the Furies the boot, you will be making space for inner peace and healing.

Please call or write me before our next appointment if you have any thoughts about this. I look forward to seeing you and your husband.

Sincerely,

Steven Friedman, PhD

Two days prior to our scheduled meeting I received the following letter from Barbara:

Dear Dr. Friedman,

I have been doing a lot of thinking since our last visit. This is the list I have come up with regarding "the Furies."

I am afraid to ask for help outside the immediate family. There was an instance during Christmas that I needed to borrow something from my sister. I was really scared to ask, but I told myself I would not be scared. In the end I couldn't do it. I can remember whenever I asked my father for something, he would usually yell at me and put me down, even in my adult life.

I find fault with everything in the house. At Christmas time I wasn't happy with the way my house looked with all the decorations. I moved the tree three times and still wasn't satisfied. I found myself at one point unwrapping a few gifts because I wasn't happy with the way it looked. I have to have everything perfect if we entertain but will procrastinate to the last minute to get the work done. In my head I know I have the work to do but I always set myself up.

A few weeks ago a person at work gave me a beautiful compliment. I couldn't believe what she said about me could be actually true.

I want my children to be perfectly behaved. Especially when we go visiting. I get very uptight if the boys wrestle on the floor. I remember this because my sister called this to my attention. I can recall that growing up, my brothers, sister, and I were always perfectly behaved. It was expected of us.

Dr. Friedman, these are just a few that I could zero in on. I hope this helped you.

Sincerely,

Barbara Reynolds

## THE THIRD SESSION

The third session took place a month after the second and included only Barbara and Matthew.

T: I got your letter . . . and it was a very helpful description of the way what I was calling the Furies push you around.

B: When I put it on paper it looks so stupid. It's like trivial stuff.

T: What were your thoughts about my letter, how I was thinking about the Furies? It seems like there are these forces that make you feel guilty.

B: Right, right.

T: Did that fit for you?

B: Yes, definitely.

T: I don't know if you had some other words to describe this force. One of the things I put together, and I'll give you a copy, is the laws of the Furies.

[I proceed to read the laws which are reproduced here (adapted from Esler, 1987; White, 1986), and then begin a process of asking questions so that Barbara can begin to re-author her story in a way that places her in control, not the Furies.]

The Laws of the Furies

1. THE FURIES feed on attention.
2. THE FURIES like to find a home with people who are experts in self-torture.
3. THE FURIES look to escape from places where they're ignored.

4. Since THE FURIES are always hungry, it is possible to starve them by not letting them dominate your thoughts or influence your actions.

5. THE FURIES have one fear (which they try to keep secret). This fear is that people will give up believing in them. When this happens they lose their power and disappear.

T:  What I'm wondering is when you think you're going to be ready to push these Furies out of your life.

B:  I want them out now.

T:  What do you think it's going to be like to have your life back, without these Furies pushing you around ?

B:  Like you said, inner peace. Just accepting me for who I am and letting all that old stuff go. My sister Sharon told me that she remembers our parents telling her she'd never be anything but there was always something in her saying she will be something.

T:  She fought it then and you're fighting it now . . . and the Furies have had more time to take hold. Does she have some ideas when you tell her about what's going on with you?

B:  She understands. It was a dysfunctional family, I know it was. She came out of our childhood hating more that I did.

T:  She was more angry.

B:  Angry, but able to get out of the house, while we *(glances at her husband)* stayed in the house.

    [Barbara explains that she took care of her alcoholic father after he had a stroke. During this period he was very angry and irritable.]

T:  What are your thoughts about how you've prevented the Furies from taking over completely?

B:  I don't know.

    [Barbara explains how her husband helps by telling her to calm down when she gets upset.]

T:  With some people I would expect their whole life would be dominated by the Furies.

B:  Yes, right. No, it hasn't.

T:  What would you anticipate if you let the Furies stay with you into the future?

B:  A miserable life. He *(looks at husband)* would be unhappy.

T:  What does it mean "being miserable"? What is your picture of this, of letting the Furies dominate your life?

B:  Maybe getting more depressed. I can remember a couple of years ago when I was in treatment, I was sleeping all the time [after her father's death]. But now I have a job. I have to work.

T: So you made some positive changes.

B: Yes.

T: But you could imagine that if you let the Furies continue you could go back in that state.

B: Could be.

T: *(to Matthew)* What sense do you have about that, if the Furies continued pushing her around?

M: Well, like she said, she would just go back into her little shell and start sleeping all day and lose her job.

[Barbara describes a change she made in her work hours that allows her to be home when the children return from school. It was necessry that she ask her supervisor for the change, which she was able to do. This change also relieves John of some baby-sitting responsibilities, and Barbara reports a positive change in the household with this arrangement.]

T: *(to Barbara)* What kind of compliment did you get that you mentioned in your letter?

B: I was doing my work. It was just before Christmas and one of the temporary staff stopped me in the hall and said, "Barbara, I just wanted you to know that you're a beautiful person, the way you take care of these people and the way you treat them." I had tears in my eyes. I told her I didn't feel that way. How people perceive me, I don't see myself, though. I said, "Thank you," and gave her a hug. But when I went home and thought about it I said to myself, "I don't see myself like that."

T: That's where the Furies come in with their negative messages. You see what I mean?

B: Uh huh.

T: So a good sign would be your being able to accept compliments . . . and in a way you did accept the compliment.

B: Yeah. Right, right.

T: But you still had some doubts. And that's the Furies coming in and getting in the way.

B: For example, at our last meeting, I was getting upset about how Ted [the youngest child] was behaving. Because in our childhood we were like this *(demonstrates sitting straight up, prim and proper)*.

T: That stuck with you. One of the ways that you will know that the Furies are going away is when you're able to tolerate those situations in a different way. And these situations will come up again. I was asking before what your picture would be if the Furies stay with you. And I'm also interested in what the picture will be like when the Furies disappear and you have that inner peace. What will life be like at home?

B:  I think a better marriage.

T:  When you stop cooperating with the Furies, what else will be different?

B:  The relationship with my children. I would feel closer to them. Joyful and being happy to be up in the morning.

T:  What other changes will happen in the family when you decide not to cooperate with these Furies?

B:  I would enjoy my children more, accept them for themselves.

M:  Probably there would be a lot less yelling and more cooperation from the kids.

T:  What needs to happen now is to look at the ways—and I know it happens now—when you don't let the Furies win out. I think the times when they do are powerful and you tend to notice that, but there are also times when you handled a situation calmly.

B:  I think John has calmed down a lot over this past month, don't you think, Matthew? There haven't been as many confrontations.

M:  I haven't yelled at him in a while.

T:  I think that's a sign that somehow you are getting control over these Furies. What I would be interested in is asking you to keep track of the times when you haven't cooperated with the Furies, when you and not the Furies, are in control of your life. That's the aim here, for you to experience that inner peace, to get a compliment . . .

B:  And let it absorb.

T:  Right, let it sink in. And it's going to take some active efforts. You mentioned your sister and how she would say no to your parents' demands, would express herself very clearly, and you may need to say that to the Furies, not let these outside forces control your life. Because you deserve that kind of inner peace.

B:  I know I have four beautiful children.

T:  Yeah. I was very impressed with them.

B:  And there again, when you sent the letter, the opening said how you enjoyed their playfulness. And I couldn't accept that. I thought they weren't behaving themselves.

T:  I took Ted's exuberance very positively, that he was feeling comfortable being here. It's going to take a little work to let the Furies know they're not needed anymore, that you don't want them around. Your sister is a support to you, as is your husband. And maybe there are some things your sister learned how to do that can be useful to you in gaining control over these forces.

B:  Maybe.

T:  Another idea I have is for you to note, to put into a sentence, what the messages are that the Furies send. For example: "Question the validity of all compliments," "Expect the children to behave perfectly," "Don't ask help from others," et cetera.

B: Okay, okay.

T: And with that, make me a list of the ways that you've *not* cooperated with the Furies' messages, when you're calm, even momentarily, and find some inner peace. And I would also suggest you look over the list of the Laws of the Furies as a way of getting the upper hand and getting these Furies out of your life.

## AFTER THE THIRD SESSION

Four days after this session I sent Barbara the following letter:

*Dear Mrs. Reynolds:*

*I wanted to write to follow up on our last meeting. I was impressed with the commitment of your husband to helping you rid your life of the influence of the Furies. Working together as a team, as you seem to do so well, is an effective way to gain the upper hand on the Furies. It also sounds like you have the help of your sister Sharon who understands the struggle that you are undertaking to gain inner peace and calm. Your sister seems to have taken on the Furies earlier in her life and maybe her anger served in some useful way in winning over them. This might be interesting to discuss with her.*

*Considering your very structured upbringing I am impressed with your flexibility in creating a different and more open family environment than the one you knew growing up. This is not easy to accomplish, especially in light of your great loyalty to your parents.*

*Your shift in work hours so you can be home in the afternoon for your children is a wonderful gift that you are giving them, that is also working to gain inner peace for you and the family.*

*You described your ideas for what would happen if the Furies were to take over completely (i.e., you would become depressed, sleep all the time, "go back into a shell," etc.). I wonder how you have prevented this from happening. As I mentioned in our last meeting, it might be useful to make a list of those <u>situations when you do not cooperate with the Furies'</u> messages, but make choices for yourself. This may be experienced as feeling some of the inner peace you desire, feeling some happiness getting up in the morning, enjoying your children more (and accepting them as they are), feeling closer to your children and feeling more joyful and self-confident. One way I can tell that you are winning over the Furies is that John was described as calmer over this past month and that you and your husband were yelling less.*

*In addition, as we discussed, it might also be helpful to make a list of the messages that the Furies send (e.g., "Don't ask for help from outsiders," "Question all compliments as unworthy"). By doing this we can have a better idea of how to counteract the power of the Furies. By the way, by coming to see me you are already not cooperating with one of the Furies messages!*

*I look forward to seeing you and your husband and hearing about the steps you've taken to gain inner peace and calm.*

*Sincerely,*

*Steven Friedman, PhD*

## THE FOURTH SESSION

In the next session, 2½ weeks after the last one, I began by asking questions that opened space for Barbara to re-author and expand her previously limiting narratives and to begin to experience and express an increased sense of personal agency. She was beginning to talk to herself in ways that were leading to a new sense of empowerment.

T: You got my letter.

B: And I made my lists *(hands them to therapist).*

T: These are the messages—"anger, negative thoughts, self-pity; unworthy as a person."

B: I put "self-pity." Sometimes I feel sorry for myself and cry. And I think sometimes they [the Furies] feed off of that.

T: Yes. That's exactly right. That makes you vulnerable. . .

[The remainder of the session is devoted to reviewing Barbar's successes, that is, the occasions she listed when she did not "cooperate" with the Furies' messages.]

The list is entitled "Don't cooperate with the Furies" and included the following:

> I calmly approached a situation and remained in control;
> I tried to tell myself I am a worthy person;
> I looked at the positive things I have done for my children all their lives;
> Defending myself against someone who puts me down;
> Deserving"

B: *(smiling)* The first one I'm the most proud of.

T: Tell me about this.

B: It was a couple of days after we saw you. And I could have just walked away and let him [Matthew] handle it. And I said to Matthew, "No Matthew, I'm going to handle this." And I told myself, even before I went to John, "I'm going to be in control and handle this"—and I did!

T: How did you take that step?

B: I just said to myself, "I want to handle this and I'm not going to be in control of him. I'm not going to holler at him . . . and make me want to have the last word." And it worked. Wonderful. We compromised.

T: So it wasn't just an imposing . . . it was a negotiation.

B: I was so proud of myself.

T: How did you manage to not let the Furies control your behavior in this situation?

B: I didn't want to holler at him.

T: What were you doing that was allowing you the freedom to not let the Furies push you around?

B: I talked to him like a human being. I don't know. It just worked out.

T: You worked with him in a way that felt like a resolution.

B: Instead of me controlling and telling him "you've got to do what I tell you to do."

T: I'm trying to understand how . . .

B: How I did it. A month ago I would have probably dragged him out of the bed.

T: What were you thinking that was helping you not cooperate with the Furies?

B: Was I calmer or feeling better about myself? I don't know. I did it instantaneously.

T: You were feeling ready.

B: Right. I was determined. I wasn't going to lose my temper with him. And I did it!

T: You surprised yourself about that.

B: I've been proud about that for two weeks.

T: That's wonderful! Taking this step, in this one situation, a positive step in a situation where you've, in the past, gotten into some difficulties with the Furies. So in what ways does taking that step make you more confident about future steps?

B: *(bright smile)* I feel like him and I have a better relationship together. I feel it already.

[She then describes another example where she dealt calmly with John.]

T: It sounds to me that some of that inner peace and calm is coming through. You're finding it in dealing with John. Who do you think would be least surprised at your taking this step at this time?

B: *(looking confused)* Surprised?

T: *Least* surprised.

B: I don't know. That's a hard one. My sister Sharon maybe. What do you mean?

T: Who would be least surprised?

B: That I was able to accomplish this?

T: Yes.

B: Sharon has confidence in me.

T: What is it that she's seen in you that would allow her to predict that you would have a successful interaction with John?

B: *(pauses)* Gosh . . . I don't know. Sensitive?

T: So she may see some sensitivity that you have, caring.

B: Deep down she knows I'm a caring person, and I'm sensitive. We weren't close as siblings. She treated me like dirt. And she recently apologized for taking advantage of my being sensitive. And now we're close. We talked about this about a week ago.

T: She may see you as sensitive, caring. Being able to work things out without conflict, may be something she would see.

B: Yeah.

T: If you think back in your own life, what would have allowed you to predict you would have handled this situation with John in the positive way you did?

B: *(pauses)* I was always a dreamer . . . as an adolescent. I was going to tell my children, when I had children, that they were special and unique.

T: Being a dreamer, then, you were always a hopeful person . . .

   [I use the idea of Barbara's being a "dreamer" to help her further amplify and consolidate the changes she has begun to make.]

B: Right, right.

T: And putting in some effort to create better times.

B: Our children are not like the way we grew up. I think you put that in the letter. One thing I thought of after I read your letter: My father used to come home drunk practically every night, and I remember hiding in the closet. And I was determined that I would never have a father to my children who didn't come home at night after work. And he *(looks at Matthew)* always has. So I controlled that; I didn't let it happen.

T: Yes. That's right.

B: Matthew's always been there for me.

T: That's certainly working at trying to change those patterns, and very successfully. Well, I'm impressed. I wrote in the letter about the flexibility that you have that's different from your family growing up.

B: It is different. It is.

   [Barbara describes the restrictions in her childhood: For example, she was never allowed to talk on the phone until she was in high school, and she was not allowed to sleep over friends' houses.]

T: You've made a different life for yourself and your children. I want to get to these other things on the list.

B: I was writing them down as I thought of them.

T: *(reads next item)* "I try to tell myself I'm a worthy person."

B: Lately, I've been thinking about when my children were born. That I was a wonderful mother when they were born, holding them . . .

T: You remember all the care you gave.

B: *(proudly)* I am a good mother! *(laughs)* I still have those thoughts about the past but I have to let it go. I'm almost forty-two.

T: *(returns to the list)* "I look at the positive things I've done for my children all their lives."

B: How proud I am of our children. Our oldest is off to college in the fall. She was accepted to her first-choice school and with a scholarship. She's a wonderful person. She's turning out the way I dreamed that she would. We must have done something right.

T: You obviously did something to allow her to get to this point, to take these steps.

B: We always paid attention to her needs.

T: You listened and it paid off. She seems to take after you in being such a caring person.

B: And motivated. Ted comes in from school smiling and I say, "Ted, you're always smiling. How come you're so happy?" He says, "I'm just happy," and I said, "What's special about you?" and he said, "Me."

T: So, he's got a real positive sense of himself, and there are things the two of you have done to instill that in the kids. Let's go back to the list. "Defend yourself." Tell me about that one.

B: There's a nurse that I work with and she can be very demeaning. And she did it to me. It struck a chord in me and very nicely I told her off—and that's not like me. But the way she talked to me was the way my father did. And I'm not going to let anybody do that to me.

T: You asserted yourself without letting the Furies get to you.

B: Or cry or or feel bad about myself. I'm the type of person who would cry and go in a corner and feel sorry for myself. But I didn't do that. I'm not going to let her talk down to me.

T: You took a stand with her.

B: And I think she got the message because she was more friendly afterwards.

T: You wrote the word "deserving."

[Barbara then describes having had the assistance of two aides, which is unusual, one evening at work and thinking to herself, "I deserve this. I work very hard . . . which is unusual for me to say to myself . . . I don't need to work hard tonight."]

T: Wonderful! How does taking these steps—and you've taken quite a few over the past two and a half weeks, affect your picture of yourself as a person?

B: You can tell. Today I feel great. *(beams)* I feel better. I feel positive about myself. I can go home and handle any situation with John or the others. I feel confident.

T: What do these steps tell you and tell your husband about what you're wanting your life to be like?

B: Happier, closer. Sarah gave us a book as a Christmas gift when she was in the fourth or fifth grade called *The Family*. And it's a beautiful poem about what a family is. They forgive each other, they share. That's what I want us to be. For her to have bought this in the fourth or fifth grade, she must have thought our family was like this.

T: Yes.

B: My oldest one noticed me being a little different. I asked her.

T: What did she say?

B: She notices a calmness in me. Sometimes I'll get a little upset but catch myself.

T: The Furies come in but they don't overtake you.

[Barbara then describes a recent situation in which she made a turkey dinner and left all the dishes piled up. In the past she would have found this worrisome: "I would have gotten mad at myself for leaving them sit." But this time she just laughed and felt comfortable looking at the piles of dishes.]

T: You didn't let the Furies get to you . . .

B: I have to concentrate, especially to fight the messages from the past.

T: I suggest you continue to keep a list of when you don't cooperate with the Furies. Keep adding to the list. It takes concentration, and your actions are already making a difference. In how many weeks would you like to set the next appointment?

B: How about four weeks?

## AFTER THE FOURTH SESSION

About a week after this appointment I sent Barbara the following letter:

*Dear Mrs. Reynolds:*

*I wanted to write to share some thoughts I had after our last meeting.*

*As a fortune cookie recently informed me, "The first step to better times is to imagine them." Being a dreamer, as you described yourself, seems to have allowed you to imagine a better life for yourself and your family. Not only did you imagine that positive future, you have acted to create it.*

*Your ability to move from self-pity to self-love is a major step. The examples you presented at our last meeting—how you approached a situation with John, calmly, how you experienced yourself as a worthwhile person, how you saw and accepted the positive things you and your husband have done for your children over the years, how you asserted yourself when you felt demeaned by another person, and how you saw yourself as a deserving human being who is entitled to a life unburdened by self-pity and self-torture—showed me that you are letting go of the past and have made a new future for yourself and your family.*

*Just to be sure the Furies are on their way out of your life, I would suggest you continue to write down the ways you do not cooperate with their demands. By so doing you will free yourself to step more fully into the future. As you experience the inner peace and calm of this step, your life will become your own again.*

*Thanks for allowing me to come along on this journey of liberation.*

*Sincerely,*

*Steven Friedman, PhD*

## FOLLOW-UP

In the fifth session, a month later, Barbara reported that although she had suffered some setbacks at the hands of the Furies over the month between sessions, she also experienced more positive days when she felt in control. As she put it, "I'm having feelings . . . like . . . I can't explain it . . . just happiness inside . . . inner peace . . . a feeling like I could deal with anything. It was a good feeling." She also reports day-dreaming about the future in a positive way; seeing herself going to nursing school and imagining herself and her husband "growing old together" with the children off on their own. I normalized the setbacks as "hiccups on the road of life" (Elms, 1986) and encouraged Barbara to continue to track the positive feelings of calm and inner peace. At the end of the meeting she said, "What I like about calling them the Furies is, it's not blaming anyone. I am an adult and I have to be responsible for myself." What follows are excerpts from two letters I received from Barbara after the sixth session:

*I thought I would let you know how I am doing. . . . I feel like I am handling each situation calmly and being supportive of my children. I have been experiencing more times of inner peace and calm. There was one day the two younger children and I had the radio on and we started dancing together. We were laughing and having fun. There are other times when I just have warm and happy feelings flowing through me.*

*John has been very good. He seems more happy and content. He did some baby-sitting for me a couple of days. He really did a good job. I wanted to do something special for him, so I bought him a new baseball comforter for his bed. He was really surprised. I wanted to show him I appreciated what he did for me.*

*There were a couple of times the Furies did try to surface. I did not let* them take complete control. I left the situation for a few minutes, calmed down, and returned to do what I was doing.

Matthew and I are grower closer together. We communicate more. I am very lucky to have had a husband who stuck by me and who didn't give up on me. My family is the most important thing to me. A family just doesn't happen, you have to work at it. Thank you for all your help.

                              ★    ★    ★

I wanted to share some thoughts and feelings while they are still fresh in my mind. The other day I realized for a while now I have not been thinking about my past. I am not as emotional. I know there will be times in my life when my thoughts and feelings will surface. I think I have learned to experience them and let them go. They are part of me.

I may write again before our next visit. Thank you for being part of my Journey to Liberation.

Sincerely,

Barbara Reynolds

I am continuing to meet with Barbara and her husband, at their request, on an intermittent basis (every 6 to 8 weeks).

## EDITORIAL QUESTIONS[1]

Q:  *You describe your approach as an integration of both solution-focused methods and the narrative perspective. Could you delineate more specifically some of the principles, ideas, and assumptions that inform your current clinical work?*

A: My clinical work reflects an integration of several domains of thinking. Since I was originally trained in structural/strategic therapy and in the brief treatment model of the Mental Research Institute of Palo Alto, CA, my work tended to be brief and problem-centered. More recently, I have incorporated solution-focused thinking and the narrative perspective into my clinical work. Basically, I am a pragmatic integrationist, tailoring various models to the clinical situation at hand. Being an experimentalist by training, I enjoy trying out different approaches and observing their impact in a variety of clinical contexts.

I think of myself as a "possibility therapist" (Friedman & Fanger, 1991), that is, one who approaches the client with a naive, curious, open, and inquisitive mind; keeps assumptions simple; avoids elaborate explanatory thinking; takes seriously the client's request; respects the client's resources and creativity; thinks in terms of solutions rather than problems; takes a hopeful, future-oriented stance; looks for opportunities to introduce

---

[1]I wish to thank Sally Brecher, MSW, and Jonathan Simmons, PhD, for generating ideas and questions for this section.

novel ideas or perspectives; and views language as the key to therapeutic change. Therapy is a conversation in which dialogue between therapist and client leads to the generation of new meanings, understandings, and options for action. The goal is to engage in conversations with the client in which alternative views of the "self-in-context" become possible and even inevitable.

My major aim in therapy is to stay "simple," especially in dealing with complex clinical situations. Since clients and therapists can easily become immersed in "problem-talk," I maintain my focus on those aspects of self and relationships that point to change. With the therapist searching for and amplifying *exceptions* (de Shazer, 1988) or *unique outcomes* (White & Epston, 1990), the stage is set for clients to become more vigilant and observant about their resources and competencies and less mired in discourses of despair. Since meanings in language are inherently unstable (i.e., negotiable), opportunities exist for co-creating ideas that support client competence and allow for the construction of new more empowering stories. As Parry (1991) puts it so well, "A narrative therapist seeks to raise into the foreground of the person's attention, alternate stories . . . in order to challenge the received text or life-story in its constraining role" (p. 52).

Q: *In the initial interview, but even more clearly in the second session, your attention shifts to the mother's self-perceptions even though the parents come in originally with concerns about their son John. Why did you choose to move in that direction and what enabled the focus of treatment to move away from John as the primary concern and toward the mother? I would imagine that some parents would not be so amenable to looking at themselves when they came for help about their child.*
A: This is an interesting question. The shift from the son to the mother as the main character in this therapy occurred quite naturally as a function of my initial conversations with the parents. In my work with families I respect the parental agenda and work from there, being careful not to stray too far afield from their original request unless this is openly negotiated. In the situation with the Reynolds family it became evident very early on in the initial interview that Barbara harbored some negative self-perceptions as a parent and as a person. When I engaged in discussion about these areas Barbara seemed amenable and open, actively encouraging the conversation.

The initial session was primarily devoted to a discussion about John. What I have chosen to share in the transcript narrows the lens to focus on Barbara since she ultimately became the main character in this story. In the second session it was Barbara who took the lead in talking about herself. I brought the conversation back to John since I did not want to ignore the parents' original concerns. Barbara very quickly and easily moved to refocus on her self-perceptions, and this then became the agenda we pursued in our subsequent contacts. We did continue, from time to time, to discuss how John was doing, even though it was clear that Barbara had accepted the responsibility to make changes in her own life and that she understood that those changes could positively impact on the well-being of all of her children.

Shifting attention from child to parent in therapy is not typical of the work that I do. I usually focus my attention on the parents' concerns about their child and actively engage them in a process of helping their child overcome the difficulty. This clinical situation illustrates for me how we need to be open and flexible in shifting gears depending on the flow of the conversation, how we need to develop the ability as P. Hill (personal communication, November 1986) puts it, "to be distracted by important information."

Q: *In your clinical example you ask Barbara to notice and track certain behaviors (e.g., the ways she keeps herself from being directed by the Furies). Your letters also contain task assignments. How do you reconcile being a neutral participant-facilitator of the therapeutic conversation with having clear goals for the therapy and using "strategic" methods to achieve them? How do directive approaches fit with a language-based collaborative model?*
A: This is a very important question. I think there are some real differences in how people view this issue. My belief is that you cannot avoid having goals. I don't believe the therapist can be neutral. One of my goals is to join with clients in the pursuit of *their* desired outcome. By so doing I align with the client's wishes and hopes for change. I feel it is my job to facilitate a process that enables clients to take actions in their lives that will allow them to experience more satisfying futures. It seems most respectful if we join together with our clients in a process that leads to some achievable outcome. The route to achieving a positive outcome may be circuitous but having some well-constructed goals in mind prevents the therapist from wandering off on some interminable journey without direction.

The tasks that I suggest are ones that I believe will enable clients to generate, out of their own observations and experiences, exceptions to the old constraining story, thus creating opportunities for new descriptions. I don't see a discrepancy between a collaborative language-based stance and using directives or tasks. Obviously, therapists need to be respectful of the client and to sensitively match their suggestions with the wishes and goals of the client. Any conversation has the potential to be one of imposition or of mutuality. The use of directives or tasks, when approached in the context of mutuality, becomes just another form of therapeutic conversation that works to enable the client to achieve their desired outcome.

Q: *I wondered about the father's role in the therapy process. Although he attended each session, his role seemed very peripheral. If the mother was the main character in this story, the father was certainly in a very minor supporting role. How did you involve the father in the therapy process, and how did you envision his role?*

A: Yes, the father was very much in a supportive role—in both senses of the word. Barbara seemed to find Matthew's presence helpful. She would look to him for reassurance and validation. He actually did more talking than the transcript shows, but this was usually in the way of social conversation between him and me. Most importantly Matthew served as a witness to the changes his wife was making.

Q: *This clinical example reflects a significant investment of the therapist's time and energy in the letter-writing process. How can a therapist manage to invest such time and energy in light of resource limitations that exist today in most human services agencies?*

A: My aim in letter writing is to make concrete the ideas discussed with clients and to further amplify and highlight unique outcomes (Friedman, 1992; Menses, 1986; White & Epston, 1990). Although letter writing can be a very time-consuming task, I find it helps me to articulate my ideas more clearly. Since preparing letters does require an investment of time and energy, I don't write to everyone I see. Often, I simply write one letter after the initial visit to summarize and expand upon issues discussed. I heard Michael White (1991) say that a letter is worth five sessions. If that is so, the time put into such pursuits seems well worth it. In the clinical situation discussed, Barbara's response to my initial letter was so positive that I felt compelled to continue. That doesn't always happen. In addition, my writing to her inspired her to begin writing to me. This was something I neither anticipated nor initially encouraged. In fact, Barbara also began writing to her son John as a way to allow herself to be heard without getting a defensive response from him.

Q: *Do you focus on making your treatment brief or is brevity simply a by-product of your theoretical orientation?*

A: Paradoxically, the less time I spend worrying about doing brief therapy and the more time I spend listening to my client's stories and accessing narratives of strength and competence, the more time-effective my treatment becomes. Although I work in a setting that has established limits on the number of sessions that clients can access, I rarely discuss these benefit limitations with clients. Rather, I direct my energies to the client's goals and engage him or her in conversations that enable those goals to be reached. I have a great deal of faith in the client's ability to regulate their time in therapy (Friedman & Fanger, 1991).

My therapy is sometimes brief in the traditional sense (i.e., one to three sessions over a short period of time), and sometimes occurs intermittently over longer periods of time (e.g., 6 months to 5 years). I may see people every 3, 4, or 6 weeks or for several sessions over brief periods of time that are separated by intervals of noncontact. The use of tasks, letters, and telephone calls all provide continuity across periods in which there is no face-to-face contact.

## ACKNOWLEDGMENTS

I wish to express my appreciation to "Barbara Reynolds" for allowing me to present her story in this chapter and to Donna Haig Friedman, MS, for her constructive and thoughtful comments on the manuscript.

## REFERENCES

Anderson, H. (1991, Oct/Nov). *A collaborative-language based systems approach to therapy*. Paper presented at the meeting of American Association of Marital and Family Therapists, Dallas.

Anderson, H., & Goolishian, H. A. (1988). Human systems as linguistic systems: Preliminary and evolving ideas about the implications for clinical theory. *Family Process, 27*, 371–393.

Budman, S., Friedman, S., & Hoyt, M. (1992). Last words on first sessions. In S. Budman, M. Hoyt, & S. Friedman (Eds.), *The first session of brief therapy* (pp. 345–358). New York: Guilford Press.

de Shazer, S. (1985). *Keys to solution in brief therapy*. New York: Norton.

de Shazer, S. (1988). *Clues: Investigating solutions in brief therapy*. New York: Norton.

de Shazer, S. (1991). *Putting difference to work*. New York: Norton.

Elms, R. (1986). To tame a temper. *Family Therapy Case Studies, 1*, 51–58.

Esler, I. (1987). Winning over worry. *Family Therapy Case Studies, 2*(1), 15-23.

Friedman, S. (1989a). Brief systemic psychotherapy in a health maintenance organization. *Family Therapy, 16*, 133–144.

Friedman, S. (1989b). Strategic reframing in a case of "delusional jealousy." *Journal of Strategic and Systemic Therapies, 8*, 1-4.

Friedman, S. (1992). Creating solutions (stories) in brief family therapy. In S. Budman, M. Hoyt, & S. Friedman (Eds.), *The first session of brief therapy* (pp. 282–305). New York: Guilford Press.

Friedman, S., & Fanger, M. T. (1991). *Expanding therapeutic possibilities: Getting results in brief psychotherapy*. New York: Lexington Books/Macmillan.

Friedman, S., & Pettus, S. (1985). Brief strategic interventions with families of adolescents. *Family Therapy, 12*, 197-210.

Hoffman, L. (1991). A reflexive stance for family therapy. *Journal of Strategic and Systemic Therapies, 10*, 4–17.

Kowalski, K., & Durrant, M. (1991, Oct/Nov). *Foolish constructions: Co-dependent vs. competent*. Paper presented at the meeting of American Association of Marital and Family Therapists, Dallas.

Menses, G. (1986). Theraspondulitis and theraspondence: The art of therapeutic letter writing. *Family Therapy Case Studies, 1*(1), 61–64.

Parry, A. (1991). A universe of stories. *Family Process, 30*, 37–54.

Real, T. (1990). The therapeutic use of self in constructionist/systemic therapy. *Family Process, 29*, 255–272.

Weiner-Davis, M., de Shazer, S., & Gingerich, W. J. (1987). Building on pretreatment change to construct the therapeutic solution: An exploratory study. *Journal of Marital and Family Therapy, 13,* 359–363.

White, M. (1986). Negative explanation, restraint, and double description: A template for family therapy. *Family Process, 25,* 169–184.

White, M. (1991, October). *Re-authoring lives and relationships.* Workshop at Leonard Morse Hospital, Natick, MA.

White, M., & Epston, D. (1990). *Narrative means to therapeutic ends.* New York: Norton.

# 12

## In Pursuit of a Better Life: A Mother's Triumph

SALLY BRECHER
STEVEN FRIEDMAN

*Looking at the family apart from its social context is like studying the dynamics of swimming by examining a fish in a frying pan.*
—SALVADOR MINUCHIN

Many families in poverty experience a narrative of demoralization and hopelessness, a sense of limited control and diminished personal agency over life events. This discourse of despair is not without its impact on family functioning (e.g., Schorr & Schorr, 1988). Just as socioeconomic issues cannot easily be ignored in society, so too do they deserve our attention in therapy. To be effective, respectful, and responsive to families facing complex social problems, therapists need to view socioeconomic issues as a major contextual force.

"One [child] in five lives in a family with an income below the federal poverty level" (National Commission, 1991, p. 24). Over 25% of the children in the United States live with one parent and the "poverty rate for children in single-parent families exceeds 50%" (Ellwood, 1988, p.128). As Ellwood (1988) points out, "Single parents [mostly female] typically must balance the dual roles of nurturer and provider . . . [and] are often supported by a welfare system that humiliates, stigmatizes and isolates them while offering limited support of incentives to become independent" (p. 129). These economic hardships are too often not given the attention they deserve in our therapeutic endeavors. The contributions of Salvador Minuchin,

Braulio Montalvo, and their colleagues (1967) are an exception, as is the work of Harry Aponte (1976, 1977). These pioneers tried to understand the culture of poverty and to highlight the powerful impact of socioeconomic factors on both family life and the therapy process. More recently, Gillian Walker (1991) has been engaged in a particularly innovative effort to work collaboratively with poor families suffering with the AIDS virus.

Power in our society is reflected in one's "access to resources and the capacity to be pro-active in one's behalf" (Imber-Black, 1986, p. 32). This ability to effect change, to be pro-active, provides a basis for "feelings of efficacy" (R. White, 1959) since our actions are reflected back to us in the world. Without such contingent feedback we are left feeling depressed, hopeless, and disempowered. Seligman (1975) refers to this process as one of "learned helplessness," a demoralizing process of finding our actions without effect. In what ways can the therapist create a context for hope?

This process of creating a context for hope is intimately connected to the methods the therapist uses in helping clients reach their goals and create changes in their lives. Tomm (1990) discusses "ethical postures" that therapists can take as they make therapeutic decisions. Some of these choices serve to open space (increase options) while others close space (reduce options). How do we as therapists engage in a collaborative process of increasing options and avoid becoming a "colonial presence" (Hoffman, 1991; Kearney, Byrne, & McCarthy, 1989) such that we are acting to further oppress those with whom we work? As Tomm (1990) points out, our picture of the client is influential in determining the approach we take. If we see clients as "resistant" or "misguided," we are more likely to engage in more manipulative or confrontative interventions. If we see clients as subjugated or oppressed, we are more likely to engage in processes that assist clients to liberate themselves from these constraining forces.

In the interview presented here a family from a poor working-class town is struggling economically. And it is these economic issues that are in part responsible for wreaking havoc on their lives and relationships. It is the mother's hope to "make a better life for the family" by getting off welfare that accounts for much of the positive change that occurs.

By maintaining her focus on strengths and resources, the therapist (Sally Brecher) sets her sights on "possibilities" rather than problems (Friedman & Fanger, 1991). Viewing the family's behavior through a lens of hopefulness, she integrates into the session a therapeutic ritual of healing and helps set the stage for the family to "re-author" (White & Epston, 1990) their lives and relationships in a way that supports the mother's sense of herself as a competent and nurturing caregiver to her children and the children as capable and responsible.

At a follow-up session, 5 months after the initial meeting, a reflecting team (Andersen, 1990) serves as an "audience to change," acknowledging, amplifying, and situating the changes made in a context of hopefulness. The therapist externalizes and objectifies the economic pressures on the family

and supports and facilitates the mother's wish to win over economic constraints. By empathizing with the mother's plight while supporting her
wishes for change, the therapist opens space for her client to reclaim a sense
of hope and optimism about the future.

## THE FAMILY

Sandra, a divorced mother of three, initially sought counseling for her
9-year-old son, Matt, whose behavior problems at school resulted in a
5-day suspension. Noted were Matt's unprovoked physical attacks on other
children and his lack of respect for teachers. At home he was quick to anger
and would, at times, become violent. His brother, Carl, age 11, and sister,
Ellen, age 12, were exhibiting similar behaviors, albeit not as extreme.

After Sandra's marriage to Sam turned abusive, Sandra moved out of
state with her children. They returned to the area 2 years prior to my initial
contact with them and were receiving welfare and living in public housing
in a large urban area. When I first met with Sandra, she was about to enroll
in a nurse's aid training program. Sam eventually rejoined the family until,
as was the pattern, his violent outbursts prompted Sandra to file for a
restraining order. It was Sandra's fear that the children were becoming like
Sam that ultimately convinced her to seek help.

Prior to the initial team consultation a number of family meetings
(several in which Sam agreed to participate) were held over a 1-year period.
These sessions were crisis-oriented and involved one child or another.
Typically, the problem subsided and the family left only to reappear when
another child's behavior begged for attention. The repetitiveness of the
contacts and Sandra's desperation and frequent loss of temper led Sally to
conclude that therapy was not moving in a positive direction. A team
consultation was then arranged. Sandra and the children attended this
session, and a consulting team observed the meeting from behind a one-
way mirror.

## INITIAL TEAM CONSULTATION

As in previous sessions, the children enter the therapy room squabbling
amongst themselves. Sandra's initial attempts to get their attention are
ignored, raising the question as to who is in charge.

T: It's been over a month now since I've seen you. What's been happening?
S: Matt is getting into trouble at school. They're calling me every day.
   The school thought something was bothering him, and they wanted to
   know if it had to do with his environment at home. And of course I
   had no idea what was bothering him. He was just getting into fights
   every day.

T: Were you seeing a change in his behavior at home as well?

S: He was hanging around with an older boy again. After he's with him, he's more aggressive.

[A discussion ensues in which Matt says he doesn't get into trouble with the boy and the mother argues that he does. It becomes evident how Sandra gets hooked into a position of trying to defend herself against the onslaught of all three children (but especially Matt). As Sandra talks about things at home, she is effectively and frequently interrupted by Matt, who interjects by saying "No" or "Wrong" or "It didn't happen that way." By commenting on this process of challenging Sandra's authority, Sally attempts to open space for Sandra's alternative explanation to be heard. However, Sandra is not able to refuse her children's invitations to subject herself to their persistent repudiations.]

T: Mom hasn't gotten past the first sentence.

S: *(asking permission of Matt)* Let me just tell her what Dad wanted to do [Matt continues to interrupt, and the other children join in, saying, "No" or "Wrong, wrong."]

S: Just let me finish . . .

★    ★    ★

T: It sounds like Mom has to end up defending herself when she wants things to move in a certain direction. She gets a lot of resistance.

M: [The team calls Sally out and discusses with her how to redirect the interview and cut down on the interruptions. The idea is generated for a team member to come in as a scorekeeper to track the interruptions and Sandra's ability to avoid being distracted from her train of thought. The scorekeeper (SK) playfully monitors the flow of conversation within the family. This action serves to focus the family and allow the session to progress. Sally reopens the interview by noting that Sandra is getting depleted by her children. Sandra begins to elaborate on this theme, explaining that the combination of school, a recent operation, and the children's unceasing demands have created a gulf of ill feeling between herself and her children.]

T: The team is concerned that mother is getting worn down with the interruptions and the attention that everyone in the family wants from her . . . getting pulled in many different directions. The team thought she needed a little support in the way of an expert scorekeeper who's going to keep score of the times that people attempt to wear her down by interrupting her, not allowing her to finish her thoughts, contradicting her, and so forth. And we will also be paying attention to how Mom is doing with this, finishing what she was starting out to say. We need to slow this process down a little and try to understand how everybody can get something from mom, but maybe not everything, because there's only one mom and three kids.

S:  Well, I think my problem was I was getting too stressed out with the school, studying til twelve every night and they were wanting to go places. And then I got sick with the gallbladder and then Matt got a little resentful because I wasn't around and then when I got home from the hospital they were like "you never take us anywhere." They're constantly asking to do something of me or Sam.

T:  *(to scorekeeper after noticing Matt trying to interrupt)* Does that count?

SK: So far, I've given Matt one for an attempted interruption, but *(to Sandra)* I gave you a plus because you kept going anyway.

[Sandra then describes her feelings while in the hospital and says, "No one visited, only my father. I was depressed and when I got home it was total chaos in my house."]

T:  What is chaos like in your family?

S:  They all just wanted me to jump up and take them everywhere, and I was supposedly on six weeks' bed rest. One week was it. I just chalked it up to experience. Mothers never get a rest. That's when Matt started acting out in school and Ellen got into trouble.

[In Sandra's selection of material to report, her own needs are sorely neglected. She seriously questions whether she has the emotional resources available to nurture her three children. In order for Sandra to give to her children, she needs to feel understood and supported. Sally's goal here is to support her so that she can convey the message that she cares about her children and has what it takes to parent. Sally empathizes with her feelings of deprivation and the burden of parenting through tough times.]

T:  So it was hard for the children to actually feel what it must have felt like for you to just have had an operation, come home, have your stitches in your side. Maybe they were scared. Do you think when you were in the hospital they may have been worried about you?

S:  I think Matt was very polite to me on the phone. I was very impressed how he treated me on the phone. Carl was okay. Ellen was very abrupt with me, like, "Mommy, I don't care."

T:  Mothers are not supposed to get sick; you're supposed to be strong.

S:  It was very hard for me. I was crying many nights in the hospital. I was pretty upset. And then I had problems with Matt at school, and school was calling me every day. And then Ellen wasn't really listening when I got home, and I put my foot down. I let her know I would get a formal CHINS [a court petition for "Children in Need of Service"] out on her. She was doing things I didn't approve of and she didn't want to be told what to do. She said to me, "You're always in school, always studying. You're never here with me; you don't care about me." I was in tears the other night and I told her *I'm doing it to make a better life for us.* Then I talked it over with Sam. Maybe we could get back together, maybe we could try because I can't do this alone. I am just emotionally drained with the children . . . very tired.

T: And physically drained from all the efforts you're putting into recovering and going to school, but *it's all been to make a better life for this family*.

S: And I was also getting a lot of verbal abuse from these two *(nods to Ellen and Matt)*.

[The opportunity for Sally to highlight her strengths comes when Sandra shares how she defends herself against her daughter's reproaches by saying she is going to school to make a better life for her family. Sally amplifies the "better life for the family" theme to give the mother credibility, to establish her good motives, and to earn respect for her from the children.]

T: I think it might be hard for them to understand what it would be like for you to have a better life. You say you're wanting a better life, working to make a better life. Maybe you need to spell it out . . . what you've been working for.

S: *(to children)* When Mommy takes her state boards, I will be able to make very good money. That's like thirty thousand dollars. That's almost six to eight hundred dollars per week take-home, able to buy a house, maybe have a nice swimming pool in the backyard—something every family would like to have.

T: How much are you living on now, Sandra?

S: Before Sam came in Sunday, poverty level, six thousand dollars.

T: *(to children)* Imagine what it would be like for your mother to be working after getting her training completed.

S: It would be great. I have to do this for myself.

T: *(to Sandra)* Do you think they see you as selfish because you're doing this?

S: I think so . . . because I'm not there, because I have to be at the library. *(crying)* I can't concentrate at home, with the yelling and fighting. There's no consistency. Maybe if Sam comes back into the house, maybe there'll be a little more order.

T: You're a very good person, Sandra. You're really trying hard to meet everybody's needs and to put the family on its feet so the things that your children want you can be in a position to give them.

S: That would be nice.

[When Sally reaches out to the children and engages them in the process, it is evident that their perceived neglect by the mother remains an issue.]

T: Let me hear some responses from you kids about what your mom's been saying. You know she's been speaking from the heart. She's been talking about some important things for your family. What's your feeling about this?

M:  She says she's studying a lot but she doesn't. She goes over her friend's house, and Ellen's there sometimes and she says she doesn't study there. And when I call all I hear is laughing. That's studying?

T:  So you're not sure that when she says she's studying she's really doing it? She might be having some fun for herself instead.

M:  Uh huh.

[Sandra defends herself from Matt's charge by acknowledging that she does take a break at times.]

T:  And when you're studying, does that mean you're not thinking about the kids or caring about what's happening in their lives?

S:  Oh, no.

T:  (noticing Matt is nodding) Matt, do you think that happens when Mom is involved in her work, that she's forgotten about you?

M:  Uh huh. (nods yes)

[Sandra and Matt argue about her perceived unavailability, and Sandra must again defend herself. Sally brings the conversation back on track.]

T:  All of you children seem to get very resentful when you're (nods to Sandra) off studying. They don't accept easily a substitute for you. You're the one and only. And they resent this very much. They get very angry, and I think that sometimes the behavior that starts to show—surliness or pushing other kids—is a way of letting you know that they're out there, these kids, and they don't want to be forgotten. When you're in your books, the feeling is you've forgotten them. They're not sure your thoughts will ever come back to them.

S:  Well, how could that not be?

T:  I don't know.

S:  (to the children) I think about you. That's so silly to think that. You know I love you guys.

[Matt challenges the perception of his mother as a loving parent. He denies he feels love from her. Rather than viewing Matt's statements as a manipulative gesture or a put-down, Sally accepts his statement as reflecting his version of the family reality.]

M:  No, I don't.

S:  Oh, come on, Matt. If anybody gets more attention . . .

T:  (to Matt) What way could your mother show you that she really loves you?

M:  I've never really felt that.

T:  You've never felt that?

S:  Oh, come on, how could you never feel loved? Tell me, Matt. When did I never love you?

M:  (sad) Every day.

T: *(to Sandra)* Did your love stop when you got disappointed [in Matt's behaviors at school]?

S: He may have felt that, but it's not true. I still love him, no matter what. *(to Matt)* Maybe if you said, "I missed you," maybe I could understand it a little better. You never said anything to me. You just clammed up and were swearing at me all the time.

M: When?

S: Do you call Mommy names all the time?

M: *(interrupting)* No.

T: Can I break in here? I want to go back to Matt's statement that he doesn't feel you love him. And you wondered how could he feel that way when you do so much for him and you love him so much and he doesn't feel it. How is it that he doesn't tell you? I think he tells you in the anger.

[To defuse Matt's mother-bashing and denial of her love for the children, Sally suggests that Matt's anger gets in the way of his receiving love from his mother and challenges Sandra to reach for the love that is hiding behind Matt's anger.]

S: In the anger.

T: In the anger. Underneath the anger is the love. Underneath the anger is the love.

S: So he wants to say, "Hey Mom, this is me. Take a look or something."

T: "Mom, am I okay? Even though I get into trouble at times and cause a commotion, do you still love me?" "Can you still love me?"

S: I have to still love him. I told Ellen the same thing. I'll still be there, no matter what. I would never abandon the children. These are my only three children; this is all I have. I don't even have a mother that even talks to me, so why would I leave my children?

T: You're trying to be very different from your mother.

S: I'm trying.

M: She's meaner.

S: Why am I meaner? I hate to hear this. Before my car got smashed up, I'd take you everywhere.

M: Where?

S: I took you out to eat practically every night of the week.

M: No.

T: *(to Sandra)* You're getting into a situation with Matt in which each time he tells you you're not a good mother, you try to talk him into seeing it differently. And each time you try, it falls on deaf ears. He may not be able to see you as a good mother. What do we do about that?

[After seeing potential for repetition of conflict between mother and the children, the team decides to interrupt and consult with Sally and the scorekeeper. After this short break, Sally and the scorekeeper return to the therapy room.]

SK: I have to say you didn't make my job that difficult. I thought that I would have to write down more things. Matt, I gave you a half one time and one for a distraction when you got your mother o~~ff~~ the topic. But mostly, Sandra, you kept on going even ~~with~~ distractions, and I saw a lot of strength in your doing ~~that~~.

[Sandra's position is str~~engt~~hened by reestablishing her importance in the lives of ~~her chil~~dren, whose protestations and criticisms are re-f~~ramed~~ as indicators of their intense wishes for her love. A ritual to take them beyond the feelings of deprivation and allow their feelings of love to be expressed is incorporated in the final segment of the session. The team's suggestion that the mother reaffirm her love to each of her children in the context of a ritual underscores the seriousness of Sandra's commitment and the team's belief that through love, healing can begin.]

T: And I think one of the real strengths in this family is that the children care so much about you and they want to be loved by you. That comment was made to me by a team member. It's not like your kids are giving up, saying you don't matter. It's just the opposite, that you matter almost too much. And it's hard for them to tolerate any moments when you're distracted by other things. We thought it would be really important as a parting gesture for you to tell each of your children, in a special way, how you love them. If you could go around and say that to each of your children. I think it's important for them to know you've said it.

[In the sequence to follow, Sandra is helped to stay focused on her positive feelings for each child and not digress into the negative realm that is more customary for her and that generally triggers a counterreaction from her children. She succeeds in the end when she says emotionally, "I love you all."]

S: Ellen should know that I love her because she's my only daughter.

T: Do you want to take her hand . . . or some gesture?

S: She knows I love her. (to Ellen) You know that I love you . . . and you're my diamond and I don't like it when you do those bad things that you were doing.

T: Take her hand and let her know that that's a message of affection coming through.

S: You know that I love you and I want you to do right. You know what I'm saying? I do love you more than anything you can probably imagine. I want you to do right, to be respectful. I don't want you swearing at me either.

T: Sandra, just stay with the love part. You love her no matter what, that's the part she needs to hear.

S: I like it when you get good grades. I want you to have a happy, normal life. You are very pretty and you never smile.

T: Squeeze her hand now. Let's go on to the next child.

S: *(smiling)* I'll do Matt next.

T: Is he still small enough to put on your lap? Let's try it.

*(Matt sits gingerly on his mother's lap to avoid hurting her stitches. Sandra puts her arms around him. He is all smiles.)*

S: I don't believe you think I don't love you.

T: No, forget the believing or not. You're just making your statements now. Hold him.

S: How many times do I tell you how well you did at school? Sally knows what a good artist you are.

T: You're wanting to give them a better life . . . real feelings about love.

S: You know I love you when you're being nice to people . . . because when you're mean you get nothing in return. Good people get more things . . . that's love. When you treat your brother and sister well, that makes me feel good. I sometimes get a little disappointed in the love when you're mean to other people, but I do love you . . . you understand.

T: Give him a squeeze that says it all. Carl's next. Close the space. *(Carl's chair is moved closer to his mother's.)*

S: *(takes Carl's hand)* You know Mother loves you too. I love you a lot because sometimes you help more than Matt or Ellen. *(crying)* I think you understand a little more sometimes. You're like your mom. I think you care too a little more than they do, and that's really special. But I don't love them any less. You're trying to help me a little more than they do, and sometimes they hurt me a little more. I love you all. *(Matt and Ellen are crying as they watch their mother with Carl, and tissues get passed around to Sandra, Ellen, Matt, and then to Sally.)*

T: It takes a lot of courage to say all those feelings. *(to Sandra)* You did very well . . . and so did all of you in this lesson of love. This is a session on showing love and being loved. *(Sally is tearful.)* This is something we're going to have to work some more on. Underneath, what's really important to all of you is love . . . loving her and having her love you.

This final sequence was the culmination of an emotional journey for the family—and for us. As Sandra gradually parted with her fears, reprimands, and hurts, Sally sensed the depth of feeling she had for her children. Sally was personally moved by this transformation and its powerful effect on the family.

## THERAPY

In the interim, Sally saw the family four times. A family focus was maintained by amplifying the "better life" theme. To further positive developments in caring for one another, Sally asked questions such as, "How would doing better in your life make a difference to your family?" "How would they want that difference to show?" Simultaneously, Sally worked to help Sandra regain control with her children.

A follow-up session was held 5 months after the initial consultation.

## FOLLOW-UP SESSION

At this point the family was no longer on welfare, evidence that Sandra's efforts to provide a better life for her family were succeeding. Sandra's effort to reclaim her status as a working person was a major step whose positive repercussions exemplify the impact of economic factors on the change process. In this session Sandra recognized that her children's behavior was improving and that she was parenting more effectively. In fact, change was apparent in both the physical appearance of the family and in the respect and attention the children gave their mother, who was now clearly in charge.

T: *(to children)* Your mother came in with Ellen one time and told me that things were much better in the family, that there were new developments and new changes, and she was very excited to talk about them. I thought our team would be interested in hearing about these new developments.

[Sandra informs Sally that the father is now out of the house.]

S: Ellen is doing fine. She's had a few moments but she's much better than she was.

T: Her behavior in the home is better.

S: Excellent. She doesn't pick on Carl and Matt like she used to. She has more friends and she's doing things like horseback riding, which she likes.

T: What about other things that have changed?

[The children sit quietly and listen attentively to their mother as she describes having made the decision to switch the two boys to different schools, something she had been thinking about for a while.]

T: *(to Sandra)* How about you? What are you doing now?

S: I have a job. I work as a nursing assistant.

T: Are you on welfare anymore?

S: No, I'm not.

T: You got off of welfare.

S:  I got off of welfare. I'm struggling but I'm getting there, slowly.

[The metaphor of a better life has been experienced now by all family members. As the therapist engages the children in a discussion of the ways their mother's triumph over poverty has affected their lives, new ideas about the mother become possible. The mother is transformed from neglectful and withholding to concerned and benevolent. Moreover, Sandra has moved from a state of feeling discouraged about her life to feeling a renewed sense of personal agency and effectiveness as a parent.]

T:  Does it feel good to be free of welfare?

S:  Yeah. It's still a struggle.

T:  How has your getting off welfare affected the family? How have the kids felt about your being off welfare?

S:  Well, I think they like it better because they get more things.

T:  *(to children)* Since the family has gotten off welfare, has it been a good thing? What do you notice that's different?

C:  She gets more money.

T:  And how does more money make a difference?

C:  We can get more stuff.

T:  What kind of stuff have you been interested in getting?

C:  Nothing really. Well, a bike and a trip to Washington, D.C., with my class.

T:  Has this money made it possible for you to be in activities that you weren't in before?

C:  Yes. I'm in flag football.

T:  *(to Matt)* You're also in flag football?

M:  Yeah.

T:  And what about you, Ellen. How has being off welfare changed things for you?

E:  I don't know.

T:  Can you tell me a little about . . . you mentioned to me once about horseback riding and that was interesting to hear about.

C:  Now she horseback rides every day. She wants to save up to get her a horse.

T:  How about you, Matt? Do you think it's been a good thing getting off welfare?

M:  Yeah.

T:  How have things changed for you?

M:  I get a lot of things.

T:  What kind of things?

M:  Um . . . a bike . . . and I go more places because she has more money.

T: You get to go more places. Not so stuck at home like before. So the changes have been good.

[Sandra then describes a situation with Matt in which she successfully set firm limits.]

T: He doesn't argue as continuously with you as before.

S: Yes.

[Sally tries to amplify the positive changes reported by asking Sandra to further elaborate on what's working.]

T: Are you more effective with him, or has he matured more?

S: I think Matt has matured a lot, but I told him now when I tell him something, he's got to listen. I won't argue with him. I try to keep my composure and not argue with this child. I do try to talk consistently even if he's angry. I say, " Matt can you just come over here and sit down?"

T: So, you've stopped screaming?

S: Yeah. I don't scream.

M: You always scream.

C: No, she doesn't.

T: *(to Carl)* You've seen a change?

C: Yeah.

[Sandra expresses a clear wish to be in control of her children and shares how she now stands up to the children's challenges to her authority. This new development is an indication that the family is separating from a "problem-saturated" story (White, 1991a; White & Epston, 1990) about their lives and replacing it with an alternative story that speaks to the newfound strengths of its members.]

T: *(to Sandra)* When they try to turn you into the bad guy, what do you do about it?

S: I get very frustrated and then I don't talk to them.

T: You stop talking to them.

S: I just ignore them. If I do it the other way I might scream at them, and I don't want to do that. I think it's good that when I ignore him *(nods toward Matt)*, in his own time he'll come around and apologize. Sometimes he gets mad at me and he'll run out of the house. He thinks I'm going to chase him. I'm not going to chase him.

M: You don't let me apologize.

S: Because he always wants to talk to me when I'm angry. I'm not going to talk to any of them when I'm angry. I want to be in control, not them. That's what Matt's learning. He is maturing about that; he's getting better about that.

T: And that's a new position for you to be in.

S: If I don't, they think they can walk all over me. I'm not going to let them walk on me anymore.

T: So when you're in charge, how does that affect the interaction with the kids?

S: I think they're better. I know Ellen and Carl are much better. Matt does pretty well with it too but he's a fighter. But in the long run Matt adjusts to it.

[The changes made by the family open the door for the introduction of questions that encourage the performance of new meanings (White, 1991b). We learn that it was from her mother that Sandra derived her backbone, that she was considered the strongest among the siblings. A recent estrangement has prevented Sandra from sharing her new discoveries with her mother. A chance to visit her mother soon offers Sandra an ideal opportunity to authenticate and celebrate her family's changes.]

T: *(to children)* Let's talk about how Mom has been able to stand up to all these challenges from you because she has to make sure that you know who the boss is, and what bosses do for families to make things run smoothly, to give them what they need, to really nurture them.

S: Well, they get to do so many things now . . .

T: You do a lot of things for your family. How did you get to this point where you are so strong and capable? Who would have, in your past, not have been surprised by this development?

S: Probably my mother.

T: Your mother.

S: My mother had seven kids and she worked nights and went to school during the day for nursing to get her RN. Father worked days. So I figured if my mother could do it, I could do it too. But it's been tough.

T: Tough it is. But you've stayed with it.

S: She [her mother, Mary] gave me the backbone to do it. She always said you can do it. You'll be a better person in the end. I've always had that in my mind. I look up to her.

T: When you have moments of discouragement, is it your mother that you turn to?

S: No. After I talked to you yesterday I called my sister and I talked to her because I'm still not talking to my mother. I have an opportunity to go to Texas at Thanksgiving, and I think I'm going to talk to my mother and get some things cleared up, because I really do need some of her guidance in my life and I think that's some of my problem. I don't think the kids realize how difficult it is to be a mother to three kids.

T: They can't but your mother could understand. There's something important about trying to keep that connection with your mother.

S:   You were the strongest in having this backbone. Do the children know about how strong you were in your family, despite the problems? So mothers and daughters are alike. It makes me think that Ellen will be strong like her mother and grandmother. It goes through the generations. It's impressive that there's real strength in the family . . . that I've not heard of before.

[The therapist equates Ellen with her mother and grandmother to celebrate the legacy of female strength, thus presenting her with positive role models and an opportunity to identify with her mother.]

At this point a team member knocked on the window, indicating the team's readiness to switch places with the family. The reflecting team (which included Steven Friedman, PhD; Cynthia Mittelmeier, PhD; and Jonathan Simmons, PhD) responded to what the family considered positive developments and showed their interest in learning how these changes were achieved. The team served as an "audience" to change. As they puzzled aloud, their comments were expanded in an open and nonjudgmental conversation.

## Reflecting Team Conversation

SF:   I'm very curious about the respect that I was observing the children showing to their mother, how that evolved to that point, because the last time we saw them that respect didn't seem to be there. Something as happened that has created the possibility for the children to show that respect in the way it was happening.

CM:   I'm curious about that too. In fact, when the family came in today they looked very different from the last time I had seen them . . . but I also thought, like you were saying, that people were acting different toward Mom and treating her with more respect. She came in and said "I'm the mother of this group " . . . so I was also very curious about that.

SF:   How she got to that place . . . in spite of the difficulties, the concrete reality difficulties of her life . . .

JS:   I haven't met the family before today but it was clear to me how much respect Mom has with the children. And, as you said, she let us know who boss number one is . . .

SF:   I'm puzzled how she can maintain her composure and her consistency in the face of the demands on her time . . . how she's able to maintain that.

CM:   You said you were puzzled. What made you puzzled?

SF:   Because, after seeing the children the last time I could see how hard it would be to maintain your consistency . . .

CM:   She really had her work cut out for her.

SF: And so . . . it just threw me to see that . . .

CM: I was interested to hear the mother talking about her mother. She sounds like an interesting woman. I was interested in her comment about, that although her relationship has been tense, that she was really thinking about making the trip and maybe seeking her mother's advice about some things. This is an area where she had a lot of respect for her mother. And I wonder how she got to that point of opening herself up to that.

SF: Yes . . . So there seemed to be the reaching out to the sister and now to the mother and that takes a lot of courage.

CM: A lot of strength in that reaching out; saying "I'm doing the best I can . . . I'm doing a good job . . . but I can use some additional input . . ."

SF: "And if I reached out to my mother in some way is that going to help my children reach out to me in other ways . . ." The only other thought I had was how the children try to turn mother into the "bad guy" and whether there's any hope for her to be out of that role. In some ways, as a parent she may be stuck with the "bad guy" role but can she also be seen as a "good guy" and have the children appreciate both sides . . . if that's possible . . .

## The Team and Family Switch Places

Sandra shared her joy that the new story she had authored about herself and her children has been heard and appreciated.

T: The team was very curious about a lot of new developments. I wondered what you found interesting about their comments. Was there something that fit . . . that didn't make sense?

C: All of it was true.

[Sally tries to elicit reactions from the children without much success and then turns to Sandra.]

S: I enjoyed the observations that they made. The impression I got was that they saw me as a strong person . . . and that I'm trying to be in control of these children that I couldn't get in control a couple of months ago. So that was positive for me. It was nice to hear that the children have changed, from people looking in. That means something is working. They do show a lot more respect now. I have even seen that. I think with Matt . . . he's much more mature now and I think he's trying really hard. Ellen's changed so much it's been great.

T: *(again trying to engage the children in a discussion about the team's comments)* The team made so many positive comments about you guys having changed. Do you know what they were talking about? Did it make sense to you? Was it like from outer space? What do they mean you changed? What were they talking about . . . you made changes?

C: They were talking about us.

T: What is it that you are doing differently now that wasn't happening before?

M: Acting better?

T: How is that so?

M: Mature.

T: That's for sure. You know, what I've noticed is your not interrupting each other so much.

S: They're more courteous to each other.

T: There's more respect. This is a very tight-knit family. You've been through a lot of pain and suffering, but you've come out on top.

S: Yeah.

[As the session draws to a close and Sandra and her children are getting up to leave, the cameraman notices that Sandra and Sally are wearing matching outfits. Sandra then tells a story about herself and her sister.]

CAMERAMAN: I like your complementary outfits.

S: *(noticing)* Oh, yeah.

S: We went to a wedding and my older sister comes from the city and she's very wealthy and here I am the practical mom. And I went to Filene's Basement and I found this dress, marked down from $100 to $30. I said, "I'm going to buy this dress; no one else is going to buy this dress." And I go to the church and I see this girl in this dress, and when she turns around it was my sister! And I said this lady has more money than I have and she bought a bargain. People said, "What is this, the Doublemint twins here"? And she said, "At least we have the same taste."

[Sandra's value of herself was appreciably enhanced when she discovered that she and her sister shared something in common. In the sisterhood of women there are points of identification and connection that transcend background, class, and economic situation. The emotional rapport established between Sandra and Sally is also reflected in this vignette.]

## A LETTER FROM THE THERAPIST

Following this session Sally sent the family the following letter. Her intention was twofold: first, to review and applaud the steps family members took in gaining control over their lives and, second, to highlight new options resulting from these accomplishments.

*Dear Sandra, Ellen, Carl, and Matt,*
*I would like to congratulate you all on the remarkable changes you have made. Sandra, you shared from where your inspiration for change came*

(Grandma Mary) and the steps you and the children have taken to win over poverty, chaos, and violence. You said that in studying to become a nurse, you would have a profession you loved and an income to provide a better life for yourself and your children. I know it was not easy for any of you when Sandra had so little time and money. Before that, Sandra, you put a stop to family violence and with the children became a single-parent family. You were tested daily as their demands escalated and their behavior grew unmanageable. You attempted to placate them and to return their fire but in the end you stood your ground. You even enlisted the help of Sam, with whom you have forged a new cooperative relationship. As a result, I see a growing respect among your children as they take control of their behavior and stand up to violence, which was the way of the past.

Ellen, you have put your energy into new interests, which have taken you away from daily fights with your parents and brothers. As you are your mother's daughter, the challenges of school will be yours to win.

Carl, you sensed your mother's struggles and were won over by reason. Many times you refused to take your frustrations out on your family. Each time you succeeded, you proved yourself a stronger person.

Matt, last time we were together, I saw you take charge of your temper when you were in disagreement with your mother. I was impressed by this recent development. It made me wonder if you might get the upper hand over your temper in school.

Sandra, I look forward to hearing about your reunion with your mother. I believe the recent family accomplishments, about which you will put your mother in touch, have given you the confidence to reach out to her with pride. In discussing your past differences, you make it possible to seek advice in the future. It takes strength of character and largess of heart to extend oneself as you intend.

Finally, you dare to think of the future and the promises it holds for your children. It is clear to me that a new family story is unfolding. I will be most interested in hearing about the responses you receive after sharing these changes with family. Please keep me posted. I will see you after your trip to Texas.

Sincerely yours,

Sally Brecher

## POSTCRIPT

The family continues to be seen on an occasional basis. Sam is currently not living with the family but does have regular contact with them. There have been no further reports of his abusive behaviors. The family's economic circumstances have steadily improved, and the children's behavior at home is significantly better. Sandra remains firmly in charge. At school Ellen made the honor roll, and Carl's overall school performance is improving. Matt continues to exhibit some unacceptable behaviors in the school setting, but he is gaining mastery over them. The work continues.

## CONCLUSIONS

By amplifying narratives that support feelings of efficacy and increased personal agency, we collaborate with the people with whom we work to create more satisfying futures. By listening to the client and providing the space for new stories to be constructed, narratives of empowerment can come to replace narratives of demoralization.

## EDITORIAL QUESTIONS[1]

Q: *In the family presented, Sandra is able to get a job and off of welfare. How would you approach a similar family situation where the parent was unable to find work and remained poor and dependent on welfare? In the managed health care organization where you work, well-defined limits exist on the number of sessions that people can be seen. What are some of the ways you have found to work effectively (and efficiently) in this setting with families facing complex social problems?*

A: Families living in poverty are prone to feelings of hopelessness and despair because they experience limited control and reduced personal agency over events in their lives. This issue relates to a larger political one that has to do with the class structure in the United States and the majority control of resources by those in the top 1% of the economic pyramid (Nasar, 1992). Obviously, major sociopolitical change is required in order to create a more equitable social structure. Disincentives in the welfare system are just one of many powerful constraining forces in the socioeconomic picture (e.g., Hays, 1992). The issues of power in society and the structural inequalities that exist in available opportunities are commented on by White (1991b).

As a result of global economic changes in the last 20 years, which have resulted in reduced jobs and wages for blue-collar workers, the categories of people living in poverty have expanded. A recent census bureau study (Gosselin, 1992) showed that nearly one in five Americans who worked full-time in 1990 could not earn enough to keep a family of four out of poverty.

Minuchin (see Markowitz, 1992), in discussing his classic book *Families of the Slums,* has come to the conclusion that it is naive to expect to have a significant impact on a family simply by working with internal relationships. Minuchin (1991) believes that "families of poverty have been stripped of much of the power to write their own stories. Their narratives of hopelessness, helplessness and dependency have been cowritten, if not dictated, by social institutions" (p. 49). He suggests that the real work needs to be done at the social policy level.

---

[1]We wish to thank Judith Davis, EdD, for her helpful editorial comments and for offering ideas that stimulated our thinking about these issues.

While we can personally advocate for social change, our main function as clinicians is to serve as consultants to the persons and families who present themselves to us for therapy. As therapists we strive to notice and amplify those positive threads or developments that will allow the family to reclaim some feelings of hope and increased personal agency. Families have histories and traditions that have allowed them to survive in the face of obstacles. With this in mind, the therapist is in a position to engage in conversations that bring forth and amplify those adaptive strengths and survival strategies and to situate them in a context of possibility and hope. By viewing the families we see as adaptive and strong, rather than as dysfunctional, we create a discourse of hopefulness in contrast to one of demoralization.

Recently, I (Steven) saw a family of seven—six children and their mother. The children had all lived in foster homes for several years and now ranged in age from 10 to 18. The mother had valiantly fought against tremendous odds to get her children back. She brought the family for therapy because of recent fighting among the siblings. One of our sessions was spent talking about how this mother accomplished the task of winning back her children. As she spoke of her accomplishments in this regard, she became more confident and assertive. Her love for her children was communicated in this conversation. I kept asking her questions about how she overcame this or that obstacle in making a better life for herself and her family. The mother and I became curious together about these developments. The children were attentive and respectful, in contrast to several previous sessions, as they listened to how their mother had reclaimed her family in the face of significant adversity.

On a more concrete level, our therapy principles and methods are influenced by the context in which we work. The managed health care setting, with its limits on the number of sessions that people can be seen, challenges us to creatively manage complex situations. We have found that our work is most effective when we (a) stay focused on the client's concerns; (b) keep our expectations realistic; (c) engage in conversations that enable clients to reclaim those competencies and strengths that form a part of their cultural tradition and/or personal history; (d) find and amplify a thread of hope from the past that can be nurtured into providing a pathway to step more effectively into the future.

We have no easy answers. In approaching families on welfare we feel it is important to help them not be recruited into the view that they are to blame for their social problems. What needs emphasizing is not why persons have failed to get off welfare but, rather, how they have resisted buying into victim-blaming notions about the poor and have managed to avoid feeling totally defeated. Whether families are living on welfare or struggling to hold together their fragile households by working long hours at low-paying jobs, the family burdens are enormous and exhausting. As therapists we try to stay alert to the "trickle-down hopelessness" (Goodman, 1992) that can invade our thinking and distract us from the work to be done.

The more complex the social situation, the more we work to stay focused on manageable change or "small wins," lest we find ourselves overwhelmed and demoralized. As Weick (1984) points out, "small wins are . . . opportunities that produce visible results . . . Once a small win has been accomplished, forces are set into motion that favor another small win . . . Much of the artfulness in working with small wins lies in identifying, gathering, and labeling several small changes that are present but unnoticed" (pp. 43–44).

Our therapy emphasizes strengths, competencies, and hope, rather than deficits, dysfunction, and despair. By working under positive auspices we create a context in which clients can experience themselves as active agents of change.

On a practical level, we advocate within the system for benefit extensions and waivers of fees in order to allow the family to continue in therapy. We use the telephone as a link between sessions. If the family doesn't have a telephone, we write letters. Letter writing, of course, has therapeutic potential beyond simply making contact. For example, Sally's letter highlighted the newly discovered strengths of family members out of which emerged a story of empowerment. When it is useful to do so, we attend school meetings and advocate, with the family, for needed services. Although therapy is indeed a limited arrangement and the impact of sociopolitical issues on this population is enormous, therapists can still act to enable change on a microsystemic level.

## REFERENCES

Andersen, T. (Ed.). (1990). *The reflecting team: Dialogues and dialogues about the dialogues.* United Kingdom: Borgmann.

Aponte, H. (1976). Underorganization in the poor family. In P. Guerin (Ed.), *Family therapy: Theory and practice* (pp. 432–448). New York: Gardner Press.

Aponte, H. (1977). The anatomy of a therapist. In P. Papp (Ed.), *Family therapy: Full-length case studies* (pp. 101–116). New York: Gardner Press.

Ellwood, D.T. (1988). *Poor support.* New York: Basic Books.

Friedman, S., & Fanger, M. T. (1991). *Expanding therapeutic possibilities: Getting results in brief psychotherapy.* New York: Lexington Books/Macmillan.

Goodman, E. (1992, May 14). Twenty-five lessions for life. *Boston Globe,* p. 19.

Gosselin, P. (1992, May 12). Poverty traps more workers, study says. *Boston Globe,* p. 1, 14.

Hays, C. (1992, May 15). Welfare's limit on savings foils one bid to break cycle. *The New York Times,* p. 1, B4.

Hoffman, L. (1991). A reflexive stance for family therapy. *Journal of Strategic and Systemic Therapies, 10,* 4–17.

Imber-Black, E. (1986). Families, larger systems and the wider social context. *Journal of Strategic and Systemic Therapies, 5,* 29–35.

Kearney, P., Byrne, N. O., & McCarthy, I. C. (1989). Just metaphors: Marginal illuminations in a colonial retreat. *Family Therapy Case Studies, 4*(1), 17–31.

Markowitz, L. M. (1992). Families of the poor. *The Family Therapy Networker,* March/April, pp. 12–13.

Minuchin, S. (1991). The seductions of constructivism. *The Family Therapy Networker,* September/October, pp. 47–50.

Minuchin, S., Montalvo, B., Guerney, B., Rosman, B., & Schumer, F. (1967). *Families of the slums: An exploration of their structure and treatment.* New York: Basic Books.

Nasar, S. (1992, May 18). Those born wealthy or poor usually stay so, studies say. *The New York Times,* p. 1, D5.

National Commission on Children (1991). *Beyond rhetoric: A new American agenda for children and families.* Washington, DC: U.S. Government Printing Office.

Schorr, L. B., & Schorr, D. (1988). *Within our reach: Breaking the cycle of disadvantage.* New York: Anchor/Doubleday.

Seligman, M. E. R. (1975). *Helplessness: On depression, development and death.* San Francisco: Freeman.

Tomm, K. (1990, June). *Ethical postures that orient one's clinical decision-making.* Paper presented at the meeting of the American Family Therapy Association, Philadelphia.

Walker, G. (1991). Pediatric AIDS: Toward an ecosystemic treatment model. *Family Systems Medicine, 9,* 211–227.

Weick, K. E. (1984). Small wins: Redefining the scale of social problems. *American Psychologist, 39,* 40–49.

White, M. (1991a, October). *Re-authoring lives and relationships.* Workshop at Leonard Morse Hospital, Natick, MA.

White, M. (1991b). Deconstruction and therapy. *Dulwich Centre Newsletter, 3,* 21–40.

White, M., & Epston, D. (1990). *Narrative means to therapeutic ends.* New York: Norton.

White, R. W. (1959). Motivation reconsidered: The concept of competence. *Psychological Review, 66,* 297–333.

# III

## REFLEXIVE
## CONVERSATIONS

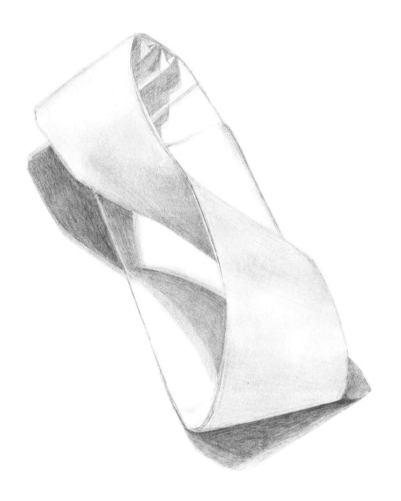

# 13

## See and Hear, and Be Seen and Heard

### TOM ANDERSEN

## PREJUDICE

When a professional—let's call him John—meets another person, say, Bill, for the first time, John already has some understanding of Bill, even if he has never heard of or met him before. John brings with him a general understanding of *what* a human being (a self) is and also an understanding of *how* he should listen and observe in order to come to know Bill in particular. Hans Georg Gadamer (in Warnke, 1987) calls this general understanding *vor-verstehen* (prejudice or pre-understanding or prejudgment). A prejudice is composed of different kinds of knowledge that come from the culture and tradition we live in and from experiences we collect over time in our own lives. Everyday expressions for *vor-verstehen* include "understanding from a certain perspective" or "seeing from a certain angle" or "looking through a certain lens." Since John has his particular *vor-verstehen*, it is impossible for him to be neutral and objective when he meets Bill. In other words, when any individual asks for professional help because of a personal problem, the professional's prejudice about such a problem will influence how it will be understood and handled.

## LANGUAGE AND PREJUDICE

We can neither describe what we see and hear and otherwise sense nor understand (come to know or recognize) without a language. The language we are *in*, according to Ludwig Wittgenstein, provides both possibilities and limitations for *what* we can understand and *how* we can understand it (Grayling, 1988). Kenneth J. Gergen (1985) mentions that persons of today are in a language that describes human traits as stable structures rather than as phenomena in process and change. Our language thereby contributes to the prejudice we are in. We are *in* a language that brings us a general knowledge (prejudice) that both limits and makes possible what we understand. This also holds true for the writing of history.

## SOME WORDS ABOUT THE HISTORY OF PSYCHOTHERAPY

In the following paragraphs I discuss what I see as the main trends in the history of psychotherapy and how I see my own professional history within that frame.

Kenneth J. Gergen (1991) has in his book *The Saturated Self* an interesting overview on how the prejudice of the "Self" (also called "person" or "I" or "individual") has evolved over time. In the Romantic period, mainly during the 19th century, a view emerged that the Self was constituted from personal depth, that is, from passion, soul, creativity, and moral fiber. One can say that in this view the Self is governed by the heart and is characterized by a deep commitment to relationships, friendships, and life purposes. In the period of modernism, beginning in the late 19th and early 20th century, another view emerged, namely, that the Self was basically constituted by rationality and cognition and governed by the brain. There is an ability to reason, to form opinions, and to deal with conscious intentions. Normal persons are predictable, honest, and sincere and can benefit from education, a stable family life, moral training, and rational choices in relationships.

Both Selves, the Romantic one and the modern one, were seen as stable over time; there was an essence that could be called either character or personality or personhood. In the so-called postmodern period, starting in the middle of this century, the idea of one Self has been challenged by the idea of many Selves. A person constitutes her or his shifting Selves according to the various relationships and conversations and languages she or he is in. That is, the multiple Selves are governed by "the togetherness with others."

Freud, as many therapists still do, bridged the Romantic and modern views of the Self. Most family therapists lean more toward the modern view of Self when they are in the theory and language of cybernetics; they see man as being part of a whole (a system) and able to make rational reassessments of his position and that of others in the system. And some therapists have begun to enjoy the postmodern view of Self, which sees a person, first of all, as creating meanings through language.

Freud, through his collaboration with his clients, searched for rational explanations that he hoped would drain the painful tension that the clients had accumulated over time. He sought to help them, through the strong emotional relationship they developed with him, generate better psychological mechanisms to protect themselves from dangerous wishes from within and from dangerous seductions in the external world.

Many family therapists act on the idea that they, through their expert understanding of a person's position in an objectively identifiable system, can intervene and change the system and the person. The interventions are understood to interfere with and change the person's (and the system's) definition of a presented problem or to change the system's own attempted solutions. I see strategic and structural family therapy as examples of this.

A smaller proportion of contemporary psychotherapists, the constructivists, seem to have a view of the Self that bridges the modern and postmodern views. A person is seen to be many possible Selves as she or he can generate more than one description and, correspondingly, more than one understanding of the same phenomenon, for example, the self or one's own family system. Therapy becomes a search for a more useful description and understanding of a problem than what the client had before coming to therapy. The reaching of this more useful understanding is, however, a result of an individual cognitive act.

A rather small proportion of contemporary psychotherapists, who hesitate to call themselves therapists, have a postmodern view of Self, in which the Self is basically seen as constituted through language and conversations. (Actually, whatever one comes to understand is, by and large, a result of the language and the conversations one is *in*.) These "therapists" offer their presence and attention so that, hopefully, a new context is created. In this new context the client will talk and think about what she or he is trying to understand differently, and a more useful understanding will emerge. The client and the "therapist" are talking *together*. Such "therapists" who are collaborators have only their own particular experiences gathered over time; they are not experts. I see Harold Goolishian's and Harlene Anderson's work as belonging here (Anderson & Goolishian, 1988), as I see my own. I have myself gone through several prejudices before coming to where I am today, and I may yet go through more.

I was educated as a medical doctor and held for a while a very physical (biological) view of the Self. It shifted toward a more psychological view when I was trained in individual psychotherapy. That training gave me a new and interesting understanding of problems, but since my therapeutic contributions did not markedly diminish the problems I worked on with my clients, family therapy became attractive to me. However, acting like the expert who knew what was wrong and what ought to happen, the expert I, in fact, attempted to be at the beginning, was very uncomfortable for me. During the period in which I used the "Milan approach" I felt better, and when I was part of various "reflecting processes," I felt much less uncomfortable. Now I see "therapy" first of all as a relationship between two parties.

Therapy is not a technique. It is a way for the "therapist" to engage in client relationships. It was a relief for me to leave the hierarchical relationships I tried to conduct before and join the more heterarchical (egalitarian) relationships that characterize "reflecting processes," where client and "therapist" talk together and work together as two equally important partners.

## OPEN TALKS

Reflecting processes, which I have discussed elsewhere (Andersen, 1987, 1991, 1992a, 1992b), are characterized by the attempt to say everything in the open. Everything the professional says about the client's situation is said so that the client can hear it.

Reflecting processes can take many forms, but a common one is for the clients (e.g., a family) to meet with a team of professionals. In this process one of the professionals talks with the family for a while while the team listens. After some time the members of the team talk, while the family listens, about what they saw and heard and thought when they listened to the family talk. Then the family members are invited to talk about what *they* were thinking when they listened to the team talk. How this is done is described in more detail elsewhere (Andersen, 1991). There are no rigid rules for how these various reflecting processes can be done, only suggested guidelines.

### Inner and Outer Dialogues

Long after they appeared, I started to think of the reflecting processes as shifts between talking about an issue in an outer dialogue with others and then sitting back and listening to others talk about the same issue. During that listening to others one is inevitably talking with oneself in an inner dialogue (*dialogue,* "through words"). The issue under consideration can therefore be said to be talked about in two different perspectives—one from the inner and one from the outer dialogue. When an issue is shuffled from one perspective to another, new ideas about the issue easily emerge (Bateson, 1979).

### Appropriate and Unusual

Two or three years before the idea of reflecting team appeared for the first time, in March 1985, there emerged in me a stronger sensitivity to the flow of the conversation in the therapeutic encounter. Sometimes the conversations seemed to stop—or actually stopped. After thinking carefully about such incidents, I realized that these intervals of silence followed conversations that were too different, too unusual, compared to what the clients were used to, with respect *what* we talked about or *how* we talked about it or both. Conversations have to be different from what clients are used to in order to bring about change (Bateson, 1972), but not too different or unusual. A major contribution to the understanding of these nuances was made by the Norwegian physiotherapist Aadel Bülow-Hansen in her work in helping people alleviate their bodily tensions (Øvreberg & Andersen, 1986). Bülow-Hansen understood that tense muscles were part of a more comprehensive physical phenomenon in which breathing was simultaneously restrained and the various parts of the body were inclined toward a closed body posture. She helped her clients stretch the various parts of the body and thereby "open it up." One way to accomplish this is to induce pain, for example, by pinching the muscle of the calf. The response is a deep inhalation. When the person exhales, some of the tension in the body dissipates. However, if the pinch causes too little pain, no change in breathing occurs, and if the pinch is too painful or is sustained for too long, the person inhales deeply but does not exhale. If the pinch is appropriately painful for an appropriate length of time, the person inhales deeply and then exhales.

In the same way, therapeutic conversations that are too unusual (too painful) make clients feel uncomfortable with the process, and the conversation tends to stop (i.e., to exhibit the equivalent of holding their breath instead of experiencing the relief of a exhalation). For therapeutic benefit it is important that the therapist be sensitive to the flow of conversation, introducing change at a pace appropriate for the individual client.

## From Either/Or to Both/And

The way our team made interventions shifted in late 1984. Before this time we basically said to the client, "This is the way to see it" or "This is the way to understand your problem" or "This is what you ought to do." After the shift we started to say, "In addition to what you saw, we saw this" or "In addition to what you understood, we understood this" or "In addition to what you have tried to do, we wonder if you might try this." *In addition to* felt much better than *instead of.*

## From Interviews to Conversations

Before the debut of the "open talks" in 1985 there was a tendency for our team to interview clients from the perspective of our preconceived ideas about how their problems could be explained. We asked questions to confirm or invalidate our ideas f.i. about certain patterns of relationships or certain patterns of communication since we believed that such patterns governed the individuals. We were in the language of cybernetics.

After 1985 a new trend developed in which we asked clients how it felt to be in a therapy session. Questions like "Who had the idea for this meeting?" and "How did you respond to that idea?" were asked in order to help us understand who should be given a chance to talk and who should be given the freedom to be quietly present without talking. Another significant question also emerged, namely, "How would you like to use this meeting?" This question comprises two questions: "*How* shall we use this meeting?" *What* shall we use if for?" *How* stands for "Let us first talk about how we might talk together." Our conversations with our clients evolved from the answers to these questions. We became more and more interested in the client's meaning of "how" and "what." I now see this as the start of the turning to be *in* the language of hermeneutics.

## From "What?" to "How?"

Now, in hindsight, I see that another shift also emerged. Before, in the cybernetic (or the constructivist) period of my work, there was great interest in *what* the various definitions of the problem might be—the descriptions of it, the understandings of it, and the possible solutions to it. Now, in the hermeneutic or social constructionist period, it has become more and more interesting to deal with *how* one reaches definitions and redefinitions.

## Conversations about Various Conversations

I have come to understand that there is no *one* certain method or technique to reach alternative definitions of a certain problem. Such definitions are reached through the sharing of ideas during conversations. Therefore, it has been of interest to us to talk with clients about those conversations in which the problem has been discussed and to ask clients which conversations have been useful and which have not. It has also been of interest to discuss with them which conversations could be made in the future (the "not yet used" conversations), with whom, at which point in time, about what, and in which way.

## The Not Yet Seen and Not Yet Heard and Not Yet Thought Of

The conversations with clients have come to be searches for what can be seen and heard in situations that were defined as problematic. Usually, there is so much happening in such situations that there is more to be seen and heard than what one can see and hear. The best way I know to reach the unseen and unheard is to deal quite specifically for quite a while with the various details of the description(s) of a situation. When something new is seen or heard, a new understanding of the situation automatically arises and new ideas about how to handle ("solve") the situation emerge.

An interesting part of the conversation with clients is to talk about the language they are *in* when they talk about what they see and hear and think. As Wittgenstein claimed, the language we are *in* has both possibilities and limitations for what we can understand.

## Being in Life Is Being in Language, in Movements, in Feelings, and in Knowledge

Extrapolating from Wittgenstein's ideas, I find it natural to say that we do not have language, movements, feelings, and knowledge *within* us but that we are *in* them, surrounded by them. If we were surrounded differently, maybe we would live differently. When dealing with what a person expresses by voice or movements or emotions, I have found certain questions very attractive: "If you look into (this or that) word, what do you see?"; "Are there more words in (this or that) word?"; "I noticed you mentioned a particular feeling [e.g., fear]. Is that pure fear or are there other feelings in that one, a kind of mixed feeling?"; "If your tears [or your laughter or your closed fist or your trembling knees] could speak, what would the words be?" I am struck by how often those who have been asked these kinds of questions seem to like them. But don't forget the overruling guideline that one should constantly look for signs that indicate that a question is too unusual!

## Informing and in Forming

When a person expresses him- or herself, through voice and movements and emotions, others (as well as the person him- or herself) become informed of what the person is thinking. If that expressing person is given the time and the freedom he or she wants to express whatever in whichever way, an attending listener will see and hear that the person is searching for the best words (metaphors) to express him- or herself and will recognize that there is a certain rhythm and a certain speed and a certain strength to that expression from moment to moment. As I see it now, by expressing oneself one is simultaneously forming One's Self. The act of expressing oneself is the act of constituting One's Self. Maybe *performing* is a better word than *expressing*. That is, when a person is performing, this *per*forming is *in*forming oneself and others and simultaneously forming One's Self.

## Sacred Place

The understanding mentioned in the preceding paragraph makes me feel that I am in a sacred place when a person comes to discuss a problem situation he or she feels caught in. The conversation is an opportunity to search for an opening out of the situation and, at the same time, an act of reconstituting the self. When I am in one of those sacred places, Harry Goolishian's words often come to mind: "You shall not be so much concerned about what you shall do, but you shall be much concerned about what you *shall not* do!" (personal communication, June 1985) One is a bit fearful at sacred places.

I believe that the therapist must not interrupt clients who are in the process of expressing themselves. Let them be given the time they need to express what they want to express in the way they want to express it. Goolishian said, "Listen to what they say!"; one might add, "And avoid listening to your inner dialogue about what you believe they mean by what they say!" It is safer for therapists to raise a question about something they heard the client say than about their own meaning of what they heard.

## Seen and Heard and Affirmed

How can we create conversations such that those who are there can be seen and heard and thereby affirmed as the persons they want to be? How can we contribute to the conversation so that we affirm that which is most meaningful for the person in the context of his or her family? Perhaps by raising the following question now and then: "Who might or who should or who can talk with whom about which issue in which way at which point in time?" Harlene Anderson, Harold Goolishian, and Lee Winderman (1986) created the powerful concept of the problem-created system. They saw that a problem could be rather small at the beginning but that it might attract attention from many different persons who then create their own meanings about how the problem might be understood and solved. *A problem creates a system of meanings;* it is not that the system creates the problem. When these meanings are appropriately different, the various holders of the meanings might listen to each other and discuss the various meanings. Under such conditions new ideas might emerge. However, when the meanings become too different, the holders stop listening to each other, the conversations close off, the various holders of the various meanings are no longer seen or heard or affirmed, and the problem grows. And all parties find themselves at an uncomfortable place. Maybe we should encourage only those who are currently able to listen to and see each other without interrupting to come to "therapy" and let those who are not ready to do so eventually join later.

## Being in Conversation

Being in conversation with oneself and/or others can be seen as a constant movement toward an understanding of oneself, one's surroundings, and one's relationships. A Self is a moving and changing being. The consequences of this for the Other who listens is to follow the person. This means that the Other listens carefully to what is said and sees how the person expresses her- or himself (i.e., how the person per-forms). If the Other looks carefully, he or she will see that something of what is expressed is particularly important for the person. Those words or movements or emotions might be a starting point for the Other's next question. The Other can only see, not hear, when the person has finished what she or he wants to express. Persons who are given all the time they need will shift back and forth between talking to the Other in an outer dialogue and, during short pauses, turning inward and talking with themselves in an inner dialogue.

I have come to believe that a normal conversation gives each person who takes part the possibility of being in a personal reflecting process, that is, of shifting between inner and outer dialogues with an interested Other present who does not disturb but only hears and sees and lets the person be affirmed.

## Being in Relationships

Earlier in this chapter I said that I see therapy first of all as being engaged in a relationship. Being part of such a relationship and the conversations that emerge in it, we as therapists should contribute something unusual for the client. What is unusual might be experienced by the client as somewhat painful. If our contributions become *too* unusual, they might be experienced as *too* painful. This we can see and hear and feel. That feeling is stirred inside us and emerges when we go beyond our ethical standards. Maybe an identification of our ethical standards ought to be the most important issue we reflect on.

## Limitations

All that is in this chapter has emerged from the prejudices and language I myself am in. I therefore believe that, basically, what is in it might be useful only to myself.

## CLINICAL ILLUSTRATION

I hope that the following material reflects my thoughts in the preceding pages. I have no practice of my own and do not belong to one team anymore. That increases my flexibility in many respects, for example, to give up a theoretical idea or a practical mode when the time is ready. Since I have no practice I go to those who wish to consult with me and work together with them as a team in their offices. This means that at present I am connected with many teams. It seems safest to meet with the local professional first to be sure that we can find a way of working that is acceptable to both of us. How I often propose a setting for such a consultation is mentioned elsewhere (Andersen, 1991).

   The following account of a therapy session includes what I saw and thought, in addition to the words I heard. The local professional, Arlene, wanted to give me the information she thought I needed in front of the couple we were to meet. Then I was to talk with the couple, with Arlene listening. Thereafter, Arlene and I would have a reflecting talk or, if the couple preferred, some of the people who would be following the session from behind a one-way mirror would engage in a reflecting-team conversation. Those were our plans.

   It turned out otherwise. I have learned over the years to notice who looks at whom in which way at the very beginning of a meeting. Those glances will often indicate who prefers to start to talk with whom.

Arlene looked at the couple and began by announcing that she had the idea of having me consult because she said, "I think Tom talks with clients differently from what you have been used to, and I believe that his presence might be beneficial for our work." The couple accepted my presence.

Meanwhile, I was engaging in my own inner talk: How can I use my ability to "talk with clients differently" to do my best in this work? Since Arlene wanted this meeting, she is the person who first of all wants something "different." And what is different would therefore be different from what *she* has been doing so far. How can I participate so that Arlene has some different ideas about how she can talk with the couple when we end this meeting? I saw that as my job.

Arlene looked at me and said that Linda initially came to the clinic 11 months earlier. Then, instead of telling me about the family, she suggested that the couple could do that themselves. There was laughter in the room, and Linda began by saying that she first came for family therapy at a time when she had been separated from George for 6 months. Linda looked at Arlene when she spoke. She explained that she and George had started to date again and that George had moved into her house 3 weeks ago since he wanted to be more in touch with the children. Linda was worried about her role as a co-dependent, she had taken part in group therapy for co-dependents. She thought she lacked self-esteem and had read a lot about such things. She also went to therapy groups for alcoholics and cocaine addicts. She wanted to try different techniques to build her self-esteem and learn not to control other people. She felt that she tried to control George and that this made him fight back. She also saw herself as compulsive with the kids. Both Linda and George were in communication with their lawyer since there had been legal questions in their marriage.

Arlene said to me that Linda had done a lot of things, including writing him letters, to get George back. They decided that they each needed to have some time alone, and they arranged it so that when one was away the other took care of the children. George said to Arlene that there had been fights about that arrangement, and he gave an example. Linda intervened during his telling of the incident, and both ended up speaking at the same time. There was laughter in the air when George said that Linda flew off to another place. Arlene interrupted and told them that that was an example of their dances, that this time it was a flying dance. Then they talked about Linda's background of nursing and George's as a pilot. All three—Linda, George, and Arlene—enjoyed the talking, and they did not hesitate to talk all at the same time when they became excited. The conversational speed was pretty high and there were small changes in the rhythm. It seemed that everybody had to speak up in order to be heard, and there was much energy in the voices.

The questions that arose in my inner dialogue were the following:

What might I bring that would be different? Could I contribute something so that one person could speak at a time?

Then Linda talked about the previous week, when she had her birth-day, which actually was on Valentine's Day, and about how disappointed she was that George did not send her flowers at work. George tried to interrupt but she cut him off. She had wanted her colleagues at work to see that he remembered her, that she was special to him. When Linda spoke of how George had not sent her flowers, her speech became even louder and faster. They had fought about it later and had worked off some steam, but Linda said she wanted them to learn to come through such difficulties without splitting up. Arlene made the observation that even if their solution was not the best, they had arrived at a solution of sorts and she again used the word *dance* to describe how they acted in a difficult situation. George and Linda both spoke at once, saying that one steps on the toes of the other.

Linda then said that some things were better, that George had taken the children to school, prepared their food, and so forth. Arlene then turned to me and said that the family had come such a long way since they first met with her:

> We talked about them learning how to dance together. There might be times when they step on each other's toes, and that they would have to learn to . . . just pace that dance. You know over time that the dance has gotten easier and easier. I still hear there are times they step on each other's toes, but there are times when they dance so beautifully together. It is . . . it is . . . it is so nice to hear that they are learning to dance together.

Linda interrupted and said that when George called some time ago and wanted a divorce, she knew that she did not want to go back to how it had been. The fighting made her crazy. I waited until Linda finished and turned to Arlene again.

From my inner dialogue: *Dance* is a word Arlene has said many times already. She seems to have used it mostly as a metaphor, and I want to deal more with it and take it literally. I want to deal with this metaphor in my "ordinary" way, which means to look for details and nuances. Hopefully, that will be something different. I have to watch carefully as I ask my questions in order to see whether or not Arlene enjoys our talk.

T: I wondered about what you said. In Norway there are very many types of dances. Was this a particular type of dance or many dances or . . .

A: This was . . .

T: What is the name of that dance?

A: It is called the two-step. *(Linda and George laugh in the background and George joins Arlene.)* It is a western dance, like an American cowboy dance. *(Linda interrupts and says something inaudible as Arlene keeps speak-ing.)* And George does it very well; he is taking lessons. And that is a dance that Linda has started to learn but she has not mastered it as much as George has. George wanted her to learn it. It is a lot of fun.

T: And where did they learn it?

A: They go to a place that gives lessons, and there are several bars and nightclubs—no, they are not nightclubs, because there are no shows—but a particular place by the name of Do Das and they have this western music and the people are dressed in western clothes and they do this two-step, which is a very fast . . . I think . . . I don't know it well enough, but it sort of makes you smile like a pope . . . makes you smile like a polish polka. It is a very lively dance, a lot of fun.

T: Did they dance before?

A: Yes. *(In the background George says yes.)*

T: Together?

A: Yes.

T: What kind of dance before?

*(In the background George says, "Rock 'n' roll." The three of them laugh heartily.)*

A: Yes, they danced before. They danced for a while.

T: Is this a dance to learn to dance or to learn to not step on the other's toes?

A: I don't understand.

T: I . . . I . . . I . . . my mind is traveling around when you used the word *dance* . . .

L: *(interrupts)* Are we supposed to learn to not step on the other's toes or learn how to dance together or dance for life?

A: Uhmm . . . I think in many dances . . . where there is a dance that you dance to music or a dance where you dance to your life. There are times when you step on others' toes. So that will bring you closer than . . . you are busy stepping on each others' toes.

T: Oh, I just wondered if this is a dance to enjoy the dance in itself or to dance so that they learn not to step on the toes?

A: That is a good question. That is a good question.

G: Oh, I see . . .

A: I would think that their answer would be dance . . . just to dance.

T: To enjoy the dance? *(Arlene echoes, "To enjoy the dance.")* What about the dance does Linda enjoy the most?

A: What about the dance?

T: Yeah.

A: I don't know. I don't know.

T: Would that be the rhythm of the tunes or moving the feet or the . . .

A: I imagine it is the holding.

T: The holding?

A: Both holding each other.

[From my inner dialogue: This conversation is slower than the one between Arlene and the couple. Linda and George are now listening quietly and they do not move. Arlene seems interested in our talk since she is listening carefully to what she hears and is taking her time in order to find the answers she prefers to give. We can just continue like this.]

T: And what does George enjoy the most?

A: He enjoys the holding too. I am sure they both enjoy many aspects of the music . . . the fun of it . . . but the holding will definitely be very important.

T: The music sort of encourages the holding?

A: Uhm. Uhm. I am sure they want to vary the dance. I am sure there are times they would like to dance the two-step, which would be very quick and a lot of movements and they would probably also like that slow, quiet dance.

T: In order to hold differently?

A: Yes. The music step back. The holding is different.

T: That will give them a chance to hold differently?

A: Yes.

T: What takes part the most in the holding—the hands or the whole arms or . . . ?

A: Probably more the hugging. The caressing of the dance.

T: The touches?

A: Yes.

[From my inner dialogue: I introduced another word for holding, *touching,* and I wonder if it is acceptable to Arlene. The way she responds indicates that it is. I introduce it because it has at least two meanings, a physical one and an emotional one. If one is touched one might be moved, and if one is moved one is immediately activated in order not to lose one's balance.]

T: So in the holding there are touches?

A: And again that . . . quick touch and long gentle touch.

T: What kind of touching does George like the most?

A: I think he prefers the long gentle touches.

T: Is it that his wishes come from his background, which is different from Linda's, or do they come from inside himself?

A: I think they come from inside him.

T: What kind of music does he like the most?

A: The melodic gentle.

T: The long line music?

A: Yes, since the touches are long and gentle, he wants the music to be long and gentle also.

T: And what about the touches does Linda like the most?
A: I think she also enjoys the gentle, caressing touches.
T: The more melodic parts?
A: Yes. I think they like the fun parts also, but mostly the long gentle . . .

At this point George interrupted to ask me how long I would be there. Arlene answered that I would be staying for 2 more days, that I was consulting. Linda commented on the "real" dance, saying that she liked the shifts of being together and going apart. Then she said to Arlene, "But you are right, in the dance of life we like to hold each other. We are kind of physical." Arlene referred to their different backgrounds and asked if that could contribute to their stepping on each other's toes.

The thoughts in my inner dialogue were the following: George and Linda have been in a listening position for a while; they have both been in their inner talks. When they now speak with Arlene, they are brought into an outer dialogue. This shift seems very natural, and I will sit back and wait until it is natural to continue the talk with Arlene, and eventually with the couple. Right now it seems natural for them to continue their conversations with Arlene.

Linda then said that her mother threw her father out several times and asked him to get out of her life. But he always came back. George's parents divorced each other three times over 16 years. Linda thinks that's why she and George split up when life gets rough but come together again when things calm down. Her mother threw her father out in anger, but he never left. So when she herself gets crazy and throws George out, she says, laughing—he leaves! But George wanted a divorce. Linda said that she was used to the fact that George would leave for a few hours or even a night to calm down and then come back the next day to make up. But when he saw that things were getting worse, he packed up and left.

Arlene then commented that even though they have different experiences with staying and leaving and different religious backgrounds, they have in common this long, slow dance and the caressing holdings, that there are things inside them that might be very similar even there are many things that are different. Linda replied that for some reason, which neither understood, they could not let go of each other. She said that they do not have long, intelligent conversations together but do enjoy going to the beach, dancing, scuba diving, snorkling, flying a kite, whatever. George listened eagerly as his wife talked. "We have to find out how to do that again. We lost that," Linda said, speaking more slowly than before. Linda then spoke about her background again, about how everyone had huge fights but then made up again. She saw the making-up part as a good part and admitted that she actually was used to being in a tense atmosphere and liked it. She said, "I do not make things smooth." Then she said that she had to learn to be without these big ups and downs.

Arlene turned to me and mentioned that she noticed that Linda sits up and talks in an excited manner when she speaks, that she speaks the way she holds her body. "She speaks with her hands like that," Arlene said, indicating with her hands. "Then when I look at George, he seems to be this very even-tempered person. I just see these things because that is the way they present themselves to us." Linda interrupted and said that she was able to make George angry the day before, that when she first met him he was so mellow.

From my inner dialogue: Arlene has obviously not finished what she wanted to say, but Linda is very eager to talk with her. If Linda interrupts a second time, I will encourage them to continue to talk.

T: *(to Arlene)* Say more!

A: Say more?

T: Yes, you said Linda is . . .

A: She holds her body how she expresses herself. And that is how she lives her life. She is either very very excited and very very down, and when she is very angry . . . show . . . and when . . . seems . . .

T: So she is showing what she is thinking?

A: Yes, definitely.

T: And George?

A: I see George as very even-tempered and very calm and basically takes everything you give him in a very quiet and very straightforward way—until you get to a point where he can't remain quiet and straightforward anymore. And then I am sure he can get a really good temper. I have heard stories abut it. I saw a small bit of it—I think the first time I met George—but since that time they have made certain decisions to work on their differences.

T: You spoke about Linda sitting up and expressing herself. What was your word? You used the word when she talked . . . "lively"? . . . no, "excited." And you said that George has another posture, of sitting back, was that the word you used?

A: Right.

T: Does that happen at the same time that he is sitting back and she is sitting up when you have met with them?

A: Yes, many times. It seems that George takes life in a very smooth and even way. He is very slow, unless something gets to him that he really doesn't like and then he too will sit up.

T: When he is in that posture, what do you notice the most, the posture as a whole or his face or his hands or . . . What can you see in front of you when you think of him in that slow position?

A: I see him as a listener to Linda's story, and I see him . . .

T: Do you see his face or his hands or . . .

A: He uses his voice. He does not hesitate to disagree with Linda, but he will still do it from that even posture. So even if he disagrees with her or comments on what she says, he maintains, generally speaking, that posture. But if he really disagrees with her, his posture will change. I have seen his posture change but not seen him very angry or excited.

T: And what is that change in the posture?

A: He will sit up. And he will become more like her.

T: If that posture could speak in the moment of change, what might the words be?

A: "I disagree with you. I have something to add to that. I have something to say myself."

T: And if Linda was able to listen to that, what would she think?

A: I think she would agree with him that he has something to say, that he does not agree with everything that she says.

T: But that might be hard to hear?

A: It was a time ago, but it has become easier and easier to hear that. And I think she recognizes it faster than she used to. And I think George does it less because she recognizes.

[From my inner dialogue: The couple is quietly listening and they do not move. They seem to enjoy what they hear. Arlene seems interested in the talk as well. I do not know if these questions are different from what Arlene is used to, but they might be. Many in Western culture think that speaking is presenting words with one's voice. Wittgenstein thought that we are *in* language and that by being in language we are in activity. That's the reason I asked, "If that posture [a static expression] could speak in the moment of change, what might the words be?" I think that all our movements are also "talking" in the sense that they are "in-forming" and those who see them see meanings in them. And what they see are their constructions of the meanings.]

T: So there might come a day when the voice takes over what the posture spoke before?

A: Um . . . maybe. Because she begins to recognize it more and more. She has become more sensitive to it.

T: If that happened, if the voice took over more—and Linda said she agrees—would that have an influence on her ups and downs? Would it be wise to let the voice take over and speak or would it be wise to let the body still speak? If the voice took over, would that have an influence on George's wish to go off and go away?

[From my inner dialogue: I am shifting my role in the sense that I am moving from a position of questioning to a position of reflecting. Maybe the thoughts I am going to share with Arlene are different from what she is used to?]

T: I ask these questions because we speak so much with our bodies. Dancing. Caressing. It might go easier that way than through all the words. Sometimes people find that more interesting. More challenging. It might be more delicate with all the small movements. Because they tell so much. What do you think about this?

A: I think I haven't thought about this before. And I think I have to think about it for a while. It is very interesting. The various touches to reflect on.

T: And if you were to reflect on it, which bit of that will you reflect the most on?

A: I would like to reflect on watching someone, the bodies, and the idea of what we talked about now about the touching . . . and . . . sometimes how we express ourselves that needs to be recognized. And I think of myself as a person who spends so much time listening to people's voices . . . and sometimes doesn't spend enough time listening to what their bodies might say. And how important that is. I have to think about that for a while. And how I might use that when Linda and George and I work together and in the work I do with other families.

T: Do you think they would accept the question, If you feel closer with the touches, what kinds of feelings are there in the touches? Is there one feeling or many feelings or shifting feelings? Do you think they might accept that kind of question?

A: Aha, I do.

T: And one could ask, Are there other touches in daily life than those which come with the dances? That speak?

A: Now that we are talking about touches in this way . . . in the conversations with them touches always seem to come out as an important issue for Linda and George. So in this family in particular it will fit very well, I think.

T: Sometimes touches move people. Sometimes touches move people so that they say, "No, no, no."

A: So a touch could be a way to talk to someone?

T: Could be. Sometimes people don't go with the words and all those kinds of things. Some people find it easier with touches.

A: As Linda says, it is the touching she likes in the dances.

T: So one question might be, Could there be other touches besides those they can have in the two-step? What do the kids think about that if mother and father start to touch them . . .

A: *(interrupts)* That I would like to talk with them about.

L: *(inturrupts)* The kids like touches. Every night they have to have a hug and a kiss and every time they go to school, the same. That's from me and from him *(glances at George)*. They like him to carry them on his shoulders. Touching is attention.

T: Maybe the kids can come and talk about touches?

A: I like that idea.

T: If they went back to each other's families and talked about the talk here about touches, what might they think? I heard they talked at the beginning that they came from two different backgrounds, different religions. How do they touch in the two families when they want to express feelings?

Arlene turned to the couple. Linda said that it might be easier to get feelings and other things across when they hug; she said that she and George used to hold hands when they watched TV, that touching is important. When Linda said that she wanted George to make up with her, he came over to her and hugged her. The session ended shortly thereafter.

## CONCLUSION

The writing of this chapter taught me, first of all, that I must try to find another way to transcribe a session, to do it so that the reader is touched and moved. It also gave me a chance to think more about knowledge. If one accepts the idea that we already are *in* a certain knowledge before we start to read, how can writing expand that knowledge so that new ideas emerge?

## EDITOR'S QUESTIONS

Q: *Some people take the position that the therapist is responsible for initiating a therapeutic process that will lead to a successful outcome. Others see the therapist's role as simply generating or seeding new ideas without a specific focus on goals. Wht is your view of the therapist's responsibility for creating a context for change within the family? Doesn't the therapist have an ethical responsibility to be outcome oriented? How do you assess you influence on the system?*

A: I see myself being responsible for contributions so that a change might occur. However, what kind of change that is, and how and when it might happen, is not my responsibility. I do not think that a therapist has an ethical responsibility to be outcome oriented, but we have other ethical responsibilities, for example, not hurting people. How do I assess the progress of a session? I try to follow the conversation from second to second to look for or hear the signs that clients give that tell me that my comments and questions are not unusual enough to be stimulating for them or that they are too unusual for them. Clients give many signs; my job is to train my sensitivities so that I can see and hear those signs.

Q: *Many family therapists have been trained in the directive/strategic model (the modernist view) and therefore assume the role of "expert" in the system. I wonder how you made the conceptual shift to postmodern thinking, where you relinquish the expert position, embrace a stance of "not knowing," and become an equal partner with the client. Perhaps you would present your thoughts on this issue.*

A: First, I must say that I don't take the "not knowing" position to its extreme. I know that it helps the process if I ask the consultee in the beginning a session, "What is the history of the idea to come here?" and "How would you like to use this meeting?" I also know that professionals very easily become too optimistic, too solution-oriented, too quick, and so on. I therefore know that I shall try to slow down.

Nor do I believe clients and professionals can become equals. Clients have "local" experiences I don't have, and I have "general" experiences they don't have. So we are different. We are also unequal in the sense that they have the final word about what we are to talk about and in which way. We are, however, equal in the sense that they and I have equal rights to refuse to take part in a particular conversation. I basically see my conceptual shift as a consequence of the relational shift that occurred after the talks "opened" during the reflecting processes, a shift from the more hierarchical to the more heterachical (egalitarian) relationship. And that relational shift was a consequence of taking seriously the uncomfortable feeling that followed my being in the superior position in a hierarchical relationship.

Q: *Your use of the reflecting position is something that grew and evolved over time in your thinking and in your work. What suggestions do you have for others who are just beginning to nurture a reflexive stance in their clinical work? What must the therapist "unlearn" in order to effectively assume a reflecting position? Also, how do you see your work evolving in the future?*

A: To those interested in adopting the reflexive stance I would say, "Try to do what you find natural to do." And I might add that what I myself found it important, but extremely difficult, to do was to try to listen to what the clients say instead of making up meanings about what they say. Just listen to what they say. And if there is something in what they say that is very important to listen to, it can be more easily seen than heard. So to listen is also to see. Maybe to see is the most important.

How might my work evolve? At present there is work going on to make the reflecting processes part of the evaluation of therapeutic work, namely, by asking the clients to be co-researchers in describing the professionals' contributions in the therapeutic meetings. This is an attempt to bridge the very wide and very unhappy gap between academia and practice and to bring research back to the people.

In what other directions might my work evolve? Maybe working together with people from very different fields. Maybe reviving my interest in medical conditions in order to try to understand them in terms of the humanities. Maybe stop it all and say, "It is over. No more."

Q: *From the illustration provided, the reader might wonder how the therapist can pay attention to both his or her own inner dialogue and the*

*comments of the family members present. How much attention must be
paid to the family's descriptions and how much to one's own silent
thoughts?*
A: I would say to that reader, "Try to do your best. That will be good
enough." I am not sure that one *must* do any particular thing. However, I
think it is all to the good if the clinician is able to listen and to see and to
think about what is seen and heard so that he or she can contribute comments to keep the conversation going.

## ACKNOWLEDGMENTS

I wish to thank Arlene Brett-Gordon and her team—Lee Shilts, Candy Hartman,
Alan Jablonowitz, Mark Shubert, and Sandy Zelleck—who worked so hard to bring
the couple to the place they came to.

## REFERENCES

Andersen, T. (1987). The reflecting team: Dialogue and meta-dialogue in clinical
    work. *Family Process, 26,* 415–428.
Andersen, T. (1991). *The reflecting team: Dialogues and dialogues about the dialogues.*
    New York: Norton.
Andersen, T. (1992a). Relationship, language and pre-understanding in the reflect-
    ing processes. *Australian and New Zealand Journal of Family Therapy, 13*(2),
    87–91.
Andersen, T. (1992b). Reflections on reflecting with the families. In S. McNamee &
    K. J. Gergen (Eds.), *Therapy as social construction.* London: Sage.
Anderson, H., Goolishian, H., & Winderman, L. (1986). Problem-determined
    system: Toward transformation in family therapy. *Journal of Strategic and
    Systemic Therapy, 5*(4), 1–14.
Anderson, H., & Gollishian, H. (1988). Human systems as linguistic systems:
    Preliminary and evoking ideas about the implications for clinical theory. *Family
    Process, 27,* 371–394.
Bateson, G. (1972). *Steps to an ecology of mind.* New York: Ballantine.
Bateson, G. (1979). *Mind and nature: A necessary unit.* New York: Bantam.
Gergen, K. J. (1985). Social pragmatics and the origins of psychological discourse.
    In K. J. Gergen & K. Davis (Eds.), *The social construction of the person* (pp.
    111–127). New York: Springer-Verlag.
Gergen, K. J. (1991). *The saturated self.* New York: Basic Books.
Grayling, A. C. (1988). *Wittgenstein.* Oxford, UK: Oxford University Press.
Øvreberg, G., & Andersen, T. (1986). *Aadel Bülow-Hansen's fysioterapi.* Tromsø,
    Norway: Tromsprodukt.
Warnke, G. (1987). *Gadamer: Hermeneutics, tradition and reason.* Stanford, CA: Stan-
    ford University Press.

# 14

## On a Roller Coaster: A Collaborative Language Systems Approach to Therapy

### HARLENE ANDERSON

Thirteen-year-old Anna and her family were referred to family therapy by her school, which had just "checked her out." Anna had a history of school and family problems, including running away, drugs, violence at home, and medical problems. The family's therapist, Nikki Theisinger, who had presented the case to her supervision group, said that despite the group members' helpful ideas and what she described as a "sincere effort" by the family, the situation was "uphill and downhill." The therapy supervision group had been especially helpful with ideas for helping the mother follow up on Anna's medical problem, which is believed to be idiopathic thrombocytic purpura (ITP), a blood platelet disorder of unknown origin. But Anna was continuing to run away from home, and she continued to have physical battles at home with her mother, Dorothy, as well as with her 19-year-old sister, Christy. The therapist feared that someone might get seriously hurt.

The therapist had met with the mother and daughter together and separately in six sessions. Anna attended reluctantly. Her sister, Christy, attended one of the sessions and then refused to return because, as she said, it wasn't her problem. The therapist's work with the family included telephone conversations with the school counselor and with Anna's physician. Although the therapist's attitude toward the family and their work together was positive, she expressed a feeling of great frustration about her experience with the uphill-downhill nature of the case.

The therapist requested consultation to help her and the family "get some fresh ideas." She invited mother and daughter to come with her to the consultation interview, which was held during a workshop she was attending with 14 other therapists; I, the consultant, was a workshop leader. The workshop concerned a collaborative language systems approach to therapy, which is the name for the clinical theory and work developed by Harold Goolishian and me, work previously referred to as a problem-determined system and a problem-organizing, problem-dissolving approach (Anderson, Goolishian, Pulliam & Winderman, 1986; Gollishian & Anderson, 1987; Anderson & Goolishian, 1988).

## PREMISES

Language and conversation are the core concepts of the collaborative language systems approach (Anderson & Goolishian, 1988, 1990; Goolishian & Anderson, 1987, 1992a, 1992b). These core concepts are rooted in contemporary hermeneutics and social constructionism, or what may be referred to as a postmodernist interpretive perspective (Gadamer, 1975; Geertz, 1973; Gergen, 1985; Rorty, 1979; Wachterhauser, 1986). Although all hermeneutic and social constructionist concepts cannot be lumped into one, they do share a common thread: They emphasize meaning as an intersubjective phenomenon, created and experienced by individuals in conversation and action with others and with themselves. This assumes that human action takes place in a reality of understanding that is created through social construction and dialogue and that we live and understand our lives through socially constructed narrative realities, that is, that we give meaning and organization to our experiences and to our self-identity in the course of these transactions.

From this perspective, human systems are language-and-meaning-generating systems: we create meaning with each other. A therapy system is a language system in which the client and the therapist create meaning with each other. It is a system in which people coalesce around relevant discourse, around a "problem": something or somebody that someone is worried about and wants to change. I enclose *problem* in quotation marks to emphasize that there is no such thing as *a* problem. The problem has as many descriptions and explanations as there are members of the system, which is why this discourse is sometimes referred to as the "problem system."

The process of therapy is a therapeutic conversation, a dialogue, a "talking with." The conversation entails an "in there together" process, in which the therapist and client engage each other, through dialogue, in co-exploring the issues at hand—the problem—and in co-developing "newness" that is, altered or novel meanings, realities, and narratives. In the therapeutic conversation, newness is continually evolving toward "dissolving" the problem and cultivating a new sense of agency and freedom for the client. Problems are, therefore, not solved but dissolved. Dis-solution of the problem may be born of the client's newly acquired sense of agency and self-capability. This sense can evolve from an altered understanding of the problem, which is then no longer viewed or experienced as a problem and may actually be dissolved through actions. Change, whether in the cognitive or behavioral domain, is a natural consequence of dialogue.

This conversational therapeutic process is best accomplished by the therapist's expertise in creating a space for the client's story, maintaining a "not knowing" position, and asking conversational questions. These set the stage for collaboration; they create a space for dialogue and facilitate the conversational process.

Implicit in this way of working is that each client, each problem, each therapy session, and each course of therapy is seen as unique. The approach does not rely on preconceived knowledge such as commonalities of problems or on across-the-board skills and techniques. This does not mean that "anything goes" or that this conversational therapeutic process unfolds simply by maintaining an atmosphere of nondirective and empathetic conversation. Instead, the process becomes a source for a wide range of thinking and action that is distinctive to the people involved and the issues at hand. Nor does it mean that therapists do not know anything and enter the therapy room as a *tabula rasa*; quite naturally, they bring with them who they are and all that that entails. It means that the therapist's pre-experiences and pre-knowledges do not lead. In this process both the therapist's and the client's expertise are engaged to dissolve the problem.

Does the therapist have to monitor what she or he says? Can the therapist offer an idea, have an opinion, ask about anything? Of course! What is important, however, is that what is asked and what is offered is done from a tentative attitude, that is, one that does not imply judgment, blame, or a fixed hypothesis. The therapist must be willing to change just as he or she expects the client to be willing to change.

I have selected excerpts from the aforementioned consultation interview—pieces of the conversations, the stories—to illustrate and highlight therapeutic attitudes and actions considered critical to creating, maintaining, and dissolving the kind of therapeutic conversation associated with a collaborative language systems approach. This is not a way of working one can learn in a workshop on Friday and then do on Monday. Working in this way entails not only shifts in one's professional and theoretical perspectives but in one's way of being in the world as well. Translation of this philosophical stance and its premises to the clinical arena will vary, depending on the case and the therapist's style. The interview excerpted here represents one translation; it epitomizes my style at the moment.

## MULTIPLE CONVERSATONS ABOUT "UPHILL AND DOWNHILL": THE CONSULTATION INTERVIEW PROCESS

The process of the consultation interview and its conversational steps evolved during the interview itself and began with the therapist's presentation of the family and her work with them to the workshop group. Issues such as who should be in the interview room, the therapist's role, the question of breaks, and whether a reflecting team approach would be enacted were determined along the way; they were specific to the case and the context of the interview. The interview included these steps:

- Therapist presents family and therapy situation to the workshop group.
- Consultant interviews therapist, mother and daughter.
- Consultant talks with mother while daughter and therapist listen from behind a one-way mirror.
- Consultant talks with therapist (while mother and daughter take a break) and touches base briefly with the workshop group.
- Consultant talks with the daughter while the mother and the therapist listen behind a one-way mirror.
- Consultant invites the mother and therapist to join the daughter, and consultant and therapist listen to participants' reflections.

The interview lasted 1½ hours. The interview was rich in language and content, and the story may easily seduce therapists to a too-rapid understanding of this family's drama and its characters (including the therapist). Leading the family and therapist in a unilaterally determined direction is tempting.

I found it difficult to decide which excerpts of the stories to select for this chapter. I chose to focus on three of the interview's conversations, thus illustrating my work with verbal transcripts, summaries, and retrospective reflections.

### Therapist Presents Family and Therapy Situation to the Workshop Participants

To begin the session I said the following to the therapist: "Tell us [The consultant and the workshop participants] what *you* think *we* need to know about the family and your work with them so that *we* can be helpful to you. and "Tell us your and the family's expectations of today's interview." I asked the participants simply to listen as the therapist told us what *she* thought *we* needed to know. If they had questions or comments, they were to note and hold on to them. In this manner the therapist told *her story* as *she* wanted to tell it without being interrupted or guided by what others wanted to know or thought was important. Neither I nor the workshop participants discussed the family or the therapy with the therapist; she simply presented her story, her dilemmas, and her agenda.

The therapist summarized the family's situation and her work with them (as described in abbreviated form at the beginning of this chapter). She said that she, as well as the mother and daughter, needed some new ideas. To organize the interview to meet her and the family's needs and expectations, she asked me to interview the family while she remained in the therapy room, as she had promised the family she would do.

Usually, my preference is to learn about the family in their presence, what I call "publicly." In this case the workshop agenda influenced us to learn about the family "privately," in their absence. But since I had not discussed the case with the therapist before the workshop (except for matters of scheduling and videotaping), I knew only what the workshop participants knew.

## Consultant Talks with Therapist, Mother, and Daughter

The interview began with the therapist, the mother, and the daughter with my introducing the mother and daughter to the workshop participants and summarizing for the family what we had learned from the therapist about them and their agenda.

H: Hi, I'm Harlene Anderson. Please feel free to call me Harlene. And let me introduce the two of you to the folks who are behind the mirror, via the video. This is Dorothy, who is the mother in this family, and this is Anna. And (*to Anna*) you're fifteen?

A: Thirteen.

H: Oh, thirteen. I just aged you a couple of years: you're thirteen. Okay. Nikki was sharing with me and our colleagues—who are observing a little bit about the two of you and a little bit about the work that the three of you have been doing together—some of the talking, and also that Nikki has been talking with Harry Goolishian and some of her colleagues in the Galveston office, and kind of in a nutshell what she was saying—(*addressing Nikki*) add what you think I'm leaving out—is that she's known the two of you since some time in October, and that you all have met six or eight times, and that you originally had met through the youth worker [counselor at the school] . . .

A: Probation.

H: Through probation, okay. And there were some concerns about *you* (*to*

*Anna*), that you were running away, for one, and the possibility of some other kind of things, but I think that Nikki mentioned the running away. And Nikki said that her experience was that things in the session would seem like things were okay and then she would find out later that something else had happened and it was kind of uphill and downhill, uphill . . .

D: Like a roller coaster.

H: Oh, like a roller coaster, okay. And she felt that all of you had really been sincerely, sort of, putting your shoulder to the wheel and working really hard at this and trying to get a handle on this, but somehow nothing seemed to really work in the long run.

N: That was for a long period of time.

H: And in talking with Harry Goolishian, the idea was, well maybe we can just look at some of the things *you folks* are concerned about, some of the talking that *you all* have been doing, and see where to go from here. But I would be interested in *your* sharing with *us* kind of what *you* currently see as things that *you all* are concerned about or that *you* see as problematic, and maybe where things are now compared to when you first met Nikki, as a way of trying to get a handle on things, and where to go from here.

[I shared what I learned about the family members "privately," before their arrival. My misunderstandings were open for correction. I did not begin the conversation with a preconceived idea concerning the family, the therapist, or their work together. Instead, I made clear that I—we— were to learn what *they* thought *we* should know. I showed my interest in each client and invited each viewpoint, making room for their stories, their familiar experiences.

Making room for the familiar and maintaining coherence with the client's views is a critical step to dialogue. This openness to the other is similar to an idea attributed to Gregory Bateson, namely that entertaining new and novel ideas requires room for the familiar. Sometimes therapists express distrust of this notion, fearing that accepting and maintaining the other person's reality risks reifying the problem, participating in the client's denials or delusions, or abdicating social responsibility. Quite the contrary. I have found that maintaining coherence and showing an openness to the other person moves beyond merely honoring the client's reality and transcends fixed positions. The therapist's curiosity and excitement about the other's reality, shown in a sincere and earnest manner, begins to peak the other person's curiosity as well. It invites the other person to join the therapist in a shared inquiry, a co-exploration of the issues at hand. As the therapist begins to learn about and tries to understand the client's view, the therapist's learning process naturally shifts to a mutually puzzling process engaging therapist and client.

Setting the stage for collaboration, I used collective, nonhierarchical language. By using *us* and *we*—saying to the therapist, for example, "Tell us what you think that we need to know"—I included myself with the workshop participants. Using *you*, I referred to the individuals and to the collective group (mother, daughter, therapist) as a working group. I also acknowledged that others had participated in the conversations (the supervision group). And I used words like *talking,* not therapy.]

D: *(beginning her story)* We still have problems . . . Anna is trying but still wants to determine what she can do and what she can't do.

[The mother then describes the problems at home between Anna and herself, the conflicts between Anna and her sister, and Anna's temper.]

D: I am a very opinionated person: "Just do it my way." I'm a dictator type, I guess. I want things done my way, and if you're not doing things my way the temper starts to flare. So she's got things against her. It's not all her.

H: So you're describing a kind of *Mutiny on the Bounty,* or what?

D: That's basically what it is: "I'm thirteen years old; I'm ready to leave; I'm ready to make a life of my own; I don't need an education; I don't need anything else."

H: So we've got two women in this family with very strong opinions and minds of their own.

D: Very much so. Well, three of them, but one of them just sort of goes her way.

[The therapist tells about an event the mother described in a recent telephone conversation: When the lights went out one night during a storm, mother and daughter had a talk by the fireplace.]

D: When they turned the lights out it was fantastic. We lit the fireplace and we lit the candles and we sat and talked and we talked about a lot of different things. And I sat and listened to her talk to her friends on the phone. And that was the first time that she was not so secretive—so you don't talk to me, you talk to your friends and let me hear what you're saying that way. Then, with the fireplace going and no lights and no television and no VCR and no radio, then it was like it was a time we could sit and get closer and talk a little bit, but that's only a small amount of time. It took two or three hours to turn the lights back on.

[I want to make room for and validate all views and be what I call "multipartial."]

H: Anna, where are you with all of this? How would you describe what's happening now and . . .

A: Confusion.

H: Confusion, okay. About . . .

[Incomplete sentences and hanging words invite the client to verbalize.]

A: I'm just real confused about all of this. I mean about the home fighting and then I only get to see my friends for weekends . . . talking to them for the last few days . . . and my personal life and my family life. There's a lot of things that are confusing.

D: This is like an old cliché, but when I was your age if I were to pull the things that you could pull I wouldn't even be seeing my friends on weekends.

A: But I'm not you.

D: So you've got a lot of different . . .

A: I'm not you.

D: You've got a lot of different things happening for you.

A: I know, but I'm not you.

H: (to Anna) Well, let me ask about the . . . you said confusion about the fighting at home, things happening at home. Can you say a little bit more about that? Fighting between whom and about what?

[Here I asked about something (the confusion) that Anna mentioned earlier. The therapeutic conversation involves learning a little about one thing and then becoming curious about something else. It is a touching on this and that, never staying with any one thing too long. I don't want to give the impression that I believe that one thing is more important than another; I don't want to find myself on a narrow path.

The telling of a client's story involves a multiplicity of things the therapist can respond to and show interest in. What taps one therapist's curiosity may bore another. Choices of questions, comments, or other utterances by the therapist may limit the client's story because they may, implicitly or explicitly, convey a position, an agenda, or an expected response. I want to make choices that widen both my and the client's room for maneuverability, not narrow it. I want to demonstrate a *"not-knowing"* position. I want to be a *responsive, active listener* and to ask *conversational questions*. Not knowing refers to a general therapeutic attitude and belief that the therapist does not have access to privileged information, is not operating on preconceived ideas, can never fully understand another person, and always needs to know more about what has been said and not said

Conversational questions come from a position of not knowing and are the therapist's primary tool. They involve responsive or active listening, which requires attending to clients' stories in a distinct way, immersing oneself in clients' conversations, talking with them about their concerns, and trying to grasp their current story and what gives it shape. The immediate dialogic event, the developing narrative, informs the next question; the questions are not formed by the therapist's preconceived theories of what the story should be. I am not, for example, gathering information to sort out on my therapist's map, a map that then would inform me about the problem (diagnosis) and guide my actions (strategies and interventions). Nor is it my aim to validate or nullify a hypothesis. Conversational questions are, therefore, not generated by technique, method, or a preset template of questions.

No one question represents a conversational question, nor can any one question influence a dialogic or nondialogic space. Each question, each utterance by the therapist, is an element of an overall process and comes from an honest, continuous therapeutic posture of not understanding too quickly, of not knowing

In summary, I heard both Anna's and her mother's views on Anna's running away, problems at school, and fights at home with the sister and mother. The interview continued with Anna and her mother telling stories about fights between Anna and Christy over a ring and over chocolate candy. Strong, discrepant opinions emerged quickly; each client repeatedly interrupted and corrected the other. Anna was in tears.]

N: This is similar to what usually happens.

H: (*to the mother*) You said a moment ago when I asked you what you thought was happening and where things are now, I think, that you thought Anna was afraid of something?

[The mother then tells about how Anna is "afraid of school," about Anna's "finding out that she's all right". . ."and how Anna doesn't want to be sick." She describes the details of Anna's medical problem and the difficulty of obtaining a diagnosis, of how it was necessary to rule out lupus, leukemia, and AIDS. The mother says that she believes Anna's medical problem may be part of, or causing, her other problems. "There are still a lot of unknowns," she says, emphasizing that the doctors advised Anna not to use drugs. Anna interrupts and wants to finish a story she began earlier about blacking out during a fight with her mother.]

A: One of these days I'm afraid that I'm going to get so bad that I'm going to try to kill her (*looks at mother*). When I black out, I can do anything because my temper gets so high and I get so mad that I don't know what I'm going to do. I see guns all around, her body lying there, and I had a knife in my hand.

N: This kind of brings up the point as to why they are here.

[Nikki is referring back to concern she shared with the group, namely, that someone in the family might get hurt.]

H: Let me tell you about an idea that I have. I was just thinking that since we are all (*referring to myself, the family, the therapist, and the workshop participants*) gathered here, maybe we could take advantage of what we can take advantage of. I'm wondering about Dorothy and me staying in here and talking some and having you and Anna behind the mirror. Would that be agreeable?

[I often use what I think of as more cooperative, softening, indefinite, and tentative words and phrases such as "wondering," "kind of," "maybe." Such words and phrases are more inviting of dialogue and the co-exploration of issues. They show more interest in the other's view and less interest in a therapist-held view.]

## Talking with Mother While Daughter and Therapist Listen from behind One-Way Mirror

Nikki, Dorothy, and Anna all happened to agree with my suggestion. Had any one of them not agreed, however, I would have been ready to talk with that person about her view and willing to take back the suggestion. Talking with the mother and daughter separately—while each, along with the therapist, observed the other—was not preplanned. The idea emerged from the immediate conversational process. Mother and daughter had become heavily engaged in correcting and interrupting each other. Absorbed in these dueling monologic[1] views, each was unable to listen nondefensively to the other. To be able to do so is an important step toward both internal and external dialogic processes. In retrospect, my suggestion to talk with Dorothy while Anna and the therapist listened was probably influenced by a combination of factors: I felt that I had the luxury of time, and the availability of a one-way mirror, and that this approach could also serve to demonstrate to the workshop participants one way in which to try to engage in a dialogic mode those who are caught in a monological gridlock

I began with the mother, as if I were saying to her "Let's start over with *your* story." This was not a strategy. I was interested in what was on her mind as a mother.

H: Can I back up just a little bit? I feel that this sounds like such a complicated situation and sounds like it has certainly escalated recently . . .

D: No, it hasn't been recently.

H: It hasn't been recently. So this is what I was wondering. This is something that's been going on for a long long time in terms of your concerns about Anna, and you're sort of experiencing her as a very headstrong child with a mind of her own. Sort of fill me in on when your concerns began, and sort of a real shift. When did those shifts start occurring?

[The mother continues her story, telling of her own personal struggles. She tells of how, in the seventies, she felt inadequate and didn't have the "capacity to handle two growing children, taking care of them, and

---

[1] *Monologic* is used here in the sense that one idea or one group of ideas dominates to the extent that there is no room (either internally or externally) to entertain another's view or to alter one's own. This, in contrast to dialogue that allows room for and multiple ideas and their crisscrossing.

making things right for them." She talks about how she got into drugs, lost her job, finally found a job in the kitchen and as a waitress at a country–western dance hall, became depressed, and had "a breakdown of sorts." Her life situation grew so critical that child welfare authorities took custody of her children for nine months.]

H: Okay. So you and the girls' father . . .

D: They don't have any fathers. I was married for seven years, and he didn't want his daughter. And when I got pregnant with the second [by another man], I said "No, there's no way." And so they're mine.

[She continues to tell her story about the downhill parts: being a single mother, working long, strenuous hours at the dance hall; and the financial stresses.[2]]

H: How did you get yourself back to where you are today?

[She told of how one day a customer's husband came in the dance hall and offered her a job with his company. She beams as she tells of the new job, her accomplishments, how her salary quadrupled, and how her life has been so much easier since then. She says it is like going "from bean bags to couch and chairs." I grew curious about the children.]

H: Let me just ask you to help ground me. When all this was happening and you lost your job, were doing the waitress work, and the long hours and having so many difficulties . . .

D: Anna was on her own.

[Dorothy tells how Christy, who was 12, would not help with Anna, who was about 9, and says Anna was "on the streets." She says Anna has always defied authority and has tried drugs, been bored, run away, and missed school. "She would rebel. She had already gained her independence and didn't want to give it away. I can get angry, but I can't make her."]

D: When she wants something, there's not much that she couldn't get. If she really wanted it, she could accomplish it. But as long as there is authority over her, she has problems with it.

---

[2]When I showed an edited version of this interview at a workshop, women who identified themselves as feminist therapists became exceptionally critical because they felt that I was unresponsive to the mother's financial difficulties. This insensitivity to gender and political and economic position, they suggested, placed me in the position of one who was further marginalizing women. Not only was my experience during the interview quite the opposite, but I have a long history (personally and professionally) of siding with those who are oppressed and victimized by the dominant political, economic, and social systems. I felt genuinely sensitive to the mother's financial plight as well as to her circumstances of single motherhood. In addition, I felt that the mother was proud of how she had overcome her difficulties. I use this as an example of how easy it is to have multiple interpretations of an excerpt from any conversation or story. What is important is how the mother experienced the interview and whether she felt heard or unheard.

H: So that part of her personality, you are saying, sort of clashes with the everyday rules of life in terms of school and . . .

[The mother agrees and quickly gives examples. Then she turns to Anna's medical problems.]

H: So you think that all of this has been complicated by the medical problems.

[I always want to make sure that I hear what the client intends for me to hear, I check it out with them. Often, I repeat to client's what I think they said, letting them know that they have been heard, that I'm trying to understand, and giving them a chance to correct me if I'm wrong.]

D: For years she was told by all of us . . . that she was just lazy and didn't want to go to school. (*shifts back to talking about herself and how she gets angry with herself*) I close doors . . . something has to be done. Anna has no respect for me, no belief in me. There's not much I can do to help her because she won't accept it. And it makes me angry too because there are so many things I could do . . . very angry because any authority I have had has been taken away.

[She was speaking of the childrens' protective service and the law. She continues talking about how she "can't handle it" when the daughters fight and how in the last few weeks she has "just let it go." She describes her older daughter as a "snot, an intellectual snob and slob."]

H: If Christy had been here today?

D: She would probably say, "If Mother would butt out of it, then things wouldn't be so bad and Anna would start going to school."

[Tearfully, Dorothy gives examples of conflicts between her daughters and tells more about the blackout that Anna mentioned earlier in the interview. She talks about how her feelings for Anna have changed, likening the change to birds leaving the nest. "I've just flat given up."]

H: Dorothy, what do you think will happen if you and the folks down in Galveston can't get a handle on this . . . down the road?

D: We'll keep fighting, keep trying, and we will find one way or another—something will work. She feels like she's an outsider . . . doesn't accept the mother–daughter relationship. I don't know what to do. There's only so far I can stretch, so I start closing doors. It would be easy just to go to sleep. But I know that it's going to turn out okay, maturity is going to come.

H: (*responding to a combination of events the mother has described*) So you're kind of three gutsy ladies. Is that hereditary?

D: Yes.

H: Let me ask you what may sound like kind of a crazy kind of question. If some of the things had not happened, like the economical and emotional downturns you and the children had . . . living with your mother, and Anna being, as you were describing, kind of on the streets and into drugs—what do you think would be happening with her these days? She's thirteen. What about the ITP, the medical issue, would she be handling that differently?

[These questions represent a curiosity about the issues from another angle; I am talking about the familiar in an unfamiliar way.]

H: Nikki had mentioned earlier, and you had also mentioned, the fireplace . . . a special occasion . . . sort of a glimpse into the future. And what do you think it would take to allow some of that to happen more? Not necessarily sitting in front of the fireplace but more a sense of peace, less conflict.

[Dorothy talks about wanting to enjoy the company of her children. She and Anna are alike, she says, and tells how adventurous she was when she was a young girl.]

H: Two peas in a pod, both adventurous. So in a way, it's how to maintain this spirit of adventure, this spirit of independence while at the same time not being self-destructive or dangerous. (*Dorothy nods in agreement.*)

[Since the interview was now into its second hour, I suggested a coffee break.]

## Brief Conversations with Therapist and with Workshop Participants

After my conversation with the mother, I talked briefly with the therapist. My sense of needing to touch base with her and my awareness of the time, not a clinical agenda, influenced my decision not to talk with her in the family's presence. Nikki talked about the change taking place in her internal dialogue. She explained that the content and details of the story were the same but that she was putting it together, moving it around, differently. She was beginning to have a new sense of agency.

H: What's going on in your head now?

N: Well, first, just before the break, I leaned forward and it's come to me. It's almost like watching and listening to this family, maybe it was like starting at the middle of the book. Now it's kind of like it's in a sequence, and things being said are not information. That is different. I heard a lot of this before, but watching and listening and being here in the room this way . . . it's very different, it's very sequential. The story is very much more organized. So that's one impression.

H: You have more of a sense of grounding just in terms of who these folks are and what's happening with them. Is that fair?

N: Yes. It's not so much who they are. I felt like I had that before . . . more grounded, more a sense of who they are.

H: But the pieces fit together in a way that makes more sense?

[I asked about Anna behind the mirror and Nikki says that in the beginning Anna acted as if she were trying not to listen. She acted annoyed and called her mother a bitch, but she soon shifted to listening very intently, "very tuned in." Then I explain about my suggestion to talk with the mother and daughter separately, with each listening to the other.]

H:  I just felt that, given the time that I was imagining we had today and that this was sort of a one-shot deal, it was going to be easier to talk with them separately, and maybe I was thinking in terms of it being more efficient and easier for me to get a sense of them because of the thing that was going on between the two of them. I had you go behind the mirror with Anna because I did not want Anna to feel that we were throwing her out of the room, and my thought was—just my very quick take on the mother—there were probably not things she was going to say differently whether Anna was in the room listening or not listening. So I felt it would be best to have Anna listen.

N:  But listening back there was very different, very enlightening: being out but in at the same time, if that makes any sense.

I decided to then speak briefly with the workshop participants. I was aware of the fact that they had been held captive in a room observing, for an hour. The workshop had a duel agenda: training and clinical work. The participants were a part of the language system that I needed to be in conversation with. I told them that I was curious about their thoughts and suggested that each participant give a quick observation in the form of a question, an opinion, or a suggestion. I listened to them without discussing their observations and then returned to the therapy room to join Anna. This time the mother and the therapist were behind the mirror.

## Conversation with Anna

Now I wanted to give equal room to Anna's story, to learn what occupied her. I started by acknowledging that there were several views: hers, her mother's, and her sister's. Anna was now the expert and was free to talk nondefensively, no longer needing to correct her mother's distorted view or promote her own. Being behind the mirror had relieved her of the opportunity to interrupt and correct her mother and had served as a small step toward an external and internal dialogue (as opposed to monologue). She talked in a much calmer fashion than before, and with less edge. She first responded to my mention of her sister's view and then shifted to her own ideas of herself.

H:  So we have your mom behind the mirror this time. Okay? Well, obviously, this is a very complicated situation; it's been going on for a while. There are many many pieces and there are many many opinions, it sounds like, in terms of what's going on. I'm only hearing your and your mom's today, and I'm sure that Christy has another slant.

A: Christy would just say that I have no consideration, I have no manners, and I need to get polite, or something like that.

H: Oh, she would think you're a rude person with bad manners, that that's what it's all about?

A: Yeah.

H: What else might she tell me?

A: Uh, I don't know. That I need to calm down. I have a very big temper, and that she doesn't like me.

H: And that she doesn't like you.

A: Uh huh.

H: Well, if I were to ask her how come Anna is so rude and has bad manners and has such a big temper, what would she tell me, what . . .

A: Knowing her, she'd probably say something like: " 'Cause she gets attention and she feeds on attention, so that's the reason she's so rude and everything, 'cause she thrives on attention."

H: Oh, she would tell me that part of the reason is . . .

A: I thrive on attention.

H: You thrive on attention.

A: I don't think that, but she does.

H: You don't think that, but she does. What do *you* think is going on?

A: I don't know. I'm just here.

H: You're just here.

A: I don't know. I'm not going to run away anymore, at least I'm going to try to make sure I don't run away any more. So I don't like running away. One reason why I want to do it is to get away from it all. I mean I'm not exactly running away from it, I'm just trying to get away from it so I can figure things out in my own way without having to stay at home and listen to all the fighting. At least, whenever I go for about a week at my friend's house, I can concentrate on something else and start thinking. And then all my friends talk to me and everything, and it's like it helps me a lot.

H: So when you run away, is that similar to when your mother say she closes the doors to kind of get away from it, and when the doors are closed it gives her an opportunity to kind of—I think she used the word "relax"—or it sounded like maybe get some energy to try to tackle the craziness again?

A: That's what I think it is.

[Attempting to learn more about her views, I invite Anna into my wondering. Curious about what she thinks her mother should do differently but reluctant to risk putting her in the position of criticizing her mother, I asked her a what-if, a speculative, question. This, as well as using cooperative rather than blaming language, allows Anna to make a less defensive response and gives her more freedom to be creative, to access the "new." I do not try try to lead her to positive thoughts about her mother or positive solutions. My aim was merely to learn about and explore her views with her.]

H: Let me ask you a totally different kind of question. What if you were a mother and you had a thirteen-year-old daughter and some of the same kinds of things were going on, what, as a mother, would you do to solve this problem?

A: Well, I'd understand.

H: How would you understand?

[As the conversation continued, I became even more curious about Anna's thoughts.]

H: How does a mother understand a daughter? Say more about that. You're saying to some extent she understands you because she's done a lot of the same things maybe you've done. Then there are some other ways she doesn't understand you. Is that what you're saying? Okay. If you were the mother, how would you handle those kinds of things with your daughter—the respect issue? How would you show your daughter respect and love? So you are each good at trying to punch each other's buttons? So, when you say "mad," is that sort of the same thing as you get frustrated very easily. Do you puff up? What do you do? How would I know you were mad if I saw you?

[As Anna talks about how she thinks it's in her blood, it's the way she lives, it's the way she eats, I remember that during the coffee break workshop participants expressed curiosity about Anna's medical problem and its influence on her behavior. I then tell Anna about my private conversation with the group.]

H: When I went back and talked to the group, they had a lot of questions . . . one, about the ITP and the complications. They were wondering what it must be like to be thirteen and to have something like that?

A: It's scary. It scares me a lot. That's about the only thing I'm afraid of except that I black out when I fight.

[She goes on to say that the doctors told her that she doesn't have leukemia, lupus, or AIDS, but that she's at risk . . . a lot of unknowns.]

A: That's what scares me the most. Bad enough having the fear of dying in my mind, but having the fear of a real disease, it frightens me.

[If she had AIDS, she says, she couldn't look her sister and mother in the face. She says that she wouldn't kill herself, though, running away is in place of killing herself, that it's a way of saying that she hates the world. In running away she understands that other people have problems. Referring to running away, she says, "I was feeling sorry for myself. I don't like pity." She returns to the attention issue.

A: If I do eat up attention like my sister says, I don't recognize that I'm doing it. I don't understand it. I don't ask for something unless I need it . . . because I get attention but I don't always want it.

H: You have a lot of pride.

[Anna began to talk about her father and how her mother "doesn't want to tell me about him until I'm twenty-one." She says her sister always calls her "a bastard child, not wanted"; she adds, rolling her eyes, "When I was calling her a whore."]

Approaching the end the conversation, I summarize and offer an appreciation of its complexity: "A lot of very complex, complicated pieces to this puzzle. Maybe sometimes the three of you aren't even working on the same puzzle." I ask Anna if her sister would come in to see Nikki. "No," Anna responds. I continue to show that I respect Anna and am taking her seriously when I ask, "Any questions you want to ask me or the group?" Anna has many questions and shows no sign of leaving even though I had intimated that we were out of time.

A: I just want to know if I'll ever get better, be a perfect person to where I don't fight, I don't yell, and my life would be straighter and forward rather than backwards and upside down.

H: An important question, one we need to write in capital letters. Sounds like all of you are quite miserable about the situation.

[Anna continues to talk. I acknowledge other things she has said that perhaps need to be in capital letters, such as "And take the bait easily. I have a lot of pride just like my mother. Will I ever get better or will I just be like this—misery?"]

H: I know that each in your own way are working to make this work. Must be awfully discouraging and frustrating and, as you say, "angry-making" that at least to this point in time that no matter what you do, that this sort of thing just comes right around and hits you in the face again and it's like you're back to zero.

[Anna continues talking about school and problems with the principal. She talks more about her medical problem, wondering what parts of her come from her father.]

H: So, lots of questions about yourself, your physical condition, your emotional condition, learning who you are, what parts of you came from your dad, lots of questions that you have.

A: I'd like to meet my dad—or meet the man who says he's not my dad—see how he acts, just to see him and say hi. I guess you can't always have what you want. My sickness, my system—I know there's a lot of pain in my system. If the doctor says no sickness, my mom and sister will say I'm a liar. They will be against me. My mind can't cause that much pain . . . bruises and headaches.

[Anna was fully engaged in the conversation and still shows no signs of leaving. I once again acknowledge her concerns and once again say we must conclude our conversation. I thank Anna for participating in the particular setting of today's interview. I want to assure her of future conversations. All conversations—conversations among the workshop participants, myself, and Nikki; future therapy conversations; and of course, those in between—are platforms or springboards for those that follow.]

H: So you have a lot of questions. It sounds like it would be really important to talk about more and to find out how to get answers to some of those questions, if there are answers. Well, thank you very much for coming in today and putting up with our format, of multiple ears and eyes listening to you and watching you, and letting me talk to you and ask you all of these questions and have you go over your story—that I'm sure you've told many times. I wish both you and your mother the very best with this. If I have thoughts later I'll certainly share them with Nikki so that she can share them with you.

[I then invited the therapist and the mother back into the room and offer some summary remarks.]

H: So I thank you for coming in and as I said, it's a complex situation and a lot of effort has gone into it and concern from different angles. We'll [the group] be talking and sharing any further thoughts with Nikki. She'll be meeting with you. We'll see what we can do help you folks get a handle on this and try to get it turned more in the direction that you're trying to get it turned into. As someone in the group said, "Now that this independence is out of the bag, how can you steer it in a safe direction?"

The therapist and I continued the conversation with the workshop participants, collecting their observations, questions, comments, and suggestions for the therapist to consider and share with the family. Offering these to the therapist *and* the family keeps the therapist and the family as collaborators in the therapy system. That is, the therapist and the family are recipients of the group's reflections. In her next conversation with the family, Nikki can join them in exploring the offerings that each finds inviting and discarding the others. In this way, she avoids choosing or preselecting what is useful or not useful to the family.

## WHAT WAS THE PROBLEM? WHAT HAPPENED?

What was the problem? There was no one problem, there was a multiplicity of problems. The therapist said she was concerned about people's safety and the uphill-downhill course of therapy. The mother said she was angry, exasperated; she felt the situation was hopeless and had no more steam to deal with her daughter. The daughter said she was confused and fearful of the unknown, of what was going on with her. The workshop participants said they wanted to see the theory in action, and I wanted to demonstrate my work and hoped to have conversations that would loosen or, at the very least, set the stage for loosening and easing the gridlock this family was in. Most importantly, I wanted to give the therapist a new sense of agency.

What happened? Did the therapist and the family get any fresh ideas? Did the problem "dis-solve"? At the end of the workshop, Nikki said she felt as if a burden had been lifted from her shoulders: She had a better grasp on the situation and was feeling quite optimistic about the future outcome for this family. Follow-up from her some months later revealed that the mother reported that the experience had given her "renewed energy to tackle the job of motherhood." Anna began initiating her own therapy appointments and was soon back in school.

## EDITOR'S QUESTIONS

Q: *As a therapist you appear to be a nondirective co-participant in the client's story. You make space for family members to present their stories without imposing a direction on the process. You talk about the idea of not wanting to find yourself "on a narrow path" that would constrain the client's narrative. These ideas are at variance with what many therapists learn about the need to home in on a specific focal issue and engage the client in more in-depth dialogue around this focus. Would you comment on the usefulness of "never staying with one thing for long"?*

A: I agree that this is at odds with what most therapists have learned to do. Behind this therapist learning are the premises that the therapist is the expert in the human story, the content expert; that the therapist *knows* about normalcy and pathology; and that such knowledge should determine what to select as central issues to be interested in and to ask questions about. The questions are usually rhetorical or serve as pedagogic devices; that is, the questions' intent, or the homing in that you suggest, is usually an attempt to progressively maximize and fine-tune information that is used for a particular purpose, usually one that confirms the therapist's knowledge. Thus, the interview tends not to be collaborative, in the sense that the therapist's knowledge leads the discourse.

In a genuinely collaborative conversation—a dialogical conversation—it is impossible to stay with one thing too long. Participating in this kind of conversation—in which one is trying to learn about and understand the other, to hear the client's story as he or she wants to tell it—assumes that one is open to new experiences. Thus, it is possible to move beyond (or at least examine) the historical experiences (i.e., the professional and personal knowledge and biases) the therapist brings along. When one is open to another person, one is authentically interested in what he or she has to say. Such openness and authenticity allows the therapist to pay attention to the client's story, to accept it as worthy, and to wonder about the nuances of that story, nuances to which *knowing* often blinds both of them.

Staying with one thing too long may be a cue to the therapist who wants to work in a collaborative conversation that she or he may have unwittingly become the content expert. For an elaboration of the notion of a therapeutic conversation and its intent—a dialogical space and process—see Anderson and Goolishian (1992).

Q: *The notion of "dis-solving" a problem through dialogue sounds magical. What is it about a conversation that gives it the power to create change in families?*
A: The essence of a dialogical conversation is to allow for change or, rather, for what I prefer to think of as the emergence of newness to allow the participants, to envision or arrive at newness. The essence of dialogue, according to Wachterhauser (1986), in discussing Gadamer's work, is that "the play [the give and take] between different linguistic accounts generates new meaning" and therefore "in a genuine dialogue the meanings that emerge in the dialogue propel each participant toward understandings that were not foreseen or intended (p. 227). Thus, in the kind of therapeutic conversation I am talking about, both the therapist and the client are at risk of change, of newness.

Q: *In the material presented, you had a dual role as consultant and workshop leader. What modifications would we see in your approach if you were working alone as the primary therapist with a family rather than as a consultant? How often do you usually see families in therapy and over what periods of time? How are decisions made about scheduling and spacing appointments? Do you consider yourself a "brief therapist"?*
A: The differences are difficult to speculate about. If the interview had not taken place in a training setting, would I have separated the mother and daughter in the same fashion? I don't know. What I and the family members bring to a conversation on any given day will vary, and will influence the direction of the conversation. Each conversation determines the next: whom that conversation will include, when that conversation will take place, and what it will be about.

I might see people once a week, every 2 weeks, once a month, three times a week, or twelve times a month. I do not sign people up for 1 hour of therapy on every Tuesday for a specified number of times. The time allotted to initial sessions is usually $1\frac{1}{2}$ hours, but it may be longer, other sessions usually last 1 hour. I do not call myself a brief therapist, although this way of working certainly tends to be briefer than most therapies. The average number of sessions is usually between six and twelve and, as mentioned earlier, the sessions may occur over a short or an extended period of time.

Q: *Most of us have been trained to be "experts" or at least present ourselves as having some special experiences or skills that determine how we structure the therapeutic interview. Your approach puts the therapist in an equal partnership with the family and requires a shift in philosophic perspective. How do you develop and nurture a collaborative position and avoid leading the family in a "unilaterally determined direction"? Can we really avoid an "expert" position as therapists? What are some ways therapists can develop the thinking required to approach families in the respectful manner you suggest? How did your work evolve in this direction?*

A: These questions call for another paper! This still-evolving way of working has grown from the flow of countless therapy conversations and conversations about therapy that Harry Goolishian and I took part in over the years. As we tried to describe and explain our work to our selves and others, and as we listened to clients' stories about successful as well as unsuccessful therapy, we kept returning to *language and conversation* as the central parts of therapy. The early focus was on speaking our clients' language (metaphorically and literally) to learn about their values and worldviews. The aim was to work within the client's ordinary language and use it as a therapeutic tool or technique to produce change. The belief at that time was that the client would be more amenable to the therapist's intervention (whatever form that might take), and less likely to resist it. The client's language gave the therapist clues to develop *therapist-determined* directions, for example, problem definitions, corrected beliefs, interventions, or disruption of faulty-solution behaviors. Over time and for many reasons too lengthy to discuss here, we shifted from regarding language as a function, a rhetoric-like *tool*, to regarding language as generative, as the essence of dialogue, and therefore the *essence* of the therapeutic process. This demanded that we pay careful attention to our own language, words, and stance so as to signal respect, mutuality, and humility—all critical ingredients of a collaborative relationship.

In this conceptualization of language the therapist is no longer a narrative editor of the client's story, (the expert) who uses language as an editing tool; rather, the therapist is more like a co-author (a co-expert). The therapist no longer needs to be the expert who structures the therapeutic interview; that structure is determined by both the client and the therapist. This does not mean that "anything goes," that the therapist throws all her or his knowledge and preconceptions out the window. It does, however, suggest that the therapist's knowledge, experience, and values are no truer than the client's—nor more final.

## ACKNOWLEDGMENT

My thanks to Robin Trusty for transcribing the videotape and for her helpful comments.

# REFERENCES

Anderson, H., & Goolishian, H. (1988). Human systems as linguistic systems: Preliminary and evolving ideas about the implications for clinical theory. *Family Process, 27,* 371–393.

Anderson, H., & Goolishian, H. (1990). Beyond cybernetics: Some comments on Atkinson and Heath's further thoughts on second-order family therapy. *Family Process, 29,* 157–163.

Anderson, H., & Goolishian, H. (1992). The client is the expert: A not-knowing approach to therapy. In S. McNamee, & K. J. Gergen (Eds.), *Constructing Therapy: Social Construction and the therapeutic process* (pp. 23–39). London: Sage.

Gadamer, H. (1975). *Truth and method.* New York: Seabury.

Geertz, C. (1973). *The interpretation of culture.* New York: Basic Books.

Gergen, K. J. (1985). The social constructionist movement in modern psychology. *American Psychologist, 40,* 266–275.

Goolishian, H., & Anderson, H. (1987). Language systems and therapy: An evolving idea. *Psychotherapy, 24*(3S), 529–538.

Goolishian, H., & Anderson, H. (1992a). Strategy and intervention versus nonintervention: A matter of theory. *Journal of Marital and Family Therapy, 18,* 5–16.

Goolishian, H., & Anderson, H. (1992b). Some afterthoughts on reading Duncan and Held. *Journal of Marital and Family Therapy, 18,* 35–37.

Rorty, R. (1979). *Philosophy and the mirror of nature.* Princeton, NJ: Princeton University Press.

Wachterhauser, B. R. (1986). *Hermeneutics and modern philosophy.* New York: State University of New York Press.

# 15

## Tekka with Feathers: Talking about Talking (about Suicide)

### LYNN HOFFMAN-HENNESSY
### JUDITH DAVIS

This is a story about an encounter with a family at the Brattleboro Family Institute.[1] It is told by Judy Davis, who was the interviewer, and added to by Lynn Hoffman, who was a member of a reflecting team[2] (Andersen, 1991). The story is commented on by members of the family, who read our version, and still further expanded through answers to questions from the editor.

We understand this experience not as a coherent story but as a fragment of a less tidy process. The narrative view, popular in psychotherapy nowadays, implies that therapy is like a story, with a *beginning* (recently hospitalized daughter and distraught parents come in for a consultation), *middle* (they engage in a conversation with therapist and team), and *end* (in the process they learn how to talk differently to each other so that daughter no longer needs to know herself or be known by others as "strange"). Our view is that therapy is more like a canoe trip on a river. It starts when we "put in" and ends when we "put out." There is no necessary structure to the

---

[1]Special thanks to William D. Lax, PhD, Director of Training, Brattleboro Family Institute, for his generosity in offering us this research site.
[2]Team membership fluctuated from session to session, depending on individual schedules. William Lax, PhD, was present for all four sessions. Randye E. Cohen, PhD, in private practice in Norwich, Vt., was present only for the first session, and Brian Lewis, PhD, in private practice in Montpelier, Vt., joined the group for the last two sessions, as did Lynn.

events at all except the ones we invent ourselves. Thus, we can only claim to present some disparate points of view about an experience in this family's life and in our own lives as they intersected for a few hours over time. Our hope is that in putting these several versions down on paper we will be, as Mary Catherine Bateson (1992) put it, "surprised into new learning."

What seems most different about this work is that it is not attached to outcome, even though it represents an experimental approach. For the most part, family practitioners write up cases and show videotapes of experiences that went well. This case leaves some doubt, and certainly the opinions of the participants vary significantly on that score. However, our idea is to model a new kind of openness in having even controversial work scrutinized by the family and by the wider clinical audience. The family here, being unusually informed consumers, were well able to provide their own comments at a level of critical attention seldom found in studies of this sort. It is we as professionals, our work, and thinking that are at issue here, not the lives and problems of the people in the family.

## JUDY'S STORY

## THE FIRST SESSION

Before we met them, all we knew about the family was that the 21-year-old daughter had just been released from a psychiatric hospital. She was being brought to the institute by her mother and stepfather. They had been referred by the mother's friend, a graduate student in a family therapy program: "If she were my daughter, that's where I'd go."

At Brattleboro we were working with a "reflecting team" approach, an idea pioneered by Tom Andersen and his colleagues (1991) in Tromsø, Norway. Since I had been wanting more experience in the role of interviewer as contrasted to that of reflecting team member, it was agreed that I would be the one to work in the room with the family. The therapy team met weekly to explore the notion of separating the therapist's traditionally intertwined tasks of inquiry and comment: What we were questioning was whether such separation of functions—where the interviewer's role was simply that of eliciting or making room for the family's stories while the team did whatever commenting was done—would open more space for new ideas. So my head, as I entered the waiting room to greet the family, was filled with thoughts about *not* reflecting, about being in the conversation as nonintrusively as possible, about following ideas rather than offering new ones. We were also interested in the concept of the "unsaid"—the possibility of allowing for thoughts that were not chosen because other thoughts had come to the fore.

Sarah and David, the man with whom Sarah had been living for 11 years, greeted me graciously but with obvious anxiety. Sarah's daughter, Tekka, a beautiful university art student, remained seated on the couch, hungrily eating a yogurt and drinking from a large bottle of spring water. Most striking about Tekka was her hair. Long and strawberry blond, it was piled high on top of her head and cascaded down around her face in a combination of curls and matted dreadlocks that were interspersed with beads, bits of colored ribbon, and feathers. Dressed in a tie-dyed jumpsuit with a fingerless black glove on one hand, and her nails painted with black polish, Tekka looked, to me, both exotic and exhausted.

Our first meeting was taking place on the day after Tekka's release from the hospital, the day after her 21st birthday. She had signed herself into the hospital (and was then kept there against her will) for 2 weeks following a spring break that had culminated in her attempting to walk into or through the side of a subway car. She described the hospitalization as a nightmare that included thorazine, isolation, and a sense that her parents had betrayed her by not getting her out and by not helping her refuse medication. Tekka was now back at school but was still on lithium. When I asked the family why they had come, they all said they wanted help getting Tekka off the medication safely. They wanted another way of dealing with whatever was going on, a way that didn't involve drugs. I saw the family four times over a period of a month and a half.

Early in the first meeting, I learned that Sarah was a music therapist. She had divorced Tekka's father when their daughter was 6. She described her ex-husband as alcoholic, violent, and possibly manic-depressive. David was a teacher who described his ex-wife as "a certifiable schizophrenic." Their 25-year-old son had been hospitalized 4 years earlier for depression and suicidal thoughts. Almost incidentally, we learned that Tekka had been married for 2 years to a young man from Italy. They had been separated (apparently amicably) for over 6 months, and Fredrico was now attending school in another state.

Tekka described herself as a recovering drug and alcohol addict. David volunteered that he had also stopped drinking some years ago and that he still attended meetings. In the '60s he had "done drugs" and was once in "an induced paranoid state for three, four, five days." Continuing the description of the past in ways that pointed to their identification with Tekka's pain, Sarah added that when she was her daughter's age she too had gone through a difficult period. "I wasn't hospitalized but I did leave school and I was very depressed."

Exploration of ideas about the subway episode revealed Tekka's explanation that "things had gotten too good." Although she could "stay grounded" during the school year, when she went on spring break, she "let out" more than she could handle. It was her first vacation on her own, and it was a kind of "vision quest." It was Tekka's thought, however, that her recent behavior was not much different from that of her usual self, "only a little more so." Tekka's mother disagreed, although hesitantly. It was her sense that Tekka had "really lost contact with reality."

It was all I could do to resist the impulse to explore this avalanche of intriguing statements. But as I remained quiet a conversation took place here between Tekka and Sarah about what they each thought was "scary," a word Sarah used to describe her feelings about Tekka's behavior. The conversation revealed a long history of conflict between Sarah, who saw herself as inadequately trying to protect her daughter, and Tekka, who saw Sarah as trying to "break" her strong spirit. Both agreed, however, that there had been less conflict between them when Tekka was married. During that time Tekka seemed to fight more with her "protective" husband than with her mother. Indeed, Sarah and Tekka had become closer during that period.

It seems important to mention here that our conversation throughout this and subsequent sessions was marked—despite the seriousness of the content and the difference in opinions—by a surprising amount of good humor and a kind of laughter that was rather bewildering to me. It was as if the family all shared the same private joke, or at least all relieved tension in the same way.

## Team Reflections (Bill Lax and Randye Cohen)

Toward the end of the session the family and I switched places with the team and listened as they talked about what they had just heard.

The reflections included comments on the amount of concern and humor the family demonstrated and on the possible role of the hospitalization: Was it to signal for help or was it Tekka's way of taking care of herself? Bill wondered where Sarah got her idea about being inadequate, of not being able to speak up. "Is she dealing with messages from *her* mother?" he mused. Randye, on the other hand, was curious about the paradox of things getting "better and better" in Tekka's life and getting out of control at the same time. Both were interested in Tekka's plans for the summer and the family's plans for this therapy. "In other words," said Bill, "how do we draw the boundaries around even this?"

## Family Response

When the family returned to the therapy room, it was clear that their primary concern was the immediate future and getting Tekka off the medication. They took the name of a psychiatrist with whom the institute worked and scheduled a second appointment for the following week.

## THE SECOND SESSION

Early in the morning of the second appointment Sarah called the institute, sounding very upset. Tekka had missed the bus to meet her parents, and the family would not be able to get to Brattleboro on time. Since our schedules permitted it, the appointment was reset for later that morning (only Bill, however, was available to represent the reflecting team).

Much of this session was devoted to the meanings each family member made of Tekka's having missed the bus. For Tekka, it was a simple act of having misread the schedule. For Sarah, it meant that Tekka wasn't capable of being responsible for herself and reinforced her idea that there was a lot of "old stuff" between them that hadn't been resolved. Tekka interjected here that she'd been wanting to talk about this old stuff but that her mother kept getting "hung up on the *way* of talking, and then it's too late. I had to have a psychotic state to get here."

In response to David's explanation of what had happened during spring break (Tekka had had "an overload of energy"), Tekka talked about having known the limits of her depths (alcoholic blackouts) but not the limits of her highs, and it was those highs which she was exploring during the break. She admitted that the hospital was more than she'd "bargained for" and was worried now that anything she did would make her mother think she was crazy.

When the conversation turned to plans for the upcoming summer, Tekka talked about buying and living in a school bus on Cape Cod. When Sarah expressed her concern about these plans, Tekka became angry and recalled an essay she'd written in high school. It was about feeling paralyzed between being "responsible" and being a "rebel." Either choice was a "giving in." Even today, she went on, she was struggling between these two ideas of herself. "Who do I want to be right now?! I am being responsible. I'm making wise choices for who *I* am. But *I am not you*," she said to her mother. Here Sarah acknowledged that perhaps she was over-involved but at the same time wondered if she should, in fact, be taking even more responsibility. "Maybe my responsibility as your mother now is to make decisions for you, to be responsible for you even though you are twenty-one." "How?" asked Tekka, challengingly. "I don't know," answered Sarah. "It scares the shit out of me."

## Reflections (Bill Lax)

Bill came into the therapy room and talked with me while the family watched from behind the mirror. Our talk was about issues of responsibility and about changes over time for a child and then for a 21-year-old woman. Bill wondered aloud about who (or who else) should be in the conversation: "Who should be talking to whom and how much?" He also commented on his changing perceptions of the family: The parents did not seem as "timid" as they had been the week before. "Maybe they're somehow less scared of Tekka now. After all, she *is* a strong woman. 'Don't ruffle my feathers!'"

I was grateful for Bill's questions and for his perception that something had changed. That view and his joking about the feathers felt, to me, somehow encouraging.

## Family Response

When the family returned to the therapy room, Tekka resonated to the comment about who should be in the conversation. "I *do* want to choose who I talk to," she said. "I don't want to say 'Fuck off,' but it would be easier. Too often I try to please everyone. I'd rather say 'Fuck you' and see what would happen." "And who else would be in the conversation?" I asked. "Lots," she answered. "My father, his mother. Big family intervention. But not necessarily right away."

Sarah responded to Bill's comment about the parents being less timid. She agreed with Bill and talked about a conversation she and Tekka had had after the last session, which both agreed felt very different: "less timid, and nice."

## THE THIRD SESSION

Our third session, a week later, began with talk about a phone conversation Tekka and her mother had had during the week. Tekka had called to say that she wanted to cancel the appointment because she had so much school work to catch up on. According to everyone, Sarah "freaked" at this idea and handed the phone to David. In her conversation with David, Tekka was able to figure out a way to make the meeting and still get to her work. In describing that discussion, Tekka talked about wanting her mother to be less reactive and more objective, "more like a friend than a mother." It was, she said, easier to talk to her stepfather than her mother at this stage of her life.

T: My mother can be objective before and after a conversation but can't step out and look more clearly [while] in the conversation. I can't talk about what's going on; I begin checking out the dynamics of what's going on and that becomes the conversation.

J: So there's a different response with David?

T: It's easy for me to be more mature.

As a teenager, Tekka went on, she'd felt forced to lie to her mother a lot. She always wished she could tell her mother the truth about where she was going and what she was doing because, she admitted, "Often what I did *was* dangerous." But Tekka felt that her mother was overprotective and that this overprotectiveness was an attempt to "squash her energy."

Sarah disagreed about being overprotective and, in fact, felt she had been neglectful. After more of this exchange, I asked how this conversation was for the two of them. Sarah answered that it was useful because one of the things that was most painful in her life was that she hadn't been able to talk to her mother about what she was doing. Her mother was "completely naive." This, she thought, was part of why she used to get so angry when she felt Tekka was lying to her. All she wanted now, she said, was for Tekka to live her life safely. "Positively! Not safely!" Tekka exclaimed, correcting her.

## Team Reflections (Bill Lax, Brian Lewis, and Lynn Hoffman)

Opening the team's conversation, Lynn, who was meeting the family for the first time, talked about mothers and daughters. She likened what Tekka was doing to going out on thin ice. She felt that Tekka wanted to have her own life but also wanted to know that her mother was there in case she needed to be rescued. The problem, Lynn said, was that "if Mom gets too upset, communication breaks down." Lynn also wondered about "karmic issues" and the idea of danger. Was Sarah's mother unable to rescue Sarah? Perhaps there was a whole conversation from the past, a conversation with other generations. How do mothers allow daughters to have the experience of getting close to danger without everybody getting so upset that no new experiences are allowed?

Brian wondered why this family appeared so jovial, and he wondered what danger actually meant to them. Bill wondered if Tekka was trying to establish herself as an adult in relation to her family, and if past conversations had had similar themes about how much concern Sarah had and/or showed. Speaking again, Lynn reflected on the "mini-boomers"— the coming of age of children whose parents had been flower children themselves—and how much to repeat and yet not repeat the experiences of past generations.

## Family Response

When the family returned to the therapy room, Sarah acknowledged that, in fact, she didn't know what Tekka meant by danger. Tekka responded by talking about creativity, suggesting that her struggle between being an artist and being practical was also her mother's struggle but that her mother had taken the safe road and had become a music therapist instead of a musician: "For myself, I need to be creating my own stuff! I'm making different choices."

With this conversation the session was ending, but I could not resist adding my own response to the reflections. In reference to Lynn's idea about karmic issues, I asked Tekka about how a conversation might go in the future when she and *her* adolescent daughter negotiated ideas about safety and creativity. "I'm not going to have a daughter," Tekka declared. "I'm going to have a son . . . because the universe has a sense of humor."

## THE FOURTH SESSION

Our next appointment was scheduled for 2 weeks later, but a medical emergency in my family forced me to postpone the meeting by a week. On the phone with Sarah I shared some of the details of my son's illness, and she and I commiserated about the pain of seeing one's child sick or hurting.

When I called Tekka with the message, she volunteered that she was thinking of spending a month in a treatment center before starting her summer job on the Cape.

When the family arrived 3 weeks later for the fourth and last meeting, Tekka was less animated than usual and looked tired. I asked them how they wanted to use this last session. David answered that he wanted to talk about the future, but that Tekka didn't want to talk at all. "She's in a slump. School's over. Moving boxes."

Tekka responded by saying she was "not great, but okay." She had definitely decided on the treatment program, which had been recommended by her 12-step sponsor. A conversation about this decision revealed that David was pleased about the plan as long as Tekka didn't see it a another hospital but as "a resort with paid humans."

Sarah also thought it was a good idea but was worried about something else: When she and David visited Tekka in her dorm room on the day of our canceled meeting, they found on her door "a doll hanging herself." Sarah demonstrated with her hands around her neck. Although she was unable to comment on it at the time, Sarah talked briefly with Tekka about it the next day on the phone. Tekka had told her it was her "recovery doll" and said: "This is what she [the doll] did to herself after she got out of the hospital. But I don't feel this way really."

The doll incident had upset Sarah profoundly, and I asked about the difficulty of talking about it. Sarah responded by talking about how "strangely hard" it was to talk with Tekka in light of the fact that in her work (dealing with troubled adolescents) she talked about "such things" regularly.

Exasperated, Tekka talked about how surprised she always was that her mother responded so intensely to her gestures rather than her words. "I think I make it pretty clear where I'm at. And when I'm not doing well, I say I'm not doing well. We went through this when I was living at home and I had my mohawk. Mom freaked out because I shaved my head: 'You must be very disturbed!' "

At this point David interrupted. "I know your mother very well, and right now she is saying to herself: 'Does this mean Tekka is suicidal all the time?' "

T: That's what I mean. I don't think people listen to me!

S: So *are* you suicidal all the time?

T: Do you think I'm suicidal all the time?

S: I don't think you are.

T: So okay! I don't think I am either. *(Family laughs.)*

[Sarah went on here haltingly, trying to speak more about her confusion.]

J: *(feeling the need to help)* So the doll scared you.

S: Yeah!

J:  And it was very hard for you to express that fear, hard to mention it to Tekka in a way that wasn't offensive to her?

S:  Yeah, I don't want to offend her. And David says, "Of course she'll be offended. Of course she's not suicidal. Don't make a big deal. Why do you always react?" But the point is, if she does feel really bad and says it, maybe there's something that she could tell us . . . what she would like us to do to help.

As she was saying this, Sarah noticed that Tekka and David were looking at each other and beginning to smile. "That gets that look," she explained, as she turned to them and joined in their laughter. Deciding to give voice to my confusion, I asked if someone could please explain what "that look" meant. "It means," David said, "There she goes again." "What does 'There she goes again' mean?" I asked Sarah. "Do you know?" "It means they think I'm overpsychologizing," she answered. I wondered here if this was some piece of the private joke, another piece of the "unsaid"?

As talk about Sarah's overreacting went on, David explained that Tekka just wants Sarah to listen like a friend but not do anything. "Yeah," joined in Tekka, "or otherwise every time I say something, there's the threat that I'm going to be taken to a psych ward."

Sarah explained her hesitation to "just listen," saying that if Tekka really needed help and she (Sarah) didn't recognize it or do anything about it, it would be terrible: "In my work, when a kid has suicidal thoughts or does suicidal art work or writes suicidal songs, we set up a suicide watch. That is my framework and I know that's part of me. That's what I do. I spend a lot of time with children who are at risk. It scares me because I want you *(turning to Tekka)* . . . I wish you didn't feel that bad." "So do I," Tekka answered, and she and Sarah laughed identically.

## Team Reflections (Bill Lax, Brian Lewis, and Lynn Hoffman)

Brian began by commenting on how different the family seemed to him this time, how much less jovial. "Almost from a happy family to a sad family. But," he said, "as the session went on, the change made sense to me."

Lynn agreed that the change was striking and went on to say that even though they were talking about death she felt reassured in a peculiar kind of way because talking about it was possible. Recalling the previous conversation about danger and safety, Lynn thought that maybe it was now possible for Tekka to talk and for mother to listen and that that seemed to be an important part of the process. If they stopped being able to talk, that would be the real danger. Lynn went on: "Thinking as a mother—and I certainly have that particular piece of the territory seared in my head and my heart—that is the one reassurance I have."

Bill's comment had to do with the difference between "what you see is what you get" and "what else is there?" He asked whether Tekka's presentation to her family in the "what you see is what you get" mode was sufficient or whether there was need for further inquiry? "And what happens when sometimes the 'what you see is what you get' mode stops further inquiry, such as with the doll? How can there be talk without an alarmed reaction to the talk? How can there be conversation around danger and safety without having to move to a 'suicide watch'?" Bill added, "Often what Tekka presents is 'I show you who I am.' And I can see from mother's point of view that sometimes that can be quite strange [laughter from behind the mirror]. There aren't many people who walk around the way Tekka does. Does that require further inquiry? Like 'You have feathers in your hair. Does that mean you are thinking of becoming a bird?' [louder laughter]. 'No, there are just feathers in my hair.' That's 'what is, is.' Maybe there needs to be more of a balance of inquiry around that stuff." Bill wondered if the plan for the treatment program was sufficient to allay concern about the danger: "Is this a plan that will allow them to move forward in such a way that then more conversation can take place?"

Lynn added here a reminder that mother was not alone. "There's not just mother, but there is also David. And even though mother could never just say 'It's immaterial to me how you feel' because she has to take action if she thinks certain things, David doesn't. That seems to me to be another strong piece in all of this." Lynn paused and added, "But I'm basically *not* relieved." Turning to Brian, she asked, "What is a recovery doll?"

Brian answered that he didn't know but had made the assumption that "somehow the doll symbolized part of the recovery process." Brian then wondered about David's multiple roles in the conversation: as one who enables Sarah to speak, as one who inhibits her speech, and as one with different ideas of his own. He wondered whether at times David might join Sarah in her worries about Tekka.

## Family's Reflections

David responded first, saying that although he personally had been feeling much better about the situation with each passing week, he was most interested in knowing what Lynn meant when she said she was not relieved. He also went on to respond to Brian's comment about the different roles he plays in the family and concluded that maybe he could be helpful because he was "not involved as a mother, but certainly involved as someone who cares very strongly for Tekka's well-being . . . and for Sarah's well-being."

Sarah responded next by asking if there was any chance of finding out from Lynn what she meant "instead of just speculating and wondering?" I assured her that the team could return before the end of the session to speak to their questions and asked if there were other thoughts about what the team had said. Laughing, Sarah confessed that she'd also wondered what a recovery doll was and, turning to her daughter, asked, "Would you mind telling us?" Tekka replied, "It's a doll when I was doing a lot of [recovery] work, my child doll . . . that I don't particularly like very much. But I had it for three years."

As Sarah and Tekka seemed unable to go beyond this single exchange, I decided to try to actively take up the metaphor as a resource in expanding this piece of the conversation. I asked Tekka, "You decided a few weeks ago to hang it on your door?"

T: I felt at the time that my recovery had been squashed in the hospital. Not taken away from me, but . . . kind of violated.

S: Because they made you take drugs or the whole thing?

T: That, and because they wouldn't let me go to group. No access to talking to people. People weren't listening to me the way I'm accustomed to having people listen to me.

J: That doll was a kind of statement about that experience?

T: Yeah.

J: *(attempting to make space for a "not-yet-said" idea)* Where is she now?

T: Still there.

J: Will you be leaving that room soon?

T: Yeah. She'll have to come down.

D: She could stay there. *(Mother and daughter laugh as one.)*

J: *(to Tekka)* If you could imagine a future past the summer or past this experience, where would you *like* her to be?

T: The doll?

J: Yeah.

T: Well, I would like *myself* to be back in control, in total recovery. So the doll can be in storage!

J: Do you have thoughts about what the team was saying?

T: Yeah. I thought it was interesting, their comments about our changing. I think that there are just so many different points [of view]. When we only come here for an hour once a week, you only get just so much. We have the ability to be humorous and we also have the ability to have a lot of shit going on and we deal with it. I know one of the accusations I got in the hospital was that I kept changing my mind. Every day a different idea.

S: That was from me?

T: Yeah, that was from you.

J: *(to Sarah)* Your thoughts about the team's comments?

S: Interesting . . . they were certainly looking at it from different ways, different frameworks. *(pause)* I was just thinking as Tekka was talking about the hospital, I wish there was a way of communicating with her where she didn't feel I was accusatory, because that wasn't my perception. *(pause)* What I'm learning in this period is how I'm perceived. And

I think often my state of worryness is, in turn, turned into feeling like accusation and criticism.

J: Uh huh.

S: I wish it could be different.

J: You're seeing her reaction, her response, in a new way?

S: Yeah. I think I never really understood it. I felt bad or frustrated or whatever, but we couldn't relate somehow. But I never thought of what it was like for her. Or understood. I mean . . . what I'm learning is that what comes out of me is not what I think. Nor does it have the reaction I wish. I wish it could be different.

J: She hears you differently?

S: Yeah, like I was saying, I really have to listen to her in a more open way.

D: So that's positive.

With the silence that followed this last statement, I reminded the family that as this was essentially the last meeting before the summer began, I wondered how this time together could be made most useful. I was again attempting to open more space. I asked if there were some things they wished they could have said or questions they wished they had asked? How could we use this time best?

David answered first by saying to me that he didn't know if it was necessary to say this, but turning to Tekka said, "I am willing to help, give support *(here Tekka put her hand out to David, rubbing her fingers together)*, including some money."

T: Thank you. *(pause)* Not just for the money.

D: *(gently)* I know.

T: I'm pretty burned out on the whole thing.

J: The whole thing?

T: The whole thing. I'm just tired of talking about it, dealing with it, being here—not here specifically, but where I am. *(yawns)* Very tired . . . hoping after treatment I'll feel better.

S: I guess *(laughs)* I feel . . . hope . . . that if Tekka needs our support, she can ask for it. She can talk about it. Use us as an asset. She is grown up. At the age of stepping out on her own. But if there are things she may need from us, she'll be able to ask and not get caught up in power struggles. I know that she's hated all this stuff, but she has actually been very cooperative. Last time we weren't able to say this when we had all that trouble getting here; we didn't say *(looking directly at Tekka)* how good it was that you *were* able to get here. We don't get to say those things.

At this point I suggested that the team return to answer the questions the family had raised.

## Team Again

L:  I guess what I really want to say before I defend my position is that this family has changed again. It has all these sides to it. And it's a very tender family. And I feel also that there is one hero and two heroines here, truly. That Tekka has worked hard and lovingly, in whatever way she does it, and her mother and stepfather have been genuinely concerned. So I just wanted to say that. *(pause)* But as far as this thing about not being relieved, I wanted to say to Sarah that I know how you must feel. That nobody says to women—and I guess to men too—that every child you have is a hostage to the universe and you're vulnerable for the rest of your and their lives. So that's all I meant. Because actually I am very heartened by this meeting and the family. Tremendously impressed with how this family has pulled together.

B:  I was also primarily struck by how much love there was . . . and struck by the sadness, but maybe it makes sense. Maybe it has to do with the fact that things are changing. Tekka is definitely taking responsibility for herself and has made this decision and there's now not a whole lot that can be done . . . Just a need to let whatever is going to happen, happen. And that *is* kind of sad. A new beginning and a letting go. The sadness for the past that is gone, and not quite sure about the future.

B:  I'm viewing life from more of a philosophical position, like "children as hostages." Life is an ongoing unfolding of safety and danger. Sadness is a letting go of the idea that the rehabilitation program is going to be "it." It's another experience. It's not the perfect experience but a series of experiences—for the whole family. Tekka's experience and Tekka's recounting of the experience. And I was thinking of something that took place here that I hadn't seen before that felt, to me, great—that was David's expressing of appreciation, "I'm here to support you emotionally, financially"—and Tekka's saying "Thank you." And Sarah saying to Tekka "I wanted you to know how much I appreciated your being here." It sounds like they're moving to a different phase of interaction with one another. . .and the conversation is getting richer, more facets.

## Family Reflections

As usual, I asked the family for their reactions to the team's comments.

J:  Any final comments, reactions to their appreciation of your appreciation?

D:  I thought that this process here has been useful, actually. I've liked this crazy one-way mirror a lot because it creates a kind of artificial situation that lets you say some things that you probably couldn't say otherwise, and yet it is not so artificial that it seems bizarre. It doesn't close you up. To have all of these insightful and very different types of people give their thoughts and feelings about what they have just experienced is interesting. I'm going to start worrying whether or not Tekka is going-to become a bird. *(all laugh)*

S:  Well, I really appreciated this process. It's given us a way to touch base with Tekka through this period, and it's allowed us to have conversations that wouldn't have happened. I'm more aware of some of the areas where I make it difficult for Tekka. I think I never heard it before. I don't think she didn't say it before. I just hadn't heard it before.

T:  I've enjoyed this—I think. I liked the mirror too. The switching back and forth, like they said, an experience among many to carry with me. I think the process will happen further down, but that's okay.

D:  *(to me)* You've also been very good in terms of letting conversations develop, feeding them without intruding. Because if you had been intrusive, the conversations wouldn't have taken place.

By this time I was thinking it was my turn to respond, but I was surprised to find myself really choked up and barely able to contain my tears. I blurted out, "Happy family, sad family, I think you're a beautiful family; so much good stuff in there. I wish you the best" (through all you have yet to endure, I was thinking. Without doubt, my tears were about my child as well as theirs.).

To regain my composure, I tried to change the subject and insert some humor. When I'd called Tekka to reschedule the appointment, I couldn't make out what the message on her answering machine was: "You can't come to the phone because you're working on what?" I asked. "My basket case," Tekka answered. As I was slowly getting the joke, Sarah suggested, "You should hear what Tekka has on the machine now: "I'm working on my anger, fuck you." With laughter and hugs we ended the meeting.

Although I don't know what meaning Sarah or David or Tekka made of the phone message, I suddenly felt hopeful. Maybe in some way, Tekka was needing to please less. Maybe she was beginning to feel she had some control over "who she wanted to talk to and how." And maybe this would make a difference in what got said and what got heard.

## FOLLOW-UP

Two months later when I called Sarah to ask how everyone was, she reported that Tekka had felt good about the treatment program, was off the lithium, and was living in her bus on the Cape. Sarah also reported that Tekka had cut off her hair but that it was cropped short, not shaved. "She looks much better now, and the sparkle is back in her eyes." Despite this positive picture, however, Sarah expressed continued anxiety. "I'm trying not to worry, but Tekka still seems so fragile to me. It's fifty–fifty whether she's fine or has another episode. But there's nothing I can do about it. I just have to trust she can take care of herself."

As the conversation ended, Sarah asked about my son's health, and the two of us reflected on Lynn's comment. No, no one does tell us ahead of time about hostages and the universe.

## AFTERTHOUGHTS

As I write this account, I keep asking myself why we have chosen this experience to focus on. Clearly, we are not presenting it as proof that something "works." Instead, we are putting it down on paper as a way of looking back at the experience and asking ourselves what happened, that is, what we thought was happening at the time and what we now, in the context of writing about it, think was happening. We see this piece as an example of our notions about participating in a less hierarchical relationship with the people we see, one in which we reveal aspects of ourselves that connect us with them, that normalize their feelings, that speak from the heart as well as the head.

Obviously, we could not determine the "truth" about Tekka's potential to commit suicide. On the one hand we felt torn between responding to the threat by encouraging the family to undertake a suicide watch and, on the other, refusing to buy into their fears lest we help make them come true. What allowed us to feel rescued from this dilemma was the reflecting stance, which permitted us to hold a position of ambiguity and use the metaphors it produced.

It was this stance that allowed Randye to reflect on how things could get better and better and yet worse at the same time, Brian to reflect on the family as both happy and sad simultaneously, Bill to reflect on the "what you see is what you get" mode being both enough and not enough, and Lynn to echo David's and Sarah's differing positions, expressing simultaneously both their hopes and their fears.

What is the relationship between this therapeutic conversation and family change? It would be reassuring to believe that the conversation made space for:

- Sarah to ask questions directly first of the team and then of her daughter instead of just "speculating and wondering," as had apparently been her way
- Tekka to articulate the family's strengths (and not just their failings)
- The family to give voice to their support and appreciation of each other
- Tekka to change her answering machine's message (the message that contextualized all subsequent conversations) to "I'm no longer crazy, just angry."
- Mother to move away from the idea of a suicide watch to the idea that she cannot protect her grown daughter in this way; "I am no longer going to tell you what to do, but invite you to ask from us what you want, need."

It would be reassuring also to believe that in this family the need for strange actions or dramatic symbols was somehow lessened as the idea developed that dangerous thoughts could be expressed in words. But who can say?

## LYNN'S STORY

I had not been present for the first two interviews, so I was listening doubly hard behind the screen in order to catch up. I too was taken by Tekka's playful style of dress and her flair for exuberance; it was easy to miss her serious side until, boom, it tripped you up. When that happened I fell right down the rabbit hole to memories of frightening times with my own teenage daughter; I remembered how I seemed to be watching her struggle through a soundproof glass wall. So much for trying to be objective; during that last meeting I might as well have been Tekka's mother myself. Luckily, David, by not being as drawn in as I was, acted like a firebreak. And when I went in to reflect, it was Bill who acted like a firebreak. Even with their help I found this a particularly hard situation to be part of and at the time felt that I was not being very polished. When David drew attention to my contradictory statements, saying first that I was relieved and then that I was not, I wondered what I meant myself.

The answer, of course, was that I found myself in two places at once. One was a place of relief that the family could talk about the possibility of Tekka being in danger. My theory is that as long as people can keep talking together about something they fear, nobody will give up and nobody will die. This is an idea I got from the late Harry Goolishian of the Galveston Institute, and it is an idea I try to take as literally as he did. The other place I was coming from was that I was feeling exactly the way Sarah did: Here was her own daughter, perhaps drowning, and shouldn't she go and rescue her? When I said I was not relieved, I was simply validating Sarah's point of view. I forgot I had just said the opposite, but when David asked if I could clarify what I meant, I welcomed the chance. In the old days that would have been against the rules because the therapist was supposed to be always in control and always skillful. But my style now is to put anything that seems like a mistake or a feeling of being stuck on the table for discussion. It certainly moves matters along.

As for Judy, I was very appreciative of what she was doing, even more so after she transcribed all four sessions and I could read them. I was already clear about the reflecting process. I think of it as a Delphic commentary that is long on associations and stories and short on interpretations and problem solving. What the interviewer did, however, was less clear. It seemed to me that the interviewer did nothing, at least compared to the sleuthlike questioning and complicated interventions of the approaches I had been trained in. But there is always more than meets the eye. Let me try to lay out a few characteristics of the way I think we work as interviewers now. I'll confine myself to the fourth interview.

1. *Beginning the sessions.* We try to focus right away on the activity of talking together and what it means to people and how they would like it to go. Our hope is to set things up so that people can "take back the interview" from the professionals. Judy's question "How would you like to use this session?" is a good example. Tom Andersen's (1991) "What is the history of the idea to come here?" was the prototype for this way of starting. Before, we used to ask about the problem, and immediately it was a different ball game.

2. *Not controlling sessions.* As Judy said, we try to stay back, deliberately not asking provocative questions and not making interesting interventions. This is harder than you think if you have been "properly" trained in family therapy. Judy tended to speak sparingly and to use a soft voice, and she followed no preset schedule. This was to allow maximum freedom for family members to come up with their own ideas. Sometimes Judy made a space for someone, but that was about it.

3. *Having less exact goals.* It seems to me that in this approach the therapist does not set out to make something happen or find something out. Judy tried instead to keep the conversation going, nudging it so as to keep the pathways open between people but otherwise intervening little. For the most part, she elicited ideas from people about whatever was uppermost in their minds, often using Milan-style agree/disagree questions. However, we don't do that much circular questioning, since it can so easily straitjacket the interaction. In the past we were always hunting for a particular animal— a hypothesis about the function of the symptom that we could connote positively—but the new way of working moves away from looking for patterns at all.

4. *Not taking a managerial position.* A common doctrine in cases of violence and threat of suicide is that the therapist should be an activist. No doubt that is often the best policy, as well as common sense, but there are a significant number of situations where the threat or use of force creates a worse outcome than if nothing at all is done. And not every therapist is comfortable with being an activist. So, as I often say, there ought to be a "different voice." Gandhi, for instance, provided a different voice in the fight against the British in India. This different voice, this softer voice, does not necessarily lack impact. As in Aesop's tale of the contest between the sun and the wind, the softer voice can be very strong.

5. *Asking special questions.* Judy asked a special kind of question from time to time; it is hard to describe, although it seems to fall into Peggy Penn's (1985) category of a "future question." A good example in the last interview is when the story of the recovery doll came up and Judy asked, "If you could imagine a future past the summer or past this experience, where would you like her to be?" And Tekka answers, "I would like myself to be back in control, in total recovery. So the doll can be in storage!" This is what I call looking for the windows, not the walls. People can often find the door on their own.

6. *Not pushing a particular outcome.* We had no aims in the last interview

other than the general ones that Tekka not hurt herself, not drop out of school, and not go back to a hospital ward. What did happen was that by the end of the meeting Sarah and David were expressing appreciation to Tekka, she was reciprocating, and there was an air of relief that maybe she was out of immediate danger. I think we expect that if we address the communication so that all parties can end up feeling that they are basically good persons, things will start to work better. That partly accounts for our relentlessly affirmative framework, one that many people object to but that I think of as fundamental.

What I like about this approach is that it allows us to invite people to influence what happens in a much more creative way than we used to think was possible. Another thing: Since there is a continual process of follow-up built into the work, there is great opportunity to change course, try different tacks, or go back and start again. What you lose, of course, is therapeutic predictability and elegance. I find this approach hard to teach, and that is one reason I like using formats like the reflecting team. Asking people to comment and to listen to each other's comments interferes with the usual process of problem solving, which we are trying to get away from. However, as this way of thinking gets built into the collective unconscious of those in the family therapy field, I think the use of a reflecting team in a formal sense will drop away.

Since we are writing a "story in retrospect," I would like to end with some remarks about a few theoretical ideas that have been in all our minds, ideas that have influenced and been influenced by our practice. As of now, I consider some of these influences to be:

1. *Ideas about the social construction of knowledge* (Gergen, 1991). The viewpoint that we create or invent what we think we know—in the field of human events, at least—challenges the legitimacy of "normal social science" as it applies to psychotherapy and family therapy. When we are dealing with the area of emotional distress, the concept of treatment becomes particularly questionable and the pressure to make a diagnosis even more so.

2. *Ideas about the harm done by normative models for psychotherapy* (Anderson & Goolishian, 1988). For me, most of the beliefs that surround the concept of psychology deserve to be challenged. I personally believe that all models of therapy that posit causes for pathology, whether of a structural nature (poor boundaries, lack of individuation) or of a process nature (growth impairments, developmental lags) should be thrown out. In fact, it might not be such a bad idea to decide that psychology is a flawed field and replace it with a new emphasis on human communication.

3. *Ideas about downplaying "texts"* (which belong to a culture of literacy) *and upgrading "conversations"* (which belong to a culture of orality; Olson, 1993; Ong, 1982). Texts and formal vocabularies are what uphold the authority of the expert. Without such supports the art of therapy becomes local and perishable, like Christmas cookies or hamentashen. At the same time, I am in favor of ways in which the consumers of therapy can

themselves become authors, as when Peggy Penn (1991) helps people to compose letters to family members or when a colleague of mine, social worker Catherine Taylor, assists client groups to compose and design their own newsletters.

4. *The idea that there are no patterns intrinsic to human affairs.* If one believes this, it makes no sense to look for patterns in the therapy process, in the family, or in the individual personality—except when doing so seems useful, and then only with a disclaimer or rationale attached.

5. *An idea about a "different voice," first advanced by Carol Gilligan (1982)* After reading Gilligan's study which suggests that women value keeping relationships intact where men value right/wrong principles even at the expense of relationships, I felt that we should make room for a style in family therapy that puts connection before truth and empathy before being right.

6. *Finally, ideas about discourse from French social historian Michel Foucault* (in Rabinow, 1984). Foucault calls attention to "the micro-fascism of everyday life." He holds that it is through the discourses that are built up around our institutions (e.g., penal institutions, legal institutions, medical institutions) that the modern state controls its subjects. Insofar as family therapists are more and more part of what Kearney, Byrne and McCarthy (1989) call the "colonialism of mental health," I believe that we now have an obligation to critique and even alter our own roles.

A word about the format of this chapter. This is not the first time a family has been invited to contribute to an article (e.g., Roberts, 1988). What is different here is that Judy and I decided to break ranks with the custom of starting an article about therapy with a theoretical discussion. This article was not written to fit any current intellectual framework, unless one can say that the postmodern critique of Western thought is such a framework. In fact, we join the growing chorus of people who question whether the study of human communication can ever be a "science" at all. Moreover, we wanted to suggest an arrangement that places the "voice of the person" first, and the "voice of the text" second. If the text continues to lead the way, the automatic authority of the professional will never be challenged.

Furthermore, we decided to keep each voice individual and separate; there is no royal "we" producing this paper but a group of people with particular and local opinions. This is why we kept to a format somewhat like Chaucer's *Canterbury Tales,* where each story conforms to the mode and manner of its teller. We hope that this lack of consensus will invite the reader to contribute his or her own critical version. Let us now consider the stories we haven't heard yet, namely, the contributions offered by Sarah, David, and Tekka.

## SARAH'S REFLECTIONS

I appreciated the sessions at Brattleboro very much. They helped me get beyond my feelings of shock, panic, and helplessness, which were the result of Tekka's episode and hospitalization, which came as a great surprise to me. I also took on my own private blame for everything in her life that might have contributed to her difficulties.

The sessions at Brattleboro gave us a format for conversations that we were unable to have by ourselves. The nonjudgmental, supportive attitude of the team gave space for a larger perspective than I had at the time. I was able to take a look at my overidentification with Tekka. It would have been easier to have someone tell me what to do at the time—but, instead, I had to reach deeper inside myself.

The talk about mothers and daughters and being a hostage to the universe stayed with me throughout this year, which continued to have difficult moments. Tekka had another hospitalization, which was more benign but definitely took its toll. This time Tekka took charge of her own discharge and aftercare plans without us. I work at not following my impulses to take on her problems as my own, remembering that she is a very capable and strong woman and accepting that she has a condition that she will have to find her own way to deal with. I have also been working with my mother in therapy this year, and the quality of our relationship is improving. I am becoming more sensitive to the times when I do to Tekka exactly what I have been angry at my mother for doing to me.

My gratitude to David for being there during all this keeps deepening, as does my respect for Tekka as a person who is separate from me. The Brattleboro experience taught me the importance of daring to talk about my concerns without getting "freaked out." I will need many years of practice.

## STEPFATHER'S REFLECTIONS: COMMENTS FROM DAVID

*The following is my view of the Brattleboro Family Center as I experienced it with Sarah and Tekka in the spring of 1991. I am writing the first section of this without reading what the team in Brattleboro has written. I would rather get on paper my own views of the experience first, before making comments about the others' perceptions. For the same reason, I have not read Sarah or Tekka's comments beforehand.*

*Sarah and I contacted the Brattleboro Family Institute to look for some form of therapy that would be useful to Tekka in dealing with what had been diagnosed as manic–depressive or bipolar behavior. Looking back, I do not know if we found what we were looking for, something primarily for Tekka. What we did find was something Sarah and I needed: a way to relate to Tekka about her condition. Tekka also gained; she got closer to her family and thus I think found more support than she had expected. Our ways of relating to her on our own were frustrating, too filled with our fears and guilt, sometimes even exploding in anger. None of us could help it, even though I think we all saw what was taking place.*

*The sessions at Brattleboro presented a kind of a safety net. Judy Davis provided an extremely neutral forum for discussion. Comments later by the "hidden therapists" behind the mirror allowed for subsequent clarification* of our statements. Often what we say may not be what we mean, especially as interpreted by another. Having the chance to hear the interpretations of the "hidden therapists" gave us all an opportunity to see how we had been misunderstood, and the ending part of each session allowed for restating in clearer words and tone what we meant to say the first time.

Implications of our thoughts and feelings also came to light. The sessions were specifically helpful to me by allowing a forum where we could discuss Tekka's plans for the future. In sum, although I am writing this as a critique of an experience and certainly not as an advertisement, I think very highly of the Brattleboro Institute and would certainly recommend it to any of my friends needing ways of communicating in a crisis.

There is still a part of me, however, that wishes the sessions had been more specific in helping Tekka directly with her psychological difficulties. Nonetheless, it was refreshing to find help oneself, especially when one is looking for help for someone else! And in finding help in communicating we all gained a stronger, or at least more positive, sense of our family together.

## David's Comments on Brattleboro's Comments

*I see that the "hidden therapists" ought to be called the "reflecting team." I really have no particular comments to add after reading the narrative by Judy Davis and the comments by Lynn Hoffman. I find I view the actual situations that took place similarly. I probably do not agree with some of the theoretical statements regarding therapy but appreciate the effort to not get stuck in preconceptions of what therapy ought to be. I say "probably do not agree" because upon reflection I might come around to the same views. I will give one example: Lynn Hoffman states, "I personally believe that all models of therapy that posit causes for pathology . . . should be thrown out." At first reading, this statement implies to me that looking for possible causes is itself a mistake. I have a hard time with this notion of throwing out the search for causes. If therapy is to some extent a curative process, this in itself means that there is something that needs curing. Whatever it is that needs curing came about somehow; trying to find out what that "somehow" is seems worthwhile to me. And yet I know the problem that Lynn is addressing by her statement. Too often theories are imposed on what we see and hear, and what we get back is only what we used as a filter to begin with. With Tekka, various therapists presented to us with equal conviction conflicting theories regading her episode: Stress caused it; biological defects caused it; having an addictive personality caused it; lack of a chemical in the brain caused it; the perils of a spiritual quest caused it. All or none may actually be true. Imposing these theories on Tekka's behavior changes how one looks at her, stifles dialogue, and prevents one from dealing with the situation as it is.*

*And yet I still believe that one ought to at least be interested in what a possible cause could be. If there is a cause that can be identified then perhaps others need not be subjected to that cause; this would be preventive* mental health. Or perhaps the cause can be counteracted, and thus cured. Or perhaps nothing can be done, in which case greater emphasis needs to be put on acceptance. I realize that the therapist is in a rough position. On the one hand, the therapist must be open to what is taking place. On the other hand, past experience and the search for understanding lead to theories, even if the theory is that there should be none.

Thank you for permitting me this small indulgence of commenting on one of the theoretical points. Thinking about this stuff makes me glad I am not in your shoes.

Sincerely,

David

## TEKKA'S REFLECTIONS

Dear Judy,

Here are my thoughts and reflections on both our work together and the material written about it. I had not given that time any thought until you asked me to write this, but I have sat down many times in the past week to put my ideas and feelings into a cohesive or articulate statement. I don't think I have fully suceeded, but since time is running out I will share what I have at this moment.

Before I begin I would like to thank you and the rest of the Brattleboro Institute team for showing so much interest in our case and for investing so much energy into "it"—whatever "it" is worth.

I find myself torn between a feeling of excitement to be part of a project that focuses on going beyond existing structures of communication and therapeutic approach—and revulsion at delving into personal territory in a pointless venture into nothingness. I resent the focus on myself as suicidal or even having problems—or at least I resent it in the context it was in last spring, where I am clearly the "patient" and the pivot point of our "family gathering."

Nontheless, I love things that have to do with me (whatever you choose to call it), and I thoroughly enjoyed the process of our work and getting to hear the team's impressions of me as a person. The concept of transient realities and perceived realities has always interested me, and to voice and hear the realities of me as a person was a worthwhile opportunity, especially in relationship to my mother and David since we all clearly have different perceptions of our dynamics. It felt like a safe environment to do this because I felt that my voice was respected by the team, and I remember at times feeling as though my views were being defended and protected.

I believe the concept of freedom versus safety that surfaced is a profound one—that was seen clearly in our case and that I see clearly in society as well. I have thought about my mother's comment that "in my work, when a kid has suicidal thoughts or does suicidal art work or writes suicidal songs, we set up a suicide watch." In my life it is played out with emotional concern on her behalf—that there must be something wrong, and she wants to help, and feels powerless. Yet her approach leaves me resentfully in a "victim" role that I don't adhere to—because I see myself more as a survivor . . . I guess that's why.

I see this same scenario on a larger scale. Where do we draw the line between putting a stop to exploitive pornography and taking away the endowed rights of expression? The line quickly moves to the right, putting censorship restrictions on art.

This week I have been listening to the new Tracy Chapman tape, Matters of the Heart. The chorus of the first song is "Bang Bang Bang. He shoots you dead." It is played all the time on the radio, and people at my job are reciting the chorus constantly. I told my friend of the fear/vision I had of little kids hearing the song and running around with toy guns singing, "Bang Bang Bang, I'll shoot you dead." My friend responded that Tracy Chapman was probably concerned with singing about reality, period.

Freedom or safety? Jimmy Cliff sings, "I'd rather be a free man in my grave than living as a beggar or a slave." I think it is an issue of oppression—personal and societal, and that once "a kid" gets to the point where he/she is able to consciously think, draw, sculpt, sing, or in any other way express suicide, that they are actually in a more healthy place.

To respond to the idea of a suicide rather than the act of expression gives the suicide even more power. For example, I felt very violated to have the topic of my "recovery doll" even be a topic. To me it was a very sensitive personal thing to begin with (the doll, that is) and to hang it on the door was my way of consciously expressing how I was feeling in relation to others. To have the "others" then react to it only perpetuated the feeling: the feeling of violation, oppression, infringement. So where does one go with that? It can become a vicious circle quickly.

But what if the response was gratitude or hopefulness? What if when the black slaves sang of freedom rather than oppression, the white people said, "Wow you are human beings with a voice to be heard and respected instead of worrying about riots and revolution?" What if when ugly things are put before our eyes we can say, "Yes, they are ugly; yes, they are real, let's get on with it and do something with it"?

I can be a rebel to the point of hurting myself, and I can be responsible to the same point. But if I were the ideal—a Responsible Rebel—or especially so, it would be dangerous. My mother once taught me a song Janis Joplin sings which says, "Freedom's just another word for nothing left to lose, nothing ain't worth nothing unless it's free" . . . something like that. Anyway, Freedom/oppression/ and then safety. I don't know if there is room for safety when you are dealing with such big issues. Look at Gandhi, Kennedy, Martin Luther King, Jr., Karen Silkwood. Safety certainly wasn't their first choice and yet they were not put on a suicide watch.

If every artist that ever dealt with the issue of suicide and death were put on watch, we would be missing out on a lot of our culture. And what if Freud was questioned about his cocaine addiction, etc?

I am definitely rambling a bit—but my point is that it is a fundamental question and one that affects me personally for many reasons. The fact that my mother is a therapist makes her not only a mother—but an institution *and an approach as well—and so there are many levels to question and dis-agree with her on—of course they are also a part of me.*

*In closing, I will say that I'm opposed to the exaggeration that I "at-tempted to walk into or through the side of a subway car" since it was not the car but the wall of the station. This was the point of conflict between my family and me, because it was the incident that would determine if my episode was "a threat to myself." Obviously, if I had tried to run through the subway car, it would have been dangerous!*

*I realize this letter is long—but I don't expect you to use it all. It's the best I can do at this point. However, I would be very willing and in-terested to continue this discourse if there is an interest on your side for any reason.*

*If you have any questions feel free to contact me. Thank you again.*

*Sincerely,*

*Tekka*

## EDITOR'S QUESTIONS

Q: *Most of us learned that it is important to have a theoretical framework to guide our clinical activities. You describe the therapy process as "a canoe trip on a river. It starts when we 'put in' and ends when we 'put out.' " In a previous paper (Hoffman, 1990) you, Lynn, refer to Judy's idea of the therapist as an "accidental ethnographer." Would you expand on these ideas and compare your approach with more traditional family therapy models? Your work is a major step away from the therapist as an active, directive, more intrusive presence in the therapy process. Would you comment on how your work evolved in this direction?*

A: *Lynn:* My earliest influences came from reading Haley's ideas about "directive therapy" and watching Virginia Satir's magisterial family in-terviews. Haley defined strategic therapy as a therapy designed by the therapist. I followed this model until I became aware, just after his death, of the immense discomfort Gregory Bateson felt with the growing family therapy industry and its emphasis on manipulation and control. His book *Angels Fear* (1987) had just been posthumously put together by Mary Catherine Bateson, and the dangers of conscious purpose was a major thesis of the book. I began to feel more and more impressed by this point of view.

Then came my awareness of the unusual work of Harlene Anderson and Harry Goolishian (1988) in Texas, Tom Andersen (1987) in Norway, and Ben Furman and Tappi Ahola (1992) in Finland, which altered the therapist-driven model, giving the ordinary citizen much more say in what went on. It was I who added the ingredient of the "different voice," taking this idea from the germinal work of Carol Gilligan. This became the basis for my own protest against a managerial style associated mostly with the men with whom I had trained but adopted by many women too.

*Judy:* My first postdoctoral training was an externship at the Brattleboro Family Institute with Bill Lax and Lynn Hoffman. I had just completed a dissertation in the field of family systems that had quite accidently, by the time it was over, led me to what was then being called the "new ethnography." In contrast to traditional ethnography, this was a reflexive approach that understood the field-worker as an actor in the very drama he or she was attempting to describe. In my case, the drama centered on the way in which four families planned and experienced the bar mitzvah of a first child (Davis, 1988).

The ethical, intellectual, moral, and methodological issues with which I had been wrestling in my attempt to "write up" my experience with these families were, it turned out, many of the same issues about which postmodern ethnographers were then writing (e.g., Clifford & Marcus, 1986; Geertz, 1988; Meyerhoff & Ruby, 1982; Ruby, 1982). Their ideas gave me a language for understanding the "ethnographic" portraits I had unintentionally produced. (My goal had been to write more traditional case studies, but the nature of my immersion in the process had made that impossible.)

It was only a short time later that these issues (of voice, position, authority, text, etc.) began appearing prominently in the family therapy literature. They were, it seemed, the very same issues with which social theorists on the constructionist, narrative end of the field had themselves been struggling (e.g., Andersen, 1987; Anderson & Goolishian, 1988; Hoffman, 1985; Miller & Lax, 1988). My attraction, therefore, to the reflecting process I encountered in Brattleboro was immediate and deep. It was, for me, both a natural extension of my research and a personally more comfortable fit (vis-à-vis client–therapist positioning) than the Milan approach, in which I had originally trained.

It was in my early conversations with Lynn that I came to recognize that my idea of open-ended, collaborative research resonated with her distrust of therapies that are too tightly planned. Both my research design and the reflecting interview were nondirective: My intention as researcher was to follow the families in their journey over time and to talk with them periodically about their experience of that journey and (secondarily) their experience of talking about that experience; it was not to put them through an exercise or experiment that I had set up. Similarly, a reflecting conversation follows, rather than directs; it elicits the family's ideas about what brought them to therapy, and also asks about their ideas about the process. With such research and with such therapy, the duration of the conversation and the direction in which it moves is placed actively in the hands of the families rather than being a function of a therapist's methodological or theoretical model.

I had no preconceived notion, as researcher or as therapist, about how the family was supposed to do what they were doing. Although I had some culturally preconceived ideas about the "proper" way to do a bar mitzvah, I had none about how families use the experience to work on issues of emotional process (Friedman, 1980, 1985). I had no normative ideal against which to measure the family culture I had been permitted to enter. My only plan was to remain as unobtrusive and as nonthreatening as possible so that they'd let me stay. Likewise, as the interviewer in Tekka's family, I had no preconceived plan about how the family had to do the work they'd come in to do. My only plan was to keep the conversation going so that ideas other than the ones they had come in with might emerge. In both cases what I was hoping for was what Arthur Penn (1991) calls a "felicitous accident," a convergence of people, events, ideas such that something new and exciting gets created.

The idea of accident was not only in the research and the therapy but in the write-ups as well. In both instances I attempted to tell the story in such a way as to include as much detail as feasible and as much of the other people's voices as possible. I also wished to expose myself as much as I exposed them, all in the service of allowing readers to construct their own meanings.

Q: *As therapists you put yourselves directly into the story as equal partners with family members. You provide space for the family to offer their ideas and then have a reflecting team comment on these ideas in a recursive process of multiple conversations. In this particular situation family members are talkative and articulate and as you say "especially informed consumers." How do you modify your approach with families whose members are not as talkative or articulate as this one, families who might not so easily make use of the space the therapist provides?*

A: *Lynn:* I don't feel that families have to be articulate to profit by this approach. What is important is the invitation to comment on the *process of therapy* rather than on the *problem.* We are talking about a shift that changes the nature of the professional relationship toward a more equitable one, if only symbolically, not a technique that works better with some people than with others. Of course, there may be a good reason not to ask people to comment publicly. If people would be endangered by open talking, you would probably not see the family together anyway, so the question wouldn't come up.

*Judy:* I would add to what Lynn mentioned, that families don't have to be particularly articulate to respond to the invitation to switch positions. For instance, we ask the family how they would like to use the time rather than authoritatively choosing what to talk about. We also invite them to listen to us or to each other from new positions, thus increasing the chance of new ways of seeing.

This is precisely the situation that Bill Lax recounts in a chapter on postmodern practice (1992). In that piece he describes a family for whom the process of therapy was intimidating and who found it difficult to talk about their situation. I was the therapist in the room and Bill was behind the mirror. We asked the child to watch from behind the mirror with Bill while the parents talked in the room with me. Then we switched and the parents watched as their son spoke with Bill. From that position, they were able to, as the mother put it, see their baby grow up in front of their eyes. It was a dramatic example of the difference a new position can make.

Q: *You comment that your work is "not attached to outcome" and yet you appear to have certain goals in mind with this family, namely, to prevent Tekka from attempting suicide and from a return visit to the psychiatric hospital. Doesn't this count as a preferred outcome? Also, Tekka says in the fourth session, "I would like myself to be back in control, in total recovery. So the doll can be in storage!" Isn't this a goal of the therapy as well? How do your goals in therapy differ from goals set by more traditional family therapists? Doesn't the therapist have a responsibility to get family members to specify their goals for therapy so that you can know whether you're moving in* their *preferred direction?*

A: *Lynn and Judy:* You ask about our bias against having a preferred outcome. In a setting that demanded clearly defined goals we would always give priority to those demands, but we would share with the family our dilemma about setting up such goals. Then we would work with the families or persons on what goals we might choose to set up, including goals that might keep changing.

However, the phrase "not attached to outcome" is probably unfortunate because it has so many meanings. One meaning is that we are not attached to any *particular* outcome, only to one that would remove or diminish the reason people came to talk to us. Here we paid attention to what the family wanted, which was to "improve communication" and to help get Tekka off medication and find a plan, at least short-term, that would be acceptable to her and reassuring to the parents. In that sense we do try to listen to what family members want. Of course, sometimes there is a concern that people can't come right out with or that there is disagreement about. In this case self-harm was such a concern, and within the constraints that defined that issue we naturally paid attention to it.

But there is another meaning to "not attached," and this is the one Bateson was talking about in *Angels Fear.* If as a therapist you try to control the therapy toward some normative outcome, you may get into trouble. First, this kind of goal often hides a therapeutic or social bias; second, getting too attached to it can seriously get in the way—the more you push, the less likely it is that it will happen. That is a principle of zen, but it is a principle of therapy as well.

Q: *You met with this family only four times over a 6-week period. Is it standard practice for you to see families for only a few sessions over a relatively short span of time? Who decides about the frequency of meetings and about the duration of therapy?*

A: *Lynn and Judy:* The time intervals and length of therapy are decided by the group or depend on the circumstances of the situation. There is a flexible negotiation from session to session dictated by the logic of events and people's wishes. But by drawing on the participation of the group as we do, we find we meet less frequently and more episodically, depending on the situation. With this family, the school year was ending and Tekka was leaving the area, so that limited our contact.

Q: *When you, Lynn, talk about the importance of people "taking back the interview from the professionals," you're talking about a radical philosophic shift in perspective. In light of the prominence, power, and pervasiveness of the medical expert model, how can these new methods of inquiry grow and flourish?*

A: *Lynn:* There is a growing pile of complaints about the profession of psychotherapy, and my twig is but a small addition to the pyre. Perhaps this criticism is growing *in proportion to* the increasing importance of the medical model in justifying insurance reimbursement and simplifying managed care. The point is exactly that: to confront the trend toward professionalizing every problem.

Actually, I see the support group movement, even when I don't agree with its rationales, as a much more useful and inexpensive way of managing many common miseries than traditional psychotherapy. Where psychotherapy does seem advisable, I would want to see it become more comfortable and collaborative. I would like professionals to share far more broadly with families the techniques we have mostly kept to ourselves. I would also like to see the process of therapy demystified by the use of ordinary language, even in conferences between professionals. Finally, I would like to see banished once and for all the idea of therapists as doctors, healers, or priests. This would not mean abandoning our hard-won skills: It would mean that instead of subjecting people to them we would explain them and teach people how to use them.

## REFERENCES

Andersen, T. (1987). The reflecting team: Dialogue and meta-dialogue in clinical work. *Family Process, 26*(4), 415–428.

Andersen, T. (Ed.). (1991). *The reflecting team.* New York: Norton.

Anderson, H., & Goolishian H. (1988). Human systems as linguistic systems. *Family Process, 27,* 371–395.

Bateson, M. C. (1992, March). *Composers and improvisers.* Plenary address, Family Therapy Network Symposium, Washington, DC.

Bateson, G., & Bateson, M. C. (1987). *Angels fear: Toward an epistemology of the sacred.* New York: Macmillan.

Clifford, J., & Marcus, G. E. (Eds.). (1986). *Writing culture: The poetics and politics of ethnography.* Berkeley: University of California Press.

Davis, J. (1988). Mazel tov: The bar mitzvah as a multigenerational ritual of change and continuity. In E. I. Black, J. Roberts, & R. Whiting (Eds.), *Rituals in families and family therapy* (pp. 177–208). New York: Norton.

Friedman, E. H. (1980). Systems and ceremonies: A family view of rites of passage. In E. A. Carter & M. McGoldrick (Eds.), *The family life cycle* (pp. 429–460). New York: Gardner Press.

Friedman, E. H. (1985). *Generation to generation: Family process in church and synagogue.* New York: Guilford Press.

Furman, B., & Ahola, T. (1992). *Solution talk: Hosting therapeutic conversations.* New York: Norton.

Geertz, C. (1988). *Works and lives: The anthropologist as author.* Stanford: Stanford University Press.

Gergen, K. (1991). *The saturated self.* New York: Basic Books.

Gilligan, C. (1982). *In a different voice.* Cambridge, MA: Harvard University Press.

Hoffman, L. (1985). Beyond power and control: Toward a second-order family systems therapy. *Family Systems Medicine, 3,* 381–396.

Hoffman, L. (1990). Constructing realities: An art of lenses. *Family Process, 29,* 1–12.

Kearney, P., Byrne, N., & McCarthy, I. (1989). Just metaphors: Marginal illuminations in a colonial retreat. *Family Therapy Case Studies, 4,* 17–31.

Lax, W. D. (1992). Postmodern thinking in a clinical practice. In S. McNamee & K. Gergen (Eds.), *Therapy as social construction* (pp. 69–85). London: Sage.

Meyerhoff, B., & Ruby, J. (1982). Introduction. In J. Ruby (Ed.), *A crack in the mirror: Reflexive perspectives in anthropology* (pp. 1–35). Philadelphia: University of Pennsylvania Press.

Miller, D., & Lax, W. (1988). A reflecting team model for working with couples: Interrupting deadly struggles. *Journal of Strategic and Systemic Therapies, 7(3),* 17–23.

Olson, M. (1993). *"Conversation" and "text": A media perspective for therapy.* Manuscript submitted for publication.

Ong, W. (1982). *Orality and literacy.* New York: Norton.

Penn, A. (1991, July). *A conversation on cybernetics and film.* Public discussion between Fredrick Steier and Arthur Penn at the annual conference of the American Society for Cybernetics. Amherst, MA.

Penn, P. (1985). Feed-forward: Future questions, future maps. *Family Process, 24,* 289–310.

Penn, P. (1991). Letters to ourselves. *Family Therapy Networker, 15,* 43–45.

Rabinow, P. (Ed.). (1984). *The Foucault reader.* New York: Random House.

Roberts, J., "Alexandra," & "Julius." (1988). Use of ritual in "redocumenting" psychiatric history. In E. I. Black, J. Roberts, & R. Whiting (Eds.), *Rituals in families and family therapy* (pp. 307–330). New York: Norton.

Ruby, J. (Ed.). (1982). *A crack in the mirror: Reflexive perspectives in anthropology.* Philadelphia: University of Pennsylvania Press.

# 16

## Helping Embattled Couples Shift from Reactive to Reflective Positions

P. LYNN CAESAR

### FACT OR FICTION

One evening I was sitting with a couple who had come to me for therapy in great despair. Their marriage had deteriorated to a point where they hardly spoke to each other and no longer slept together. The only commonality in their lives was their young daughter. In all other aspects of their relationship they functioned separately. Both husband and wife felt a deep sense of loneliness and isolation. When they tried to talk about anything other than their daughter, tempers flared, voices were raised, blaming and accusatory remarks were exchanged, and someone usually left in the heat of the argument, leaving the issue unresolved. So many grievances had already accumulated that when they arrived in my office divorce was considered a viable option, given the level of anger, despair, and hopelessness the couple felt about their future together. Both felt that their daughter was the only reason to try to work out their problems. So there they sat, two people immobilized by their pain, past hurts, and anger.

The husband raised a topic he wanted to discuss. Although his wife agreed to the topic for discussion, she became more and more furious about his version of the story. She could not stop herself from interrupting him. At one point she clenched her fists, her face became red, her neck tight, her eyes intense, and her breathing shallow; she abruptly got up from her chair and moved toward the door. I asked her, "Why are you leaving?" She said,

"I cannot listen to his lies." I asked her, "Would you like to tell your story?" She said, "I will tell my story, but I cannot listen to his story because his story is a lie and I am telling the truth." I asked, "Is it possible for two people to have different versions of an event?" She said, "It is possible, but my husband has the facts wrong." I wondered aloud what the difference was between a fact and a perception. Given that my approach was to talk with both partners and elicit multiple views, I wondered how to avoid a collision of beliefs with the wife. Furthermore, when the husband responded to his wife's grievances, he had the habit of reading a deeper meaning into everything she said, thereby failing to take seriously her complaint. He believed he was in charge of determining what was the deeper truth beyond the surface of what his wife said. Both partners seemed to be embracing a philosophical position of realism in which they were searching for one objective reality. This was in contrast to my rationalist/ idealist position in which what we take to be observable is determined by the way in which we conceptualize the world. As Gergen (1986) eloquently elaborates, "To the extent that the mind furnishes the categories of understanding, there are no real-world objects of study other than those inherent within the mental makeup of persons (p. 141)." My clients and I also seemed to differ about whether reality is monistic or pluralistic. I felt like I was treading water in a delicate sea of philosophical differences.

I pondered my dilemma of wanting to broaden my clients' view of the world. I decided to abandon any attempts to try to change their position; after all, they had been arguing for years about each other's perceptions of reality. Perhaps I could best let go of my need to change their perceptions by offering them the idea that accuracy, truth, and objectivity could coexist alongside perception, multiplicity, and imagination. After the wife sat down to try to converse again with her husband, the following understandings and interchanges emerged: The wife felt that her husband's story included incriminating characterizations of her as a person, and she was compelled to interrupt to correct these false accusations. Her husband's portrayal of her did not coincide with her perceptions of herself. Nor did she feel that her husband was characterizing himself as she perceived him. She could not wait until he was finished because with each passing moment she felt depicted more and more as a villain while he remained blameless. Such a depiction did not fit with her sense of being victimized by her husband, particularly when he minimized her complaints by claiming to know what was behind them. When his wife corrected his story, he became enraged about being interrupted and soon raised his voice to such a level that she threw up her hands and said, "See, you can't talk to him when he gets like this!" Both partners seemed to be battling for their version of the truth, and neither could tolerate more pluralism.

As I reflect upon this story and my work with other couples with similar dilemmas, the following questions arise: How is it that couples stop listening to each other? How is it that one person's descriptions and explanations are experienced by the other as so aversive or assaultive that they must be stifled? Are there ways to tell stories that invite a partner's interest and curiosity? How do we introduce pluralism to monism without disrespecting a different worldview? How is it that one partner's use of language—along with familiar grimaces, glances, and intonations—can serve to ignite a familiar reaction from the other? Is there a language of anger that promotes rather than dissolves conversation? How do we as therapists respond to couples for whom the basic rules of courteous conversation have been so violated? How do we talk with couples whose orientation is to blame, accuse, and punish rather than understand, love, and cherish? How do we as therapists help couples shift from a reactive stance to that of reflection?

## THE REFLECTING PROCESS

Tom Andersen's (1987, 1990, 1992b) ideas of the reflecting process have been most influential in my clinical work. Andersen's (1990) understanding of Bateson suggests that making a picture of a situation makes certain kinds of distinctions. Since there is an infinite number of distinctions one can make, the picture one makes of the world is made by the distinctions seen by the describer. "In other words, there is always more to see than one sees" (Andersen, 1990, p. 30) since in every act of description many other possible descriptions are left out. As explanations are given about how to understand a picture, Andersen says certain meanings arise for the person that form the basis for how the person relates to the thing that is being described and explained. On the basis of his understanding of Maturana and Varela, Andersen states that people react to certain situations in whatever way is available in their repertoire at the time. This repertoire can change over time as old ways fade and new ways are introduced. If a perturbation occurs in a situation about which persons are not prepared to react because of their unique repertoire, they can either close up and preserve their integrity or disintegrate. Andersen asserts that in order to stay in a conversation with a person, one must respect the person's basic need to conserve his or her integrity. Andersen operationalizes these ideas by suggesting that the system itself defines what should be talked about and in what way this should be done.

   Andersen (1990) proposes that there are three parallel conversations going on at the same time when a client and therapist talk together. There is the inner talk of each, which preserves the person's integrity, and the outer talk, which occurs when one takes part in a relationship with others. We typically invite people in therapy to a dialogue to search for unseen descriptions and explanations about a particular issue. The reflecting process, as described by Andersen (1990), can be described as shifts between talking and listening among all participants. When talking, participants are engaged in an outer dialogue with others. When listening, they are talking with themselves. Andersen (1990) sees one goal of therapy as making room for the inner dialogue. In the process of making room for multiple conversations, clients and therapist can search for multiple descriptions, explanations, and meanings about problem situations.

Andersen has offered ideas, based on the work of a Norwegian physiotherapist, Aadel Bülow-Hansen, about how to be different or unusual enough in a therapeutic conversation to help fade out old ways and add new ways to a person's repertoire. Bülow-Hansen developed a method of working with people who suffer from muscular tensions. She sees the inhalation/exhalation cycle of breathing and movement of the body as inseparable. When muscles become tense, breathing is restricted. Andersen points out that emotions and words follow the exhalation of breathing. One way to prevent expression is to limit the breathing cycles. Limiting the act of inhalation may restrain exhalation. By manipulating certain bending muscles and stretching muscles in her clients, Bülow-Hansen induces a certain level of pain that stimulates deep inhalation, thereby helping to decrease tension all over the body after exhaling. By watching her clients' breathing, Bülow-Hansen can determine if she needs to use more or less painful touches. Andersen learned from this that the physiotherapist's touches need to be strong enough to stimulate breathing. He likens psychotherapists' questions to such touches. We watch to see if clients open or close in response to our questions.

Andersen (1992a) applies Bülow-Hansen's ideas to describe the physiology of conversation. He sees conversation as an exchange of listening and talking; one listens to another's talk. Andersen suggests that talking is a constant building up and relieving of tension. Our words and emotions come as we exhale in the breathing cycle. The words are formed from the air following exhalation. When a person stops talking, there is a pause in which the person appears to still be thinking about what was just said. Andersen prefers to wait until the person has not only stopped talking but seems more eager to participate in the outer dialogue. "By making use of the breathing as a metaphor, we have to follow another person's speed and shifts through her/his listening, thinking, and talking. If not, the conversation might suffocate" (Andersen, 1990, p. 47).

Extending Bateson's notion of difference and Bülow-Hansen's work, Andersen wondered if people stayed the same if they were exposed to ideas that were not too different or unusual. He suspected that a change might be triggered if they meet something that is unusual but not unusual enough to close them up. To quote Andersen: "What we, their supposed helpers, should strive for is to provide something unusual but not too un-usual in the conversations that we take part in with these people. This is a rule that comprises the setting in which we meet, the themes or issues the conversation comprises, and the way or the form the conversation takes" (1990, p. 33).

## A CLINICAL DILEMMA

The issues presented from the couple described in the opening story form the basis for this chapter. How do we work with couples who engage in chronic verbal fighting, couples for whom the process of talking and listening has gone awry? (Clearly, this phenomenon is not restricted to couples; parent–child conflicts can present similar dilemmas. For the purpose of this chapter, however, this discussion will focus on my understanding of the reflecting process in work with couples.) In particular, I am interested in applying Andersen's ideas of the reflecting process to couples who are reactive to each other. Couples whose pattern of fighting includes ongoing physical abuse will not be considered here.

Andersen's (1990) use of the word *reflection* is borrowed from the French *reflexion* and the Norwegian *refleksjon* and means that something heard is taken in and thought about before a response is given. The reflective process involves the creation of a format to allow people to talk about unusual, but not too unusual, things in a manner that respects their autonomy and integrity. This process allows all members to talk and to listen in a style and at a pace that breathes new life into the system. In so doing, new distinctions, descriptions, explanations, and meanings are generated for all who participate in the conversation.

Couples engaged in chronic verbal fighting rarely allow each other room to pause and think before responding. Responses given to the one who last spoke are often in the form of a rebuttal. Often neither partner is able to allow the other to complete a sentence, much less accord the other time to complete the thought process following what was said. If one goal of therapy is to create a format to give voice to all participants', including the therapist's, inner dialogue, this goal becomes an elusive one when argumentativeness and anger threaten to dissolve the conversation. Furthermore, how can we respect the manner in which partners talk to each other when it may involve contempt, demeaning criticism, and blame? How can a therapist intervene while respecting the autonomy and integrity of each partner?

If more room is created for inner conversations to develop, how can this enhance ongoing dialogue among people? Focusing on one's inner conversation can give rise to the process of imagination and the creation of new images or ideas. Philosopher Paul Ricoeur (Kearney, 1989) said that imagination is an indispensable agent in the creation of meaning through language. Couples who are stuck having the same repetitive fights have difficulty making new distinctions. This limits their ability to access their imaginations. How can we as therapists help partners react less and find routes back to their imaginations? Without new distinctions, pictures, images, and ideas, couples often play and replay familiar, and often painful, fights.

## RELATIONSHIP CONFLICT

There has certainly been a voluminous body of literature focusing on marital conflict and couples therapy (Bader & Pearson, 1988; Chasin,

Grunebaum, & Herzig, 1990; Crosby, 1989; Dicks, 1967; Framo, 1982; Guerin, Fay, Burden, & Kautto, 1987; Jacobson & Gurman, 1986; Napier, 1988; Paolino & McCrady, 1978; Paul, 1985; Sager, 1976). In addition to this body of knowledge the fields of communication, sociology, and social psychology have concentrated attention on conflict and conflict resolution. Retzinger (1991) discusses her theory of protracted conflict in marital quarrels. She believes that conflict escalates because of a threat to the social bond. Such a threat can be manifested in the form of contempt, disgust, blame, perceived injustice, demeaning criticism, rebuke, and devaluation. The person on the receiving end of such threats feels a sense of shame. Without acknowledgment from the injurious partner that he or she has helped to create these feelings, conflict escalation is likely. Acknowledgment can take the form of an apology or taking responsibility for one's own part in the quarrel. With such acknowledgment the social bond is repaired, and there is a sense of being understood. Without acknowledgment, the behavior of the injurious spouse is experienced as an attack by the other, who, in turn, retaliates in kind with behaviors of blame, contempt, and devaluation. Although each feels injured by the other, each is unaware of his or her own injury of the other and is unable to take responsibility for his or her part played in the escalation.

If conflict escalates when the social bond is threatened, how can conflicting thoughts, feelings, and ideas be communicated to a partner while preserving the integrity of the individuals and their relationship? On the basis of social exchange theory and a review of several research studies, Schaap, Buunk, and Kerkstra (1988) identified two dimensions of conflict resolution: (1) the ability to assert oneself and care for one's self-interest and (2) cooperation or showing concern for the relationship. Schaap, Buunk, and Kerkstra's review of Boyd's dissertation (cited in Schaap, Buunk, & Kerkstra, 1988) on interpersonal communication skills also identified similar features of constructive communication. Boyd's research found that expressions of respect and caring; active listening, including paraphrasing; and acknowledgment that the message is heard were important for any program in the training of communication skills.

Katriel and Philipsen (1981) have designed a ritual of interpersonal confrontation aimed to enhance feelings of being understood. One partner initiates the ritual by announcing the existence of a problem that can benefit from constructive talking. The other partner acknowledges the legitimacy of the problem by indicating a willingness to discuss the issue. Some degree of negotiation then takes place where the problem is stated and explored from several different points of view. Thus, the person who initiates the ritual discloses the issue while inviting feedback and suggestion for change from the partner, and the partner cooperates by listening nonjudgmentally and empathically.

Although couples can disagree over an infinite number of issues, it appear that the process of talking about and listening to an emotion-laden issue may contribute to an escalation of conflict and reactivity. It is likely that the conflict can be defused if the bond is secure between the couple, the manner of expressing and listening to the issue is respectful of each partner, concern is shown for self and other, the issue is treated as a legitimate concern, and responsibility is assumed by both partners for their part in creating or maintaining the problem.

## UNDERSTANDING

In the field of interpersonal communication it is believed that as relationships mature, the feeling of being understood, of perceived understanding, grows in importance as a goal for the relationship (Cahn, 1990). Perceived understanding refers to a person's assessment of his or her success or failure when trying to communicate. According to Cahn, perceived understanding correlates with increases in trust, interpersonal attraction, and communication satisfaction as couples move from courtship stages through marriage.

Baucom (1987) adds that part of developing a close and intimate relationship is getting to know and understand the partner. Part of the process of understanding involves trying to understand the basis for the other's behavior. Baucom maintains that this closeness, which includes understanding and causal explanations, is an important and gratifying aspect of relationships. Most people do not want to live with someone whose behavior they cannot explain.

Making attributions can be part of the process of explaining behavior. According to Baucom, couples who have lived with long periods of ongoing negative interaction are less likely to engage in a thoughtful logical attribution process when a partner behaves negatively. Typically, the perception of the spouse's behavior involves the interpretation that the spouse is intentionally behaving negatively to hurt or be selfish. According to Gergen (1985), descriptions and explanations are significant tools for laying blame, assigning responsibility, and giving reward and censure. Each use can invite certain conduct at the expense of others. Thus, to view others as possessing inherent sin is to invite certain lines of action and not others. Likewise, to view the other as being basically good might motivate the other to forgive seemingly unforgivable behavior.

Feeling understood and understanding why a partner behaves in a particular way are important aspects of an intimate relationship. Making causal connections and attributions is often a part of the process of developing such a relationship. Attribution theory (Baucom, 1987) focuses on who or what is responsible for some behavior, whether the actor seems to be behaving voluntarily, whether the actor's intentions are positive or negative toward the other person, whether the cause is likely to change in the future, whether the person making the attribution can change the cause, and how many aspects of the relationship will be affected by the cause. What persons attribute behavior to can influence how they think about themselves, their partner, and the relationship between them.

The concept of how people understand, explain, and make attributions need not be limited to the couple seen in therapy. We as therapists bring with us our understandings and unique way of describing and explaining the world. Philosopher Jurgen Habermas developed a model of the rational explanation of action (Baynes, 1990) that falls within the field of interpretive social science. He suggests that the social scientist belongs to the "lifeworld" whose elements he or she wishes to describe. In the process of describing and understanding those elements, he or she must be able to participate in their production. That which is being studied by the social scientist, or inquirer, is embedded in complexes of meaning constituted by the social actors. The inquirer can understand this system of meaning only by relating them to his or her own pretheoretical knowledge as a member of the "lifeworld." Andersen's (1992a,) discussion of Hans Georg Gadamer relates a similar concept of "pre-understanding." Our general assumptions, or pre-understanding, of what human beings are will influence how we come to understand a particular person. Andersen (1992a) says that "every time we understand something, we have the chance to re-search and re-arrange our assumptions and prejudices about that which we try to understand" p. 12).

What role does understanding play in helping people change problem behaviors or situations? This question can easily be the focus of another chapter entirely. For the purpose of the present discussion, let me just say that couples come to therapy very distressed about certain behaviors and associated feelings but are often eager to postpone change while searching for understanding. With understanding comes tolerance, acceptance, empathy, compromise, conciliation, forgiveness, and patience, all of which can help couples weather the most distressing problems and identify solutions. With a new understanding new positive descriptions, images, and ideas may follow. Such a framework is consistent with Lynn Hoffman's idea, borrowed from L. Boscolo and G. Cecchin (L. Hoffman, personal communication, September, 1992), that people don't change under a negative connotation. Perhaps with a pattern of understanding, people can initiate change spontaneously rather than feel change is being legislated by their partner.

## MY UNDERSTANDING OF COUPLES IN
## CONFLICT AND THE THERAPEUTIC WORK

On the basis of the ideas described in the foregoing paragraphs, I have come to believe that couples engaged in repeated arguments, couples for whom the rules of courteous talking and listening have gone amiss, have limited access to their inner talks when they come together in conversation. The repetitiveness of their argument is the playing and replaying of the outer conversation. If being intimate involves a balance of separateness and connectedness, how does a couple accommodate space for private inner thoughts to live in the relationship? Sharing one's inner dialogue with a partner may involve sharing ones' dreams, aspirations, desires, wishes, and fantasies. Alongside such disclosures may also be the sharing of disappointments, anger, frustration, and sadness. How is it that some couples can communicate their inner thoughts within a framework of love, understanding, and respect while others use the language of blame, contempt, and transgression?

Couples who blame typically feel very misunderstood. The sin or crime that is the target of blame may be an actual betrayal, such as infidelity. The accuser may feel falsely accused of some wrongdoing by the partner or may feel that the partner was unavailable in some profound way. The transgressor may be accused of mistreating the partner in some way. Often, the accuser feels that the accused is not contrite or has not accepted responsibility for whatever behavior is the subject of the accusation. Responsibility is often very important. The fight can involve a disagreement about who is responsible for what. Typically, responsibility is volleyed back and forth like a tennis ball, never landing in anyone's court. I believe that if all involved in the therapeutic conversation take some responsibility for some part played in the creation or maintenance of the problem, more room is made for understanding and new ideas to emerge. If responsibility is shared among all involved in the therapeutic conversation, then a climate of cooperation may be generated. Consequently, one focus in therapy is to help couples shift from an adversarial position to one of working in concert in the service of a mutually shared goal.

It is probably common for many therapists to work separately with partners who have a history of protracted conflict, particularly if such couples engage in fights during therapy sessions. After all, managing a session with a couple fighting feels unwieldy at times. In fact, therapies for extremely conflictual couples are often highly structured and educational (Guerney, Brock, & Coufal, 1986; Jacobson & Holtzworth-Munroe, 1986) In addition to these approaches, I would like to offer some ideas about how to help couples talk and listen differently with each other in conjoint sessions. If one talks and the other listens without reacting, what new distinctions, images, ideas, and responses in their repertoire can be made? When a person is able to access his or her inner private conversation and introduce this talk into the exchange with the partner, new descriptions, explanations and meanings can perhaps be generated by the couple as well as the therapist. In this context perhaps a shift can be made from a framework of transgression to a paradigm of love, compassion, and responsibility. In the following portion of a transcribed therapy session with a couple, I present an illustration of these ideas.

## Sarah and Jack

When Sarah and Jack came in for therapy, the problems in their relationship had reached crisis proportions. They were arguing constantly and seemed unable to resolve basic issues that emerged around the day-to-day running of their household. Jack was often anxious about getting household tasks done; he felt that he was unable to relax unless everything was completed. He felt that the onus for the worrying about and performance of such tasks was always on him, and he wanted more reliable participation from Sarah. Sarah felt excessively criticized by Jack, who in her opinion was unable to accept responsibility for his share in their problems. Sarah and Jack had been living together on and off for 5 years. The issues that brought them into therapy had contributed to a painful separation in the past. They had reunited and had agreed to try to work out their differences in therapy. Two past attempts at therapy, one of which was helpful, had not touched the pattern of escalating conflict between them. One fight, which occurred prior to their calling me for therapy, had escalated to the point where Jack had pushed Sarah up against a wall. This episode frightened them, since both had witnessed their father hitting their mother while growing up. Both felt that they could not live in a relationship that was physically abusive, and they wanted to stop this pattern before it contributed to the demise of their relationship. After meeting eight times, the couple felt that they were arguing less often and with less intensity, and they renewed their commitment to each other. In spite of the continuation of some of the issues that brought them into therapy, they decided to get married and were looking forward to planning their wedding together.

Prior to the session illustrated in the following pages, Sarah and Jack began to talk about how to lessen Jack's anxiety about household tasks. In particular, Jack wanted to extricate himself from his need to remind Sarah to take out the trash and from his preoccupation about whether there would be food in the refrigerator. Sarah agreed that she needed reminders because she did not notice the same things that Jack noticed. Together we came up with the idea of a job chart like those used in communal houses to spell out each person's responsibilities and the time by which chores would be completed. Sarah and Jack left feeling hopeful that they could, with this issue being managed, pursue other important goals in their relationship. In the session described here the couple present in their familiar argumentative mode, with Sarah (S) and Jack (J) quarreling about who initiated the idea of sitting down to create the job chart. (T indicates therapist.)

J: I got stubborn because I didn't want to initiate one more thing. That was it!

S: No, that wasn't it! In fact . . .

J: Let me finish what I was saying. I got stubborn because I didn't want to initiate one more thing.

S: Jack, I have to disagree with that because I felt I initiated it by being the only one to bring it up. In fact, you were out and out saying, "I'm not doing it!"

J: I don't agree.

S: *(louder)* Ha! Please! That's how that discussion started that night. Jack, are you going to sit here and call me a liar?

J: Uh huh!

T: Okay. Do you want to talk about the exercise in here?

J: You know, I don't want to waste our time doing it. I feel like this is a waste of time doing this exercise. It feels like such utter bullshit to me.

S: Why can't I just do what you want me to do *(pounds the arm of the chair)* and be the way you want me to be and call it a day!

J: That two adults need to waste money and time to do something that just seems so natural to me.

S: He is just resistant to it.

J: I am in some disbelief about this. This feels childish that we are spending money, time, and mental resources figuring out who is going to take the wastebasket out. You take the wastebasket out when its full. You buy milk when its a quarter of the way, or whatever, low.

S: The bottom line is I don't think the way he does. I don't see the same things he sees. Or I don't see them in the same amount of time that he does or as quickly as he does. Well, I guess I see it faster than I used to. So I shouldn't say that. But it's never going to be . . . well, frankly, I don't want it to be the same as Jack does. So chances are, it's never going to be good enough. It's never going to be just like him. In moments, he'll admit that.

J: I want to get something out in the open here. I do not want Sarah to be like me. All I want is plain and simple. All I want is for you to participate.

S: I do participate.

J: No, you participate very little.

S: I don't participate to the extent that . . .

J: Let me finish . . .

S: . . . to the extent that you want me to participate.

T: Wait a minute. I get the impression that this is going to continue to heat up.

S: Well, it has been for the last two weeks. There is a lot you don't know about what has happened in the last two weeks. I mean, I obviously am very angry and have been.

J: I don't want to live like this. In other words, I am not going to get married and live like this.

S: Let's just explain something! I want to stop right there!

J: I am going to finish this statement. I do not want to live this way. I am not threatening you. I am making a statement about me . . .

S: Let's talk about a promise that was made. Do you remember a few weeks ago when . . .

J: I am going to finish what I was going to say, Sarah. You are not going to block my words!

T: I would like to finish what I was going to say.

J: Go ahead.

T: Can we create some rules now in order for each of you to say what is important to say? I realize both of you are very angry. And I also recognize that when you both are angry, tempers can flare fairly quickly. So I'd rather establish a way for us to talk before that happens rather than afterwards. Does that sound like something each of you would like to do?

S: Yes.

J: Yeah, that's fine.

[Jack and Sarah came in assuming a fighting stance with each other. They were unable to do the assigned task, which suggested to me that a new understanding of this familiar fight took priority over attempting any behavior changes. Although they had talked about their fights, until this meeting the couple had typically controlled their interactions in my presence. I usually don't interfere with the choice of issues or the manner in which clients speak. However, Jack made a statement about the uncertainty of their future together that enflamed Sarah. There was a threat to their social bond. Sarah also felt that her integrity as a person was being threatened by Jack's expectation that she behave like him. It did not seem to be safe to speak of differences around these issues. Sarah offered an alternative picture that there may be other ways to look at Jack's grievance. Their conversation began to follow a route that is argumentative, defensive, and stifling of the other. This is familiar territory for Sarah and Jack. Each partner seems to need to talk and is unable to listen to the other. This clearly felt to be a time for me to intervene. I worried that if I did not intervene, this all-too-familiar fight might take place in yet another context, my office. l wanted to offer Sarah and Jack an opportunity to talk about the issues in a different way. I wanted to offer them the idea that "talking about talking" was as important as the issues themselves. Clearly, they seemed unable to listen to each other. I thought they might be more likely to be in the listening position if I talked. I also thought that if I talked more with each partner, they might talk less with each other and might have more room to focus on their inner conversations. I specifically chose the word "rules" to describe a process of establishing a way for us to talk. I thought the word "rule" would fit with Sarah and Jack's wish to have something or someone exercise authority over a process of talking that escalates out of control.]

T: Each of you have something important to say. And I'd like for us to figure out a way today for each of you to have the air time to talk and also to be heard. So, that means, each of you want to talk, and also each of you want the other to listen to you. So I'm wondering what needs to happen in order for each of you to have that without the other feeling you need to react?

J: What I need is that I don't get interrupted. It's as simple as that.

T: What do you need from Sarah as you say what is on your mind?

J: That I'm listened to.

T: How would you know?

J: That there is a spot of silence in between. Maybe a second or two of reflection. And that I am not immediately judged or laughed at.

T: And, instead, what other response might Sarah give?

J: Sarah might say, "Jack, can you say more about that?" or "I haven't heard that before; can you say more about that?"

T: Is there a way of saying what you want to say in such a way that it invites Sarah's curiosity?

J: Yeah, if I don't come across as accusing: "You did this or you did that." I'd say, "This is how I feel." *(long pause)*

T: I'm just wondering, how does someone express a feeling that may be an angry feeling without making accusations?

J: I have an idea about that! I just want to be able to say I'm angry and that's it. I'm angry without being accused: "Oh, you're angry, Jack."

S: No, she's saying how do you talk to me about being angry without your sounding accusatory?

T: How does someone express an angry feeling without making an accusation?

S: And blaming.

T: Yeah, and blaming. Is that possible?

J: Yes, I think that is possible. By saying, "I'm angry about this or that. I'm angry that I've taken out the trash a couple of times now and you haven't taken out the trash. I am feeling that I have been using my time this weekend by doing this and this and this. I'd like you to participate." Cite an example and say, "This is what I'd like for you to do to participate."

T: *(to Sarah)* I'm wondering if you were on the receiving end of that, if it might feel like an accusation or something else?

[By asking Jack to imagine and describe a dialogue with Sarah in which he felt understood, I thought perhaps Sarah would feel less pressured to change on demand. With Sarah and Jack less argumentative, there was more room for me to offer aloud some questions I was having about what the language of anger should be. I was also offering the idea that Jack could participate in the process of inviting Sarah's curiosity and, possibly, empathy.]

S: Everything Jack says to me at this point feels like blame and accusations. If I say something back to him, he says, "Well, I do that because of what you do. I do that in reaction to your reaction." Well, I do that because I get so angry when you make me do this; it's real hard for me not to hear things as accusations or blame. Because even the things that I complain about that he admits weren't right to do, somehow it's my fault. So I am going to have a hard time believing that Jack can come up with a way of expressing anything, much less anger, without blaming and accusing.

T: Can you help him . . .

S: I don't know how to help him, Lynn. Everything I say to him is denied and thrown back at me. Including, I mean, just last night . . .

T: Wait, hold on. When I say help him, what I was thinking was that maybe you could help him know how to let you know he is angry in ways that you can hear as nonblaming and nonaccusatory.

S: I don't know how to get through to him. He will not listen to me. He will not accept it or hear it. A brick wall goes up and he denies it all to himself as well as to me.

T: So in order for you to listen, you need to be listened to.

S: I need to be listened to. And not have the response be "It's because of you. If you didn't do this, it wouldn't happen."

[By asking Sarah "Can you help him?" I made a mistake in offering a framework of cooperation while the couple still remained quite adversarial. My suggestion was, for them, too "unusual."]

T: Right now we are trying to establish a way of talking with each other when you feel angry. How do you invite the other to listen? *(to Sarah)* You need something from Jack in order for you to listen to him. You need to be listened to. Since one of you is going to have to go first, that means one of you is going to have to wait to be listened to. How can we figure that out?

S: I don't know if I can. I'm just too upset. I don't know if I can sit and do this. I don't know that I can. I have just been walking around with this too much. It's too much. *(sad and tearful)* I just don't know what to do with it.

[I think this is the heart of the dilemma in working with reactive couples. How does a therapist respond when both partners need to talk simultaneously? Typically, the listening partner is often preparing a rebuttal, rather than listening in such a way that he or she can shift back and forth between the outer and the inner conversation. This is often a time when therapists consider physically separating the couple and meeting individually with each partner. As I was preoccupied with this dilemma, I thought that it would be best to share my inner conversation with the couple. I hoped that by broadening the conversation from the polarized issues between the couple, more ideas could perhaps be generated about how to create room for everyone's thoughts and feelings.

We continued to talk more about how we should proceed. Sarah continued to express anger about Jack's blaming her for actions for which she wanted him to take responsibility.]

S: I didn't expect to be this upset. I'm just afraid to do this. He's just going to try to hurt me if I talk about it. *(tearful)*

T: What do you need from Jack in order to feel safe to talk?

S: Not to blame me and not to throw it back at me. And not to threaten me the way you just heard him do when he feels backed in a corner. When he feels like he has no argument, except all he can do is say "You are right" or "I did that," he threatens: "I don't know that I want to do this. Go find someone else." That's what he does when he gets threatened. I need not to be threatened with rejection when he feels he has no other alternative or nothing else to throw at me than that.

T: So if Jack has second thoughts about getting married, the time to express it is not during an argument.

S: No, because he swears up and down that he doesn't have second thoughts. He doesn't know why he says that in those moments.

J: I do have second thoughts.

S: Oh shit, Jack. Then you change your mind every ten minutes.

T: Okay, if Jack had second thoughts you would appreciate if he expressed them in some moment other than during the heat of an argument.

S: Yes. It's more than that, though. It's not just been since we decided to get married. It's been forever. That when he feels I'm making a point or that he has no argument or that I'm making so much sense, it just frustrates the hell out of him, or that he gets frustrated, period, he brings me to the edge because he knows that is the worst thing he can do to me and the most frightening and scary and most hurtful thing. And he knows it! And I've said it over and over again. And I have literally begged him not to do it! And each time, each and every time, he says, "Honey, I'm so sorry. I'll never do that again. I promise you I won't." And each time he does it again. I feel like an abused wife.

T: Well, let's talk about it. In order for you to feel safe about what is on your mind, say more about what you need from Jack.

S: I need for him not to go after me. He goes for the jugular.

T: Can you say what you do need?

S: I need for him to own what he does. I need him to own and take responsibility for himself, which he won't do. I need for Jack to hear me and I need for him to say, "You are right" about things I am right about. "I did that, Sarah. I did it. I shouldn't have done it. I did it for these reasons. And the reasons aren't because of what you did. "I need for him to, once—no more than once—to be able to do that. I know I can't live that way. I get criticized enough by him. I can't take him when he does something cruel and mean and does not even own it.

[As Sarah continued to express her feelings about wanting Jack to take responsibility for hurting her, I suggested we wait to get into specific examples, which is what Jack started requesting of Sarah. We discussed how they could talk together if Jack had a different idea about whether or not he did something wrong. I asked Sarah if there was some other way she could feel heard under those circumstances.]

S: Yeah, if he doesn't blame me. I'm not saying he has to agree with me all the time. I'm not saying he has to suck up and say, "I'm sorry." I'm not even looking for an apology.

T: What you want to be able to say to Jack is "I hurt; there is something you did that hurt me," and you want him to be able to say "I'm sorry I hurt you."

S: Yeah. "I didn't mean to hurt you. I didn't do it to hurt you, or maybe I did do it to hurt you and I feel bad that in that moment I was angry and I tried to hurt you. But I was wrong." Instead I hear "Yeah, I wasn't trying to hurt you but you drive me to that. You provoke me and you get me to the point of anger."

T: So the message from Jack you would like to hear is "Sarah, you don't deserve to be hurt."

S: Yes, exactly! Not that I deserve it. That's exactly it! Somehow, I deserve this all the time. *(tearful)* Because I'm less than . . . no matter what it is, the most amazing things are justified . . . *(long pause)*

T: We have a half hour left. And each of you have something to say to the other. Is it fair or realistic to divide the time for each of you?

J: That would work for me.

S: I just don't know.

T: Well, think about it.

S: If that's the only choice, I guess, because I don't want to sit and listen to him for thirty minutes.

T: Might there be any other choices? That is one idea.

[We discussed different ways Sarah and Jack could talk together. Jack said that he preferred to have a dialogue with Sarah, rather than have each of them talk for half the time. However, he was clear that he wanted to talk without being interrupted. We also discussed how each imagined responding if the other didn't reply in the hoped-for way. Sarah and Jack decided to divide the time between them. When I asked who should go first, Sarah wanted Jack to begin.]

J: First, I want to say I am more genuinely sorry than I think you think I am. This morning I tried to say I was sorry, and I felt like you weren't hearing it. And I think, probably, because you were so angry.

[At this point I noticed Sarah starting to wince. I asked her for permission to sit closer to her. Sarah agreed. It seemed to me that Sarah was preparing herself in the event that she experienced Jack's words as attacking. I thought that sitting beside her might help her feel less alone.]

J: I came over to the bed and I tried to comfort you and I wanted to let you know I was sorry. I didn't know completely what I was sorry for. Because I was also feeling hurt, and I get mixed up in my own hurt and then your hurt. And I feel kind of wounded sometimes because of the fight we had the previous night. And so I feel like I would like you to say some healing things to me as much as you need me to say some healing things to you. I feel you have been doing a lot of tit-for-tat kinds of stuff these days because we both feel as though our boundaries are being preyed upon by the other. I just really need for you to do some things so my time doesn't feel so crunched. I have a lot of anxiety in my life right now. There's the wedding and planning for that. My business and the development of that. I have a lot of things that are unfinished. I have to call the shots in my business. There is all this change going on in my life. I really want the change. I want you in my life. I want us and our relationship to work out. I want to have a great wedding. I want to have a business that's financially sound. I am going through some personal changes in terms of my friendships. And I just find that my life in the past couple of years is extraordinarily stressful. And little things around the house. I feel I come home and I want it to feel like a home. I don't want it to feel like what I grew up in. Which was a damn mess. I am sorry that I hurt you sometimes. I am very sorry about that!

S: I wish you would do something about that.

T: Hold on.

S: I thought there was dialogue.

J: I'm done.

T: Before you respond, though, is there more you want to say or would you like to hear from Sarah now?

J: Yeah! That didn't feel good. That response, "I wish you would do something about that," is punishing me. As you feel punished by me, I have a hard time talking to you these days. I feel very punished by you. I feel punished by your critical and quick-triggered behavior. So I don't know what came first. Maybe it was me that created whatever was happening first. Maybe it wasn't me. I don't know. But all I know is we are caught in some dynamic where one is accusing the other and it keeps on going back and forth and the ball isn't landing.

T: What would feel like a response from Sarah like you were listened to?

J: Sarah would take a piece of what I said and would say, "Jack, can you say more about that?" or her saying "Gee, I didn't know that things were that stressful for you." Or " I do see things are really stressful, and I have been trying in these ways to help you."

S: (softly) Of course I understand how much stress there is in your life. As there is in mine. And I want to have a home too. I don't need to hear more or have you say more about what you are saying. Not because I don't want to hear it. But because of two things. I have heard it often. And I really do . . . I know you don't believe this, but I really do have the capacity to understand where you are and what you are feeling. I truly do. I don't always respond the way you want me to. But I really understand. So I don't think I need a better understanding of where you are. Does that make sense? I'm really not being resistant?

T: Could you say something to let Jack know you understand?

S: I understand that when Jack gets stressed, like legitimate stresses in his life, he becomes overwhelmed and he has an immediate need for order in his life in some areas, because he is feeling out of control and like there isn't enough order in other areas. It is not in his grasp enough and the home is the first place that he turns to. And he likes to have everything and most everything okay. And he likes to stay up with it. And all of that stuff. And I know how upsetting it is to him when it isn't that way. I know that.

T: *(to Jack)* What are your thoughts about what Sarah has been saying?

J: It's helpful that you say you know that, and yet there is a place that I go to . . .

S: Why don't I . . .

J: No. Please let me finish. The place that I go to is . . . that not only if you know, but if anybody knows something . . . the place I go to is "Why don't you do something about it?" I want to preface this by saying I grew up in a house that was so uncomfortable to be in and I just . . . I guess I worked hard when I was single, if you will, to have a house that was comfortable. If Sarah would say once a week or so, "Jack, its time to do the shopping" or "Jack, I've noticed that we have to do the bathroom or sweep this weekend. Why don't we split it up?" And I would like it if you say it in a straight voice and not a whining voice. That's basically it.

[Although Sarah did interrupt Jack, I was still curious to hear her finish her thought. I regret not intervening at that time. I believe Sarah was listening empathically to Jack in the way that he seemed to need. Although Jack was still in the talking position, he may have missed an empathic connection from Sarah that could have enhanced their talk. This is always a dilemma when I am talking with clients who rarely take a breath between statements. How do we create the pause or opening to interject our comments? How do we punctuate who is interrupting whom?]

S: What Jack doesn't understand is that the reason I don't do anything about it—and I think I do things about it but not nearly what he wants—is that I'm put together very differently and it conflicts greatly with my need and that's not even a conscious thing, where I'm saying, "Well, that doesn't suit me so I'm not going to do it." I have been soul searching about this. How come I'm not this way? What is wrong with me? I sat with a friend and we really talked about it and went through the whole thing. My friend asked me, "When you were a little girl, did you play house?" and I said yes and she said, "What happened when you played house?" And I said, "Oh stuff about finding out I was pregnant. I was going to have a baby . . . going to the doctor and finding that out. Or maybe decorating my house." I saw my mom doing that. Then my friend asked, "Did you ever bake bread or anything like that?" I said, "No, never." It was never role-modeled. It wasn't a priority. And I grew up just trying to stay safe and take care of myself. I didn't grow up dealing with that stuff. I grew up dealing with making my life function-al. So it's very overwhelming to me. I think what would it take to make me really good around the house. It would take not working full-time to be good around the house the way he wants me to be. It's hard for me to go and give so much at my job and at work. To take care of yourself is to be able to have my home to be a place where you come home and unwind and vegetate, and I don't mean be taken care of because I did it real well when I was single and living alone. It's different. It's about having it be a place for me to take care of. To call my own shots. And to structure my own time. *(crying)* That's what my home is to me. It isn't about having to do this and having to be there and "Oh my God, I better get this done or I'm going to be in trouble." I dreamt last night that my mother was screaming at me and telling me I was selfish and self-absorbed and don't care about anybody but myself.

T: When you hear Jack saying you need to take more initiative around the house or you don't notice when the trash can is full, do you hear him saying you are selfish and self-absorbed?

S: I hear him saying, "You better stay on top of this," and it's like I run around and say, "Shit, he's going to find this. I'd better take care of this before he gets home."

T: *(to Jack)* I'm wondering, Jack, if you can replace that message with something else. Somehow, what gets triggered for Sarah is this message from her mother that overpowers her. Can you replace that?

J: Yeah, I can. I am not saying, Sarah, that you are self-absorbed.

S: Oh, Jack, you say it all the time.

T: *(to Sarah)* He's not saying it now.

J: I feel like I've been misunderstood for a long time. And I feel like I've miscommunicated my whole intent around this. I guess I really want Sarah to believe that I don't want her to be like me.

S: I do believe that, Jack.

J: I wouldn't want Sarah to do some of the things I do around order because that's my world. I'm not calling her a self-absorbed, selfish person. *(Sarah begins to wince.)* I want to interject that right now I am feeling turned off. I want to go inside and leave because you are shaking your head and not listening, because that is the place I go to. And you know that. And I feel that you are punishing me in your way by doing some of those things. By nodding your head and squinting your eyes and twitching your face. I just want to leave. I don't want to deal with that. And that's what makes me angry and I go inside. So I want you to know that I appreciate the different way that you are than me. Sometimes, not all the time . . .

S: I believe you.

J: I am not finished yet, Sarah. And I am not asking for you to be the same way I am around the house. What I am asking is, I also work a full day. I also am absorbed by other things in the outside world. And I feel . . . the way I have been feeling in our house is overly committed to the ordering of the house. And the place I go to is our future sometimes. And the reason I go nuts sometimes is I say to myself if you and I are having a difficult time, at least from my eyes, managing a household, what is going to happen when we combine our money, when we have children. I really get afraid. Believe me, I want to take full participation in raising a child and running a household. But I need more of your help. And the help I need specifically is for you to say sometimes . . .

S: Do I have to hear this again? It is so hard for me to hear the same things over and over and over again.

T: I'm wondering if to the degree that Jack has said this over and over again, perhaps there are aspects he may feel you have not heard?

S: Oh, certainly there is. But being heard and being agreed with are different, and I don't believe Jack always sees that.

T: *(to Jack)* If Sarah was able to call the shots more around the house, what might that free up in you?

J: I would feel more relaxed. I think I would go off and read more. I wouldn't be worried about scheduling, even in my mind scheduling. A lot of the way I . . . *(sighs)* I'm a real initiator in my life. No one has to create a job description for me. I just go at it. I don't need anybody to say to me, "This is what you have to do now." Sometimes I get tired of it. Tired of thinking we can fit in grocery shopping here. We don't have enough milk in the refrigerator. You know it's my job to recognize that. It would be wonderful not to have to.

S: There are times when I see . . . I'm sitting here thinking, "Can *I* say when things need to be done?" You said at one point if I said such and such needs to be done this weekend, we can split it up. I was sitting here thinking, "Can I do that?" I certainly notice when things need to be done sometimes—not like you do—but sometimes. So, can I say that? And what occurs to me is my first reaction when I see those things is to ignore it or hide it or not say anything and maybe he won't notice, because somehow I am going to get into trouble. That's mine and I own that as my fear. But that's what goes on for me. It's "Oh God, I'm going to get into trouble. I did something wrong. I've got to get to it before he notices." And you always get to it first.

T: *(to Sarah)* I'd like to share my picture of what Jack may be asking you to help him with. He would like you to say, "I will make an effort in our lives together to do what I can to bring out the part of you that you would like me to know more intimately. And that is the part of you that is the relaxed Jack, the less compulsive Jack. The Jack who would like to develop his imagination. The Jack that would like to free up the clutter of his mind that is filled with structure, tasks, and work and play more." *(to Jack)* Does any of that fit for you?

J: Thank you. That feels right to me.

T: *(to Sarah)* As you are embarking upon your lives together, does any of that feel like something you can help Jack with?

S: I guess. It just feels so hard right now. I just have so little trust right now. It makes sense, of course. I believe Jack when he says he likes those things about me that are different from him, like my capacity to play. I know that is what he has always been attracted to, those parts of me, maybe, and what they can do for you, somewhat.

[As I was listening to Jack struggling to be heard in a particular way by Sarah, a new picture came to my mind. As I thought about how to describe this picture to the couple, I wondered if it would again be a mistake to use the language of cooperation. I was thinking that Jack was looking to Sarah for help in shedding the armor of his orderly and structured life, and I thought that Sarah would be more likely to be helpful to Jack if she could access a part of her both she and Jack valued. I also wondered if by sharing my picture of their dilemma, we could broaden their polarized struggle about who is responsible for what.]

J: I do love those parts of you. I love that you have a warm heart. You are a great person. Everybody loves you. I love you. I like all those things. And you know what? You just triggered something for me. I have spent the past year and a half . . . I was going literally crazy in my past business . . . *(Sarah winces and Jack yells)* Sarah, I have to say these things!

T: Jack, I know you do. But I'm also aware we soon need to make a shift to Sarah.

J: I know but, Sarah, why react to me the way you react to me? I don't want to be around you when you do that. I don't want to be in your presence. You don't know how often you do that. You come home and you tell me about people at work and you encourage them to talk. And you come home with me. And the littlest thing that's off, you accuse me of judging. The littlest thing that's off, you wince and you . . .

S: Honey, it would be real helpful to me if you wouldn't talk about how wonderful I am to the rest of the world but you. That's really hard for me to hear. And you do it a lot. "With so-and-so you are so wonderful, and your staff thinks you are wonderful. And I get shit." I can't hear you when you do that. Because, again, you are telling me how shitful I am with you and to you. How I mistreat you. That is not going to make me hear your point. And I know you have a good point to make. I give you that. That's not going to help me hear it.

[Sarah and Jack were beginning to make room for their inner conversations. They were introducing more private thoughts into their talk. They were sharing their fears, anxieties, worries, and needs as well as what pleased them. There were more terms of endearment offered than in the beginning of the session. They were also beginning to expand their worldview from being preoccupied with themselves to trying to understand the other. The angry exchanges that occurred seemed small in the face of the larger conversation that seemed aimed at generating new and mutual understandings. Both Sarah and Jack were interjecting more comments about taking responsibility for their share in their problems. There were also more openings for me to offer my pictures of their pictures. I didn't abandon my paradigm of cooperation, which, when offered earlier in our talks, had seemed too "unusual" for them. The partners, and Sarah in particular, seemed less repulsed by the idea of helping someone who was previously perceived as the enemy.]

J: I don't feel I get shit from you, Sarah. And I know that my creating that *(sighs)*, me doing that, isn't helpful to you. We do the same thing to each other.

S: *(sighs)* See, it's me.

J: No, no.

S: Oh, it's either my fault that I do it or I'm just as bad.

T: *(to Jack)* Jack, up until this point, how have you felt about how the conversation has gone with Sarah?

J: I feel good that I've been listened to.

T: I'm aware that it is beginning to degenerate because I failed in my job of not being a good timekeeper. I should have been a better taskmaster and stopped us sooner to shift to Sarah.

J: Okay, let's shift.

T: So I take responsibility for the fact that this is starting to degenerate. I am also aware that in the service of this being a dialogue, we didn't make the shift to get to Sarah's issue. I'm wondering what we should do because we don't have adequate time to give Sarah's issue the attention it deserves.

S: I don't know what to do because I don't want to walk around with this anymore. I don't want to be afraid of going home and having another fight. I don't know. I don't want the responsibility for deciding what to do about it. I don't know what to do. I'm just not working well now.

T: I have a couple of thoughts. I'm wondering what it would be like to wait two weeks to get to Sarah's issue.

[When Sarah and Jack first came into therapy, they had a struggle about how often they should meet. Sarah wanted to come weekly, an arrangement to which Jack agreed initially. After several months of therapy, Jack felt that he would like to meet less often. They struggled more and agreed they would meet every other week. I typically defer to clients to decide how often and how many sessions they want to meet. However, in this situation I wanted to offer an alternative framework for the next meeting to the one to which we had previously grown accustomed. I was concerned about Sarah's concern that she could not survive another fight. Although there had not been another episode of physical violence since the episode that brought them into therapy, I did not want to risk the possibility that violence could erupt.]

J: I kind of thought of that. I guess I'm torn about what to do. I don't want to come to therapy every week. I would feel that we are going back to what I don't want to do. I don't want to take the initiative. If I say, okay, let's come next week, then I feel I am doing what I don't want to do in this relationship.

T: So who should take the initiative around this decision? Should I take the initiative?

J: No!

S: What is it that you want from me?

J: I want you to tell me what you need. That's part of what this is about.

S: What's part of what this is about?

J: You say to me frequently that I don't listen to what you need. If you need something, I don't want me or Lynn to decide what you need. So, Lynn was asking what you need and you said you can't decide. She asked me and I have some ideas.

S: Fine, I want to come back next week.

T: *(to Jack)* Sarah did say what she needed. She needed someone else to take the initiative.

S: I needed to be taken care of. Which is something you are not willing to do.

J: That's not true.

T: *(to Sarah)* It's also what Jack needs.

S: I know.

T: In having you call the shots, it also seems to be a way for Jack to be taken care of.

J: Maybe I was, like, feeling a little bit of heat around that whole issue I was preoccupied with. The whole thing that I was adamant I was not going to initiate. So I was in that place as opposed to listening to what Sarah needed. 'Cause I think you hit the nail on the head. And I think a lot of this stuff has to do with one thing: both of us being nurtured. And we both grew up in homes where there was that much nurturance *(gestures with his hand to signify a zero)*. I think we look to each other in different ways for nurturance, and we get stubborn and we draw the line. And this is just a metaphor for that. And it shows up sexually, it shows up in our communication, at the dinner table. It shows up in our ability to listen to each other. It shows up in our interruption. Both of us are saying we are not getting enough.

[We ended the session by discussing Sarah's concern about the possibility of having a fight between sessions. Sarah and Jack were concerned that if they were to try to talk on their own, the discussion would escalate out of control. We agreed that they would wait to talk about these issues until our next meeting.

Given the theme of responsibility in our session, I did not exclude my own behavior in this area. I decided to let the conversation continue, without my interrupting the flow, instead of shifting to attend to Sarah. I recognized that such a decision might have consequences, but I was willing to accept responsibility for my decision. I felt it was critical to share with the couple my thinking about this decision. In a system where blame is thrown back and forth, I did not preclude myself from such a process. Although I did not see myself as wanting to shoulder blame, I did want to suggest that I should share the responsibility for certain decisions. Toward the end of the session it seemed that a shift had been made in giving new meaning to the problems. The theme of caretaking and nurturance seemed to be one both Sarah and Jack shared in common. Instead of highlighting differences, their dialogue now made their commonalties more apparent.]

## Follow-Up

I met with Sarah and Jack for six more meetings. Although there were occasional arguments, each episode seemed to be an opportunity to build on the work in progress as described in the transcript. Their marriage deepened their commitment to each other, and they became preoccupied with how to merge their new lives in ways that also protected their individuality. They felt confidant that they could negotiate their differences without causing an escalation of conflict. We ended our sessions with the understanding that they did not need to wait until their relationship deteriorated to call again.

## CONCLUSIONS

Talking with couples in a therapeutic context can be challenging. Couples who have a history of protracted conflict pose a particular dilemma for therapists who rely solely on "talking" as the main tool to generate new ideas in the therapeutic system. This chapter focused on the application of Tom Andersen's ideas of the reflecting process in work with couples who are reactive and embattled. Additional ideas from the fields of interpersonal communication and social psychology were offered to elaborate on how to enhance the process of listening and talking among all member of the therapy system. As partners react less to each other, more room is made for each partner (and for the therapist) to access and introduce his or her private conversations. Thus, new descriptions, explanations, and meanings can be generated by all who participate in the conversation.

## EDITOR'S QUESTIONS

Q: *I was very impressed with your ability to maintain your poise, calm, and neutrality in the face of the couple's very high levels of reactivity. What internal conversations were you having at those times when the couple's reactivity was high? How did you manage your own reactivity so that you could be effective in working with this couple?*
A: I was most preoccupied with the issue of my control as a therapist. As the session began to heat up at different times, I debated with myself: "Should I or should I not intervene? At what point should I intervene? How could my intervention affect the flow of the conversation? If I try to diffuse the couple's reactivity too quickly, might I interfere with their opportunity to express themselves or discover new possibilities?" Oftentimes, I intervened on the basis of the decibel level of the speaker's voice in the room. If I could no longer listen because the talk was too loud, I needed to do something in order to stay in the conversation.

Q: *Your approach reminds me of the Bowen systems model, which places emphasis on reducing reactivity by having the therapist talk with each member of the couple in the presence of the other and act as a neutral third party who works to stay "detriangulated" from the emotional intensity of the process. Would you comment on the similarities and differences of your approach and the Bowen model?*
A: Bowen developed his model to describe not only techniques of family therapy but a new natural systems theory of families. The ideas of Tom Andersen, in particular, which I have applied in my work with couples, serve to offer a "format" (Andersen, 1990) or a way of talking and listening among clients and therapist. I do see a distinction between Bowen's concept of "detriangulation" and my relationship to the emotionally reactive process of the couple described in the transcript. I recall that early in the interview the couple interrupted each other frequently and this extended toward me as well. At the point at which I became preoccupied with my thoughts and feelings about being interrupted, I knew I needed to join the intensity of the conversation and ask to finish my thought. Rather than staying out of the emotional intensity, I joined with it. I needed to introduce my internal

conversation into the outer talk so that I could continue to be in the listening position for the couple.

Q: *How would you have modified your approach had physical violence been an ongoing issue with this couple?*
A: Completely! If violence is an ongoing issue, then damaging actions are speaking louder than words. In order for talking therapy to be helpful with the issue of violence, I believe a therapist needs to first talk about taking certain actions. I would assess the degree of physical risk and determine to what extent we should be concerned about suicide and/or homicide potential. If there are children involved, I would talk with the couple about what effect the violence may be having on them. I would also assess to what extent alcohol or drug abuse may be involved with the pattern of violence. I would talk with the couple about the existence of weapons in the home. Depending upon what we learn in these conversations, I would discuss taking certain actions, if necessary, to assure the safety of the couple and their children (e.g., encouraging the woman to seek a temporary restraining order, referring the man to a group for men who batter, calling the department of social services, discussing arrangements for the weapons to be removed from the home, etc.). I think the message that the therapist is willing to take nonabusive action in order to keep everyone safe is a prerequisite to talking therapy.

Q: *What is your view of the therapist's responsibility for making the relationship work? At what point would you feel compelled to let the couple know that they are on a destructive course that may be unalterable? What factors would influence your thinking about the continued usefulness of therapy as a helpful forum?*
A: I feel responsible for trying to make therapy, rather than the relationship, work. I consider myself responsible for offering a format that allows people to express themselves in ways that can generate new possibilities and make shifts in new directions. Other than intervening in instances of physical, verbal, or sexual abuse and drug and alcohol abuse, I tend not to comment on a seemingly destructive course a couple may be riding. If they can live in or tolerate what could be perceived as a destructive course, than I will enter their world and search for meaning in such a way that I can be as free and imaginative on their behalf as possible. If I find that our talks become repetitive and restrictive in content and process, I may ask if we could have a consultation to broaden our conversation.

## ACKNOWLEDGMENTS

I wish to thank Michele Bograd for her helpful comments and suggestions. I also am grateful to "Sarah" and "Jack" for their permission in publishing our private conversation.

# REFERENCES

Andersen, T. (1987). The reflecting team: Dialogue and meta-dialogue in clinical work. *Family Process, 26*(4), 415–428.

Andersen, T. (1990). The reflecting team. In T. Andersen (Ed.), *The reflecting team: Dialogues and Dialogues about the dialogues* (pp. 18–107). Broadstairs, Kent, UK: Borgmann.

Andersen, T. (1992a). Relationship, language and pre-understanding in the reflecting processes. *Australian and New Zealand Journal of Family Therapy, 13*(2), 87–91.

Andersen, T. (1992b). Reflections on reflecting with families. In S. McNamee & K. J. Gergen (Eds.), *Therapy as social construction* (pp. 54–68). Newbury Park, CA: Sage.

Bader, E., & Pearson, P. T. (1988). *In quest of the mythical mate.* New York: Brunner/Mazel.

Baucom, D. H. (1987). Attributions in distressed relations: How can we explain them? In D. Perlman & S. Duck (Eds.), *Intimate relationships* (pp. 177–206). Newbury Park, CA: Sage.

Baynes, K. (1990). Rational reconstruction and social criticism: Habermas's model of interpretive social science. In M Kelley (Ed.), *Hermeneutics and critical theory in ethics and politics* (pp. 122–145). Cambridge, MA: MIT Press.

Cahn, D. D. (1990). Confrontation behaviors, perceived understanding, and relationship growth. In D. Cahn (Ed.), *Intimates in conflict: A communication perspective* (pp. 153–165). Hillsdale, NJ: Erlbaum.

Chasin, R., Grunebaum, H., & Herzig, M. (1990). *One couple: Four realities.* New York: Guilford Press.

Crosby, J. F. (Ed.). (1989). *When one wants out and the other doesn't.* New York: Brunner/Mazel.

Dicks, H. V. (1967). *Marital tensions.* New York: Basic Books.

Framo, J. (1982). *Explorations in marital and family therapy.* New York: Springer.

Gergen, K. J. (1985). Social constructionist inquiry: Context and implications. In K. J. Gergen & K. E. Davis (Eds.), *The social construction of the person* (pp. 3–18). New York: Springer Verlag.

Gergen, K. J. (1986). Correspondence versus autonomy in the language of understanding human action. In D. W. Fiske & R. A. Shweder (Eds.), *Metatheory in social science: Pluralisms and subjectivities* (pp. 136–162). Chicago: University of Chicago Press.

Guerin, P. J., Fay, L. F., Burden, S. L., & Gilbert Kautto, J. (1987). *The evaluation and treatment of marital conflict.* New York: Basic Books.

Guerney, B., Jr., Brock, G., & Coufal, J. (1986). Integrating marital therapy and enrichment: The relationship enhancement approach. In N. S. Jacobson & A. S. Gurman (Eds.), *Clinical handbook of marital therapy* (pp. 151–172). New York: Guilford Press.

Jacobson, N. S., & Holtzworth-Munroe, A. (1986). Marital therapy: A social-learning perspective. In N. S. Jacobson & A. S. Gurman (Eds.), *Clinical handbook of marital therapy* (pp. 29–70). New York: Guilford Press.

Jacobson, N. S., & Gurman, A. S. (Eds.). (1986). *Clinical handbook of marital therapy.* New York: Guilford Press.

Katriel, T. & Philipsen, G. (1981). What we need is communication: Communication as a cultural category in some American speech. *Communication Monographs, 48,* 301–317.

Kearney, R. (1989). Paul Ricoeur and the hermeneutic imagination. In T. P. Kemp & D. Rasmussen (Eds.), *The narrative path* (pp. 1–31). Cambridge, MA: MIT Press.

Napier, A. Y. (1988). *The fragile bond.* London: Methuen.

Paolino, T. J., & McCrady, B. S. (Eds.). (1978). *Marriage and marital therapy: Psychoanalytic, behavioral, and systems theory perspectives.* New York: Brunner/Mazel.

Paul, N. L. (1985). *A marital puzzle.* New York: Gardner Press.

Retzinger, S. M. (1991). *Violent emotions: Shame and rage in marital quarrels.* Newbury Park, CA: Sage.

Sager, C. (1976). *Marriage contracts and couples therapy.* New York: Brunner/Mazel.

Schaap, C., Buunk, B., & Kerkstra, A. (1988). Marital conflict resolution. In P. Noller & M. S. Fitzpatrick (Eds.), *Perspectives on marital interaction.* Clevedon & Philadelphia: Multilingual Matters LTD.

# IV

## THE POSTMODERN ERA
### A Universe of Stories

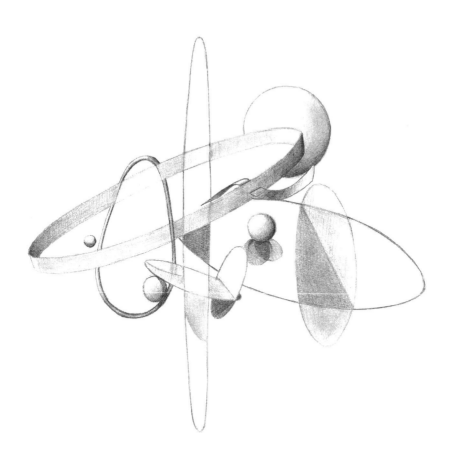

# 17

## Silenced Voices Heard: A Tale of Family Survival

### D. DONALD SAWATZKY
### THOMAS ALAN PARRY

*Every story one chooses to tell is a kind of censorship: it prevents the telling of other tales.*

—SALMAN RUSHDIE

The story that follows illustrates a central element in a narrative approach to therapy, even though it is not a therapy session. It is a dramatic account of a journey by the senior author (D. D. S.) to find the missing story of one-half of his family. His father had come to Canada from the Soviet Union in 1923 at the age of 21. Subsequent developments in that land, with the consolidation of Stalin's power, put him effectively out of touch with his family, except for occasional bits of news, for several decades. In May 1991 his son bridged that loss of contact by traveling to Novosibirsk, the capital of Siberia, to reconnect with his paternal family of origin. Once there, he heard their story and, in doing so, became part of it as they filled in the missing half of his family story.

This interview between the authors of this chapter, Don and Alan, illustrates the theme of the connection of stories, of people moving back and forth in and out of each other's stories, and the impact of this on both the individuals and the families concerned. Although not technically a therapeutic one, this interview was certainly a therapeutic experience and accurately followed the course and nature of narrative therapy, where the telling and reflecting upon the story is deemed sufficient for healing to occur.

## THE INTERVIEW

A: Don, as you know, I am interested in the consequences of people entering into each other's stories; in the impact of the discovery of parts of our own story that have been neglected, forgotten, or minimized; and in the part those hidden stories play in filling in the gaps to make possible a more complete life. When I first heard your story I was struck by Salman Rushdie's words in his novel *Shame:* "Every story is a kind of censorship: it prevents the telling of other tales." So when you talked of your odyssey across the already-crumbling Soviet Union to connect with your father's family, I was overwhelmed not only by the drama and power of the story but by what it must mean for your life and that of your family to find that there was another family story that you had had very little idea of. So let me hear the story again and what it might mean for you and for your newly discovered family.

D: I'll begin with your reference to Rushdie's statement about every story being a form of censorship. I grew up with my mother's extended family, with whom I was intensely involved. My maternal grandfather was a leader and I idolized this man. He had been for many years the primary spokesman for the Mennonite community in Canada. He negotiated with the Canadian government and Canadian Pacific to allow thousands of Mennonite people to enter and resettle in various parts of Canada. He also founded a school where teachers prepared themselves for work in Mennonite communities in Canada. He was very much a hero for me. The only family I really knew was my mother's family. My father had come over from Russia in 1923 by himself. He was 21 at the time and wanted to pursue an education in Canada; apparently, he thought that eventually his family would follow. For a variety of reasons this didn't happen, and he was here in Canada by himself while the rest of his family was, as I learned much later, going through trauma in their lives there. During my growing-up period, there was very little discussion about my father's family. For whatever reason, I didn't know how many siblings my father had or very much about my paternal grandparents. Nor did it occur to me to ask many questions. I think my father to some degree adopted my mother's family, and we simply didn't talk much about his family in Russia. When I had the opportunity a year ago to go to Finland to present a paper, I decided that this was a good time to extend my trip to include the Soviet Union and to "look up" my relatives in Siberia. I had no idea where they lived, although I did know that it was in the area around the city of Novosibirsk. Although I found the prospect of visiting this branch of my family to be exciting, I was also, before leaving, quite nervous about the prospect of spending several days with people who were, for the most part, strangers to me. I had no idea about their way of living, or how they would receive me. However, at the end of May 1991 I flew to what was then known as Leningrad and from there to Novosibirsk.

A: Do you have any idea, Don, what force moved you in that direction? Considering that there had been such a silence about your father's family, do you think there was anything that tugged at you about that silence? Did it play any part in the impetus to go there?

D: I think it did. For a number of years I have had a very strong curiosity about my family in Siberia. Given the silence I think I wondered whether there might be issues that couldn't be talked about for whatever reason. In my adult years I had spoken with my father on a number of occasions about possibly writing down some of his story or about talking about it on tape. He was always reluctant to do that. He told us a few stories about his childhood. I knew, for example, that he grew up in an agricultural community in southern Russia where there were many beautiful fruit trees. I knew that he swam in the Dnieper River and that his father, my grandfather, owned a flour mill upstream from the Mennonite community. However, I was acutely aware that I had very little information about his family. I also knew very little about my family's involvement in the chaotic events following the beginning of the Russian Revolution in 1917. I wondered, for example, to what extent long-established Mennonite principles of nonviolence might have been violated or at least compromised at a time when lives were threatened and property was lost. These kinds of thoughts crossed my mind periodically and certainly contributed to my curiosity.

A: Do you see any connection between his declared intention of bringing the rest of his family with him and the consequence of his not doing so?

D: Evidently, one of the reasons his family couldn't join him was because one of his sisters developed tuberculosis and so could not be admitted into Canada.

A: Things also became very spooky in the Soviet Union in those years, with the consolidation of power by Stalin, so I don't imagine it was the easiest place in the world to get out of, no matter what the intentions.

D: That is certainly true. During the Stalin era it was very difficult to leave the country. Earlier, when Dad left, leaving was much easier, even though the country was in a state of chaos. I'll make a few comments about the circumstances in Russia at the time of his leaving, which must have been almost unbearable. I've heard many stories about groups of bandits who stole goods and animals as well as raped women and threatened lives. One day at my grandfather's mill the employees were all bludgeoned to death. My uncle, who had been managing the mill at that time, had not gone to work that day and so his life was spared. There are stories of epidemics of typhoid fever, which affected most families in the Mennonite communities. What I was told by my relatives while I was in Russia was that my grandfather died in the same year my dad left, in 1923, and my grandmother died three years later, in 1926. My dad's younger brother died of "lung disease" in 1931, and his older brother died in an accident in 1939. In this same year his youngest sister died. So the years following my dad's leaving were difficult ones for his family. However, compared to the years that followed, they were tolerable. During World War II several factors resulted in extreme hardship for German-speaking Mennonites. Certainly, the fact that Russia was at war with Germany was an important factor. Also, Stalin's policy of "Russification" and its implementation caused extreme hardship for people in Russia whose ethnic origin was not Russian. My family, being Mennonite, was part of a German-speaking community that had functioned virtually as an independent society since the 1700s; they had their own schools, hospitals, and local governments. They had also, for several centuries, been exempted from participation in war. From 1941 until 1954 my father had no contact with his family. So, as you suggest in your question, the years following 1923 were difficult, and the likelihood of being able to emigrate diminished.

A: One of the things that I wonder about in family stories is the unspeakable. The unspeakable doesn't appear in the stories but is presented precisely in what is left unsaid. I am struck by your statement that it scarcely occurred to you to inquire about grandparents, aunts, uncles, cousins, and so forth. I was wondering if your father's family just wasn't a reality to you, given the power and presence of your mother's family, or whether there were unspoken messages not to ask.

D: I don't know. I don't know the answer to that question. It didn't occur to me to ask. There was some curiosity there but it was more like the kind of curiosity that you might have about your great-grandparents. You know, they were not in the picture, they were not physically present, and so it was as if they didn't exist.

A: By your father not volunteering information there wasn't a message of "Don't ask," just simply a further instance of their non-presence.

D: That's right. On the wall of our house when we were growing up there was a picture that my mother had had enlarged that Dad had taken with him of the flour mill. So we had some awareness of the fact that my grandfather had owned a flour mill. And there were some stories that were told to all of us children growing up and later to all the grandchildren. There was the story of Surqua (the word *surqua* means "vicious") my father's dog, a guard dog. As I remember the story, Dad was leaving his house never to return. As he closed the gates to the yard to leave for Canada, he could see a tear in Surqua's eye as if the dog were grieving that he would not see his master again. From my present vantage point as a psychologist it would appear that it was easier for my father to deal with his sadness by projecting it onto Surqua than by accepting it as his own.

A: The tear may have been in Surqua's eye, but there was also a tear in your father's eye that he was less comfortable with acknowledging.

D: Yes, and I think that this story, to some extent, says something about who he was and who he still is in terms of talking about his own feelings about the family he left in Russia.

A: When I try to understand my own parents and their generation—and I think that your father is of the same generation, almost the same age as my parents—it strikes me that the climate that must have almost pervaded the entire Western world, maybe especially Eastern Europe, was that this was a time of opportunity, of individuals and sometimes families pulling themselves away and going across an ocean to make it. Although leaving was a great act of will and heroism there seems to have been a remarkable absence of worry about the emigrants' inner selves. It's almost as if they were more than simply reticent; it's as if they just didn't think in those terms. They must have had inner strength but they were very outwardly directed and didn't think a whole lot about their inner lives.

D: I think that this is very true of my father and probably true more generally of his generation. There must have been incredible internal dissonance in leaving family as well as familiar surroundings for an uncertain future. Yet the anxiety and sadness were put aside and goals were pursued without a lot of focus on the emotions. I think that for my father there is a current dissonance when he compares his relatively prosperous life and the opportunities he has had with those of his siblings and their children. He has a strong need to believe that they are doing well; when he sees them "doing well," the dissonance—or perhaps guilt—is resolved somewhat.

A: It sounds more like existential guilt rather than a guilt of connectedness. These were people that he was connected with, and although the connection was severed physically and geographically, the sense of obligation and connection wasn't severed emotionally and spiritually.

D: That's true. My hypothesis would be that throughout his entire lifetime he has wondered about what was happening back there and has, whenever possible, made an effort to send them whatever might be most helpful. Certainly, a strong connection was there even though the physical tie had been broken. The connection may have been at least partly maintained by obligation, but I think it extends well beyond that.

A: Do you believe that your going there means that that sense of obligation was transmitted to you?

D: To some extent I see my trip as the completion of the trip my father began in 1986. At that time he intended to travel to Novosibirsk along with my two sisters and my brother-in-law to see his one remaining sister, Maria, to meet the children and grand children of his other sisters and of his brother, and to see where they were living. When they got to

Moscow, it was not possible, for a variety of reasons, for them to travel to Siberia. The doors were closed to him. As a result, my father sent a telegram to his sister, inviting her to come to Moscow. When she arrived, with her daughter, there was an incredible reunion between a brother and sister who had not seen each other in 63 years. Evidently, for 2 days many stories were shared, as well as laughter and tears. My father was disappointed, however, about not seeing his many nephews, nieces, and their children. Also, he very much wanted to see where they lived and how they lived. This is where I came in. One aspect of my motivation to go was to become his eyes and ears. He was very interested in my trip, and even though he is almost 90 he was at the airport to greet me when I got back from the Soviet Union and was very eager to have whatever information he could about his family in Siberia. Although I went largely on my own behalf, I also went on his behalf and, more generally, on behalf of my siblings.

A: To back up a moment, you mentioned that between 1942 and 1954 there was no contact with the family in Siberia. Do you have any recollections of what the fate of your father's family was thought to be? Was there an assumption that they were surviving, or were they thought not to have survived the war?

D: Well, the information was available that they had been moved to Siberia and that a lot of the males had been conscripted. However, to my knowledge, neither my father nor anybody else in my broader extended family had any information about where in Siberia the family was or what the conditions were like. That information was just not known to them at all.

A: The recontact in 1954 would have been the time of the post-Stalin thaw.

D: I think Khruschev was responsible for changing some of the policies at that time. And certainly at that time the Red Cross was able to locate a lot of families on behalf of Canadian citizens, which is how my father regained contact. He became aware that two sisters and a sister-in-law were living in Siberia and a third was living in Kazakhstan.

A: It wasn't just that a letter arrived one day.

D: No, and I don't know how the information was conveyed. I remember that after we received the information there was a discussion in my home about what these relatives might need the most. For example, apparently they did not have glass for their windows. Consequently, a clear plastic material was sent over there to cover the windows so that there would be light and the mosquitos wouldn't get in. Again, I don't recall any discussions about particular individuals.

A: Can we now pick up the start of your trip to Leningrad and from there to Siberia?

D: My flight into Leningrad was my introduction to the Soviet Union. I found this first contact to be depressing. Although on the surface the city had beautiful buildings, I found the living conditions to be almost squalid in some cases. The food seemed inedible. Everything, from the burned-out light bulbs in my hotel room to the cars parked in the middle of the street, seemed broken or not cared for. The Russian people seemed depressed and aimless. The question that kept recurring for me was, "What am I doing here?" This was particularly true on the day I was to fly to Novosibirsk. I arrived at the airport early and then waited and waited. When I asked for information about when the plane would be leaving, I was just told to sit down. Finally, I was instructed to go down to a large waiting area in the lower level of the very run-down terminal building. Here I noticed people watching a TV screen; after talking with somebody who spoke English, I became aware that there had just been a plane crash on the runway of the Leningrad Airport and that eleven people had been killed. What we were seeing on the TV screen was people cleaning up the debris.

A: You learned that while you were waiting?

D: Yes, I learned that while I was waiting for my flight out. I had a lot of questions. I had experienced cars parked on the road without wheels, and I kept debating in my own mind whether the Russians had actually put a man on the moon or not. I wondered whether I should be taking this flight—it was four time zones from Leningrad to Novosibirsk. So this entry into the Soviet Union was initially quite distressing for me, and I certainly questioned whether I really wanted to follow through.

A: Was it scary? Did you experience fear, or was it more just perplexing, like "Why am I doing this?"

D: I experienced some fear. I found myself clutching my passport and repeatedly checking to make sure that my tickets were still in my pocket. I was aware of being very alone in a context that was almost overwhelming. People were speaking a language that I couldn't understand. Since I don't understand any Russian, I wondered how I would be able to make any contact with my relatives. Since I was the only tourist getting on this plane to Novosibirsk, I initially boarded the plane by myself. So I had a very strong feeling of being alone, of being in a place that seemed dangerous. I also thought of my wife and children at home and realized that I needed to notify them as soon as I got to Novosibirsk that I was all right. I knew the information about the plane crash would get back to Edmonton.

A: Are you normally comfortable with air travel? When you heard of the plane crashing, did you think, "I hope this plane makes it"?

D: I'm normally comfortable with air travel, and I do a fair amount of it. I had heard previously that Russian pilots have a very good reputation for their ability to fly a plane well. But I had not anticipated what I eventually found when I walked onto this plane: The plane was physically run-down; it was very dirty and many of the seats were broken. So

I was relieved when we landed in Novosibirsk and the Intourist person came on board to escort me out.

A: How long did the flight take?

D: It must have been about a 6- or 7-hour flight. We were supposed to arrive there at five in the morning but actually arrived in early afternoon.

A: Did you sleep on the flight?

D: No, I didn't sleep on that flight at all. It was noisy. The person next to me kept offering me vodka from the bottle he had in his pocket. I assume that others on the plane must also have had their own private supplies of vodka. What was refreshing for me when I arrived in Novosibirsk was a smiling in-service person who informed me that people were waiting for me. She led me down through the baggage compartment, where I picked up my own luggage. As I walked down the ramp I saw three people standing on the tarmac. They introduced themselves with an old family picture that included me with my siblings. Evidently, they had waited at the airport for almost 12 hours. The plane had been late and there had been some question as to when I would arrive and on which plane, so they had waited there for a long time. But they were there and they seemed really pleased to see me and I was pleased to see them. I had a reservation at the Hotel Siberia in Novosibirsk for the four nights I was going to be there. I mentioned this to my cousin, Lena, who said, in German, "While you're here you're with us and we would like you to cancel the reservation at the hotel." She also said, "And why are you staying for such a short time?" My immediate decision was to cancel the hotel reservation and arrange to extend my stay by a day. Lena signed the document that said that they would now have full responsibility for me while I was in Novosibirsk. So I rode with them in the little Lada that was owned by one of my cousin's sons, named Victor. He drove me to the apartment in which he lives with his wife and two small children. The apartment was, of course, like all the others. It was run-down on the outside and the elevator was tiny and cramped. However, when I arrived in the apartment I felt welcome and comfortable. For the first time since arriving in the Soviet Union I felt at home. It felt clean, it felt loving, I felt cared about, and they offered their bed for me to sleep in for a few hours before we were to take the big trip from Novosibirsk to Lukovka, which is where the majority of my family members now live. So that was my introduction to Novosibirsk, and I felt a warmth that I hadn't experienced since leaving Canada.

A: So they weren't inhibited.

D: Not at all. I was welcomed into their home and welcomed into what is now their part of Russia. They were very clear about that, that I was welcome. They made a lot of physical contact with me and clearly saw me as family.

A: I've heard you mention that you felt that right from the start you were welcomed as family and that that sense of family wasn't so instantly present in you.

D: I think that's absolutely true. I had made a reservation in a hotel, thinking that I would visit them periodically and always return to the hotel. They had quite a different conception of where I would spend my time: There was absolutely no question that I would be immersed with them and that I would not be staying at a hotel while I was in that part of Russia. I accepted that.

A: So they viewed it as more than a social visit?

D: I think I thought of it as a social visit. I thought I might attend the occasional family reunion but I would have my own base from which I would come and go. They certainly didn't think that way at all. There was a big car there waiting to take me to the hotel. They sent that car away. I was going with them in their Lada. I think I was viewed as being part of the family and they wanted me to feel that.

A: It's been a cliché over the years that the West represented the extreme of individualism and the Soviet Union represented the extreme of collectivism, and I wonder if it's reading too much into it to see their instantaneous sense of family and community as being present against your sense of being a more autonomous individual who had intended to look after himself and not impose and live in a hotel.

D: That may be true, that there were cultural differences between us. It may also have been a function of the way the family organized themselves. When I say "the family," I'm thinking of my father's siblings. You see, what I realized when I arrived in Lukovka, which is where most of them now live, is that the boundaries between families are almost nonexistent. They walked into each other's homes and they often ate together, so that may have been a factor too in how they incorporated me into . . .

A: So for them it was already an extended family in which you were just one more long-lost extension. A far cry from our emphasis on the nuclear family, where aunts, uncles, and cousins are family but there are some boundaries.

D: That's right and I think that with this kind of organization that as long as you remain within the family, you're accepted and treated well. If you try to move outside of those boundaries, sometimes it's hard to move back in. What I discovered is that one cousin who lives in Novosibirsk seemed to have alienated herself from the rest of the family, and the whole family was aware of that and, I think, set some boundaries that excluded her, which made it very difficult for her. For those within the boundaries, however, there seemed to be a lot of caring and good feeling.

A: We often romanticize the extended family and think of it as a good that we have lost, but there are some aspects of the traditional family that are quite binding and could even be suffocating where a spirit of individual venturing forth is concerned.

D: I think so and I think that if you venture forth too far the result is a kind of shunning process, which makes it very difficult for the person on the outside. Certainly, this one cousin was not told of my visit, and it was only when I kept asking about her that we eventually went to her home in Novosibirsk. Part of the anger that was directed at her had to do with the fact that her mother, my aunt, died a number of years ago and since her mother's death she had not visited the community a lot.

A: At what point did they begin to tell you their stories?

D: Almost immediately. On the trip from Novosibirsk to Lukovka by car I really learned to communicate with them. Victor, the son of a cousin, was driving the car and Lena, my oldest cousin, who still knew German, was in the car with us, so I communicated a lot with Victor through Lena. Victor would speak in Russian, and Lena would translate to German. By the time we arrived in Lukovka, an 80-kilometer trip, we were managing the communication process quite well. I was first driven to where my Tante Maria lives with her daughter and son-in-law. She came right to me, kissed me on the mouth, and seemed very pleased to see me. As I was introduced to the people who kept arriving at the house, I began, the very first evening, to draw a genogram for myself, to get it clear who belonged where—who was my cousin, who was my cousin's spouse, and that kind of thing. So as I was drawing this genogram, they would tell me about the people whose names I was writing down. They told me about births, deaths, marriages, etc. From the very beginning I was learning things that I had not heard before. I first heard the story about their trip over from Southern Russia to Novosibirsk from Tante Maria on the second day I was there.

A: What did your aunt tell you?

D: By way of background, I had before leaving for Russia a number of the questions that I wanted to ask, translated into the Russian language. I presented these to Tante Maria in the written format, and she answered them in German. I wanted to know, from her perspective, why my father had left and what that had been like for them. What she said to me was that he had always been more interested in going to school and had been away from home attending school for several years prior to leaving for Canada. So they had not had a lot of contact with him just prior to him leaving. She said that it was clear that the older brother was going to take over the business and that my father wanted something different for himself. So when a couple of his cousins were going to Canada, he approached the family about him joining them. It was when I asked her about what life was like for her after 1923 that she eventually began to tell the story about how they got from southern Russia to Siberia in 1942. That story had a strong impact on me, particularly when I think of it in terms of my own flesh and blood. Evidently, what happened was that military people came into the community and announced that families would have a few hours to gather up whatever small items they wanted to take with them as they were being moved out of the community. The adult men were first taken and told that they would be conscripted or sent to work in mines. Meanwhile, the women and children were loaded onto train cars.

A: Did they have any warning that something like this was likely to happen?

D: They had very little warning, apparently, that anything like this was going to happen, and their assumption was that wherever they were going it was going to be short-term and that they would eventually return. They were loaded onto flatcars that didn't even have sides on them. Tante Maria at that time had four small children, who ranged in age from two to ten. Since the flatcar was crowded, she and the other women sat on the outside so that the children wouldn't fall off.

A: So they were treated not only as the enemy but as not much more than cattle.

D: That's how Tante Maria described it. She said that they were treated worse than animals. She was on the same flatcar as her two sisters (my two other aunts) and a sister-in-law, the wife of my oldest uncle. Among them these women had a total of 12 children, and what she described to me was a frightening journey. Periodically, the train would stop and everybody would get off to relieve themselves, and several times children were left behind. The mothers would scream, but nobody would respond to those screams. She said that from her perspective it was a miracle that all the members of her family arrived safely at their eventual destination.

A: It must have been thousands of miles.

D: It was a very long distance and the trip took several weeks. When they got to the train station—that is, where Novosibirsk is now—they were unloaded and taken in groups to different places in the surrounding area. My family were taken to a place near a community that became known as Lukovka. This was in October of 1942. They had no shelter and it was starting to get frosty. The group Tante Maria was part of consisted of herself, her two sisters, and their children, eight in all. What they did to survive was to dig a hole in the ground and cover it with birch branches, which were then covered with dirt. They survived the winter in that 10-foot square hole only because the Russian peasants who lived nearby took them in when it was bitterly cold. Shortly after they were "settled" here, military authorities arrived and forced two of my aunts, including Tante Maria, to walk to Novosibirsk, where they were put to work in a munitions factory for 3 years. The third aunt, who was lame, was left to look after the 8 children.

A: How old were the children?

D: The eight children, all girls, ranged in age from two to eleven. The older children were put to work with the cattle on the collective farms that were being established. The older children had been to school in southern Russia and never again returned to school. When I reflect on the situation of these young girls, I wonder what it was like for them to be taken to the fields to look after the cattle. I found myself observing four of the women who had spent a large part of their childhood in this way. Several of them often looked depressed, as though they had deep emotional scars.

A: One can only speculate on the likelihood of sexual abuse.

D: That's what I speculated about too, that there probably was sexual abuse. If there was, I don't expect this is something they have ever talked about.

A: I guess in the context of struggling for survival, sexual abuse wouldn't even rank near the top of their horrors.

D: Not only that, but I expect that issues related to sexuality generally would not have been openly discussed in this community at that time. If there was abuse, children would have had to deal with it on their own. I can only speculate about how grim the struggle must have been, not only physically but emotionally as well. For 3 years, six of the children had no contact with their mothers. Sometime within this 3-year period the father of three of the children, my uncle, found his way back to his family. Evidently, he was allowed to leave the mine he was working in because he was sick. He died about a year later of "lung disease."

A: This was an uncle from . . .

D: This was one of the men that had been forced to work in a mine. Two of the husbands of my three aunts eventually found their families. The third didn't find his wife and child and eventually married someone else in a distant Soviet republic. He did eventually rediscover his daughter when she was 15, and he is currently living in Germany. It was the husband of the aunt who looked after all the children who did not return to his family.

A: They remained living in the hole in the ground?

D: They remained living in this hole in the ground for 7 years, although there were times when they were given some temporary homes elsewhere, particularly in the wintertime. But that was still their base. Evidently, they hoped and believed that they would eventually return to their original homes. Consequently, they didn't really try to reestablish themselves. Eventually they moved into a house. They showed me the house they moved into: a tiny wooden structure that is now abandoned.

A: It must have seemed like a palace at that time. You mentioned that on the day you started to hear this story you were taken to the meadow where the hole in the ground had been. First of all I'd like to ask what were your reactions as this story was revealed to you?

D: As the story was unfolding, I had difficulty comprehending much of what I was hearing. I was struck by how people seem to adapt to conditions that, to me, seem unbearable. I focused a lot on Tante Maria, with her leathery, lined face. Although lines are etched on her face, her body is straight and her blue eyes sparkle. She was able to somehow transcend all the trauma and, at 86 years of age, has remained optimistic and has a strong presence. She seems to have not lost her spirit. On the other hand, her daughters, my contemporaries, appear to have been deeply scarred. One of them appears to be depressed and suffers from chronic headaches. Another has swollen arthritic hands. A third appears to have Parkinson's disease. What these women have not lost is their capacity to care for each other and for their children and grandchildren. So when the story was told, I found myself focusing differently on these members of my family. I felt sadness as well as admiration.

A: As you tell me the story I find myself trying to imagine people going through those circumstances, surviving, and even prevailing. I find it stunning and I'm wondering how knowing that these are members of your own family, the family that had been such a source of mystery for such a long time, affected you.

D: I think that's a really important question. Even when I watch really traumatic events being portrayed on a television news program, I can often remain quite detached. While listening to what was happening to my own extended family, I experienced a range of emotions from anger to sadness. I found myself thinking about the tragedy as well as about the resilience of the human spirit. The tragedy took a toll physically and emotionally as well as materially. From my Western perspective and the value I put on education, those who were my contemporaries seemed like a lost generation. They have not been to school and have learned to read and write from their own children, who have had the opportunity to go to school. I also thought about my place and that of my siblings in this extended family. My father was one of six children. One died early but the other five all had families. Of those families, my siblings and I are the only ones who have not had the Siberia experience. I thought about the probability that it could have been I who went through all of this. I reflected about how different my experience has been from theirs. Even though there is a physical resemblance, our lives have been dramatically different. I reflected often on the ways in which life is a series of accidents.

A: Thomas Pynchon, in his novel *Gravity's Rainbow*, plays with the old Calvinist distinction between the Elect and what they called the Preterites, the passed-over ones. He takes this Calvinist notion and suggests that in a profound way the Preterites are especially blessed because

without the ones that are passed over there would have been no Elect.
So the Elect somehow can't look down with disdain at the Preterites but
need to be grateful for the mystery that has allowed them the lives they
had, compared to the passed-over ones. Pynchon suggests that in these
postmodern times the passed-over ones, the neglected, the wretched
really offer us something of tremendous value, and it sounds like you
received something of a gift from these people.

D: Certainly, as a result of my contact with these people I have had a more
profound appreciation of my own opportunities. However, they're not
a wretched people, and that's the part that I found uplifting. I think I
experienced some of what is also presented in a different context in the
*City of Joy*. In spite of the hardship, in spite of the struggles, what they
had there was a sense of community that I had seldom encountered
before. They laughed a lot, sang a lot, and seemed to deeply appreciate
each other. They took time to tell stories of times that they had all
experienced, and they all had a different version. So when you suggest
that there might have been a gift, the gift to me was in this context. I
didn't experience them to be generally unhappy in spite of their difficult
circumstances. There was a lot of joy and optimism, and that certainly
made its mark on me.

A: You had mentioned that one of your cousins had said, "We laugh a lot,
and we have enough to eat."

D: Yes, and they do. I experienced that with them. They obviously have a
lot more time than we do. The lunch meal would begin at noon and
finish at three, and when conversation would run out they would all
sing together. There was a lot of laughter at mealtimes, and I experienced in a profound way a real sense of community.

A: You had mentioned that when you did go with them to the meadow,
their actions there were somewhat surprising to you.

D: That trip to the meadow was probably the highlight of my time there.
We all got into an early 1940s military jeep. It was the only vehicle
owned by a member of my generation. Seven of us crowded into this
little old jeep. What I was told was that they wanted to show me the
flowers in the meadow. Most of the homes I had been in had bouquets
of flowers that had been picked in the meadow. They wanted to show
me where they got these flowers, and so we drove out over the bumpy
fields to this meadow. When we got to the general area, they seemed to
know where all the different varieties of flowers were located. There
were, for example, orange flowers that looked like fireweeds and in
another place there were small purple flowers that looked like miniature
irises. They knew where to look for the different varieties and seemed
happy in the meadow. I was reminded of Victor Frankl's story about his
prison camp experience, when he talked about the flower that kept him
focused on life's meaning beyond the prison walls. I would speculate

that something similar occurred for my family. It was in this meadow where they lived in a hole in the ground for all those years. I suppose it is possible that they found beauty, life, and meaning in the flowers at a time when these were hard to find elsewhere. While on that trip in the meadow they also showed me, as you were suggesting, Alan, the indentation in the ground that had been their home for the 7 years. I have pictures of three of my cousins sitting there on the edge of this hole, which is now overgrown with grass. The thought of all of those people huddled into such a small space made a strong impression on me. I couldn't imagine living in those small quarters and I suppose they kept themselves alive and warm with the contact of each other's bodies.

A: Did they tell you stories of what it was like living in the hole in the ground in the middle of Siberia?

D: What I regretted the whole time I was there was that we couldn't communicate directly. If there had been someone who could have translated from Russian to English, I would have managed much better. The information I got was in broad strokes, and I missed a lot of detail. They had the same regret I did about this. They did tell me that they didn't have many clothes or shoes to wear and that in the winter they would often look for warm cow dung to stand in so that their feet would stay warm. One cousin said to me that sometimes things got so bad that they almost lost the ability to love. When she said that to me she had tears in her eyes, and I really felt some of her own emotion. I also had a sense of how desperate life must have felt at times.

A: Just grim survival.

D: That's right.

A: It sounds like it was just each for oneself.

D: I think so. When people are functioning at that level of just keeping themselves alive, the primary consideration is often to fend for oneself. I would expect that this was what they were experiencing in themselves.

A: Where would Siberia be in latitude, compared with Calgary or Edmonton?

D: Where these people live is roughly the same latitude as Edmonton, although the terrain there looks more like the terrain north of Edmonton. The growth is sparser, and the trees are smaller than they are between Calgary and Edmonton. There's a lot of what looks like scrub growth. They've planted a lot of poplar wind rows because there is a lot of wind. At the time that I was there, in early June, they still had their tomato plants under glass because they would freeze if they left them out in the open.

A: After you had been acquainted with this story of unbelievable survival against terrible odds, what were those remaining days and nights like visiting with them? How did your understanding of them influence your feelings about them?

D: Much of the time was spent around meal tables. We would move from one home to another. The noon meal was barely over and we would be moving to another home for the supper meal. It wasn't that we ate a lot, it was just that that's where the conversation took place, and the people just seemed to move from home to home. I did spend some time with them in just looking over the community. The community of Lukovka is on flat and barren ground with very few trees. There is a school but no churches. Marriages and burials take place in a community hall. Near the village are two collective farming operations, one dairy and the other an agricultural grain collective. I became aware that the son of one of my cousins was an engineer and was now heading up the agricultural collective. He seemed cautious about wanting to have a lot of contact with me, and my assumption was that this kind of job was very political. My relatives asked me a lot about my life in Canada: They wanted to know about my children; they wanted to know what I did in my spare time and what I did at work. One of the questions they were a little embarrassed about, but also asked me, was about my salary. When I was pressed on this issue I told them what my salary was, and they seemed awed by the amount. It was completely incomprehensible for them.

A: Two remarkable stories were being told from each one's perspective. You were stunned and moved by their story, but to them your story must have been almost equally unbelievable.

D: I think that's true. They wondered why I hadn't brought a picture with me of the house that I live in and of the cars that I drive. They were curious about all of this. They were amazed that I might have two cars and that several of my children have their own cars. They couldn't believe this since they share one old jeep within this whole extended family. Some of the younger generation have vehicles, the son of a cousin, for example. But from within the ranks of my contemporaries they really had only the one vehicle. Often they seemed startled with my answers and I was embarrassed. I would have preferred to not touch on these subjects!

A: Did you get any impression that there was envy? I'm sure there must have been envy in some sense, but did you get the impression of any resentment of your greater good fortune?

D: I don't think so. They seemed startled but I don't think they responded to me any differently after having this information.

A: I'd like to return with you to the image of the hole in the ground. We talk in these times about a reconnection with earth, and here's the example of people who rose up out of the earth.

D: That's an interesting observation. They very literally lived in the earth, and the beauty that they experienced in the flowers was a natural product of the earth.

A: So once again this theme of just living.

D: It was interesting to me that Victor, my cousin's son said, with a lot of pride, as he drove me to the town of Lukovka, "This is my Lukovka." It was windy that day and it was dusty. From my perspective the town looked primitive, desolate, and barren. However, he was proud of it and liked to be there, and it was in this town where they had, as you put it, risen from the earth. The younger generation had the opportunity to be educated and to work at jobs that require training and expertise. They again have more of the kinds of opportunities that my father's generation had in his community on the Dnieper River. In the process of growing out of the earth, they also seem to have crystallized a set of values related to the importance of caring for each other. I don't want to idealize what they have, but my impression was that they are much more focused on attending to basic human values than we are. These values have to do with kindness, generosity, and consideration for the needs of those close to them.

A: You are sharing this story with other Westerners who live in affluence, where so much is made convenient for us that it is easy to surrender to a passivity about life, of expecting and it shall happen, of flicking switches and making things happen. From this story of being put down and rising up at the most elementary level we see what determination can accomplish; your family could not have survived and prevailed had they not drawn on resources of determination and a decision to live.

D: The tremendous determination is still there in my aunt. Some of my contemporaries there are passive observers in a somewhat different way than we are with our Western technology. For example, there is, among some of my family members there, a tendency to consume too much vodka, which may be another way of avoiding a difficult reality. In general, however, they are still an earthy group of people in their humor and their lifestyle.

A: Do you recall what your feelings were as you flew back across the steppes of Asia?

D: To start at a slightly different point, I had a lot of feelings as I walked up the ramp to board the plane in Novosibirsk. I looked across the field, and all of the relatives I had met were waving from behind a fence. Even those from Lukovka had come to see me off at the airport. They did seem like family to me, even though they were very different from me. That's the part that is puzzling when I think about it. They would not be the kinds of people that I would typically seek out as friends. We have dramatically different lifestyles. What we had in common were grandparents, of whom very little was spoken. As I flew across Russia toward Moscow I thought a lot about what it means to be family and why it was that I felt this bondedness with a group of people whom normally I would have very little in common with, if not for our genetic connection and a common history.

A: It wasn't only that you entered into their story and they into yours, but the implication was that those two stories, as disparate as they were, were already connected even though no one knew about them. What you did was give voice to that silent connection.

D: I suppose the connection of the two stories was made tangible through my being there. I was in a position to hear their story and to tell some of my story.

A: And of your family story, which essentially involved half a family, a mystery, with only glimpses of the other half. You knew it was there and suddenly it was your story as well.

D: That's right. I was able to make a better connection with a part of my roots that I had little knowledge about. This connection does represent a kind of completion for me. I have a better understanding of a significant part of my personal history. I imagine that for them this might have occurred as well. They were curious about this uncle who had left, who had gone to a new world, and I think they wondered what his family might be like.

A: I would imagine so. They have long since left behind the Stalinist story that life was miserable and squalid in the capitalist world and that they lived in a worker's paradise. They have long since begun to discover that life was pretty good in the capitalist world.

D: I think they have a pretty realistic conception of life in North America. I suppose that is one of the benefits of television and radio, to which they all seemed to have access. Since I returned from the former Soviet Union, Victor, the cousin's son who drove me out to Lukovka has been writing to me and I've been writing back to him. His assessment of the situation over there is interesting to me. He suggests that in Russia at this time there is a need to address cultural and spiritual issues as well as material issues. I was aware that within my family considerable thought was being given to what was really important in life. They seemed to consider these issues even though their involvement with structured religion, for example, is virtually nonexistent at this time.

A: They were Mennonites who had paid a terrible price for being Mennonites. And even though they hadn't had the explicit structures of the church community to keep that alive, that was part of their story.

D: Yes, that was part of their story and I'm sure that the influence of those Mennonite values is still there. My father's generation ensured that the values were passed down. Currently, my one remaining aunt, Tante Maria, has been important in establishing the story connections with where they have come from. What she said to me one morning was significant in this context. She said that her children hadn't had the opportunity to go to school and to take music lessons but her grandchildren now have that opportunity. I think a lot of what was possible and a lot of the values that she had grown up with were communicated not only to her children but also to her grandchildren. And so there is now another generation, the individuals that are my children's contemporaries, who seem to be reflecting on issues that I don't think a lot of the Russian people are reflecting on—issues that have to do with culture and spirituality and values more general than material values. I think my aunt's impact is being strongly experienced by that generation.

A: She would be the matriarch of the family in a sense.

D: She appears to be. She's hard-of-hearing and her face is like leather. She's lived outdoors most of her life and yet she's straight and strong and she goes to the *banya* most evenings. The *banya,* incidentally, is the bathhouse in the backyard of most of the little houses in the villages. It's like a Finnish sauna where you perspire and use birch branches to sprinkle yourself with cold water. My aunt appears to be a physically strong and mentally determined woman. Although she's almost 90, she still has a strong presence and is very much the pillar of that extended family. She's a remarkable woman.

A: In a powerful sense the missing story of your family of origin has been filled in and it has a different quality. The story that you drew sustenance and identity and direction from in your life in many ways, namely, the story of your heroic maternal grandfather, was heroic in one particular way—here was someone who made things happen, a patriarch in the positive sense—and then you become acquainted with the fact that on the other side of the family you are also connected to, and are now a part of, a story of a different kind of heroism.

D: Your summation has some powerful implications for me, Alan. Certainly, my maternal grandfather's legacy to me was that of a man who derived a lot of his satisfaction through providing leadership and accomplishing important goals. He was a patriarch in the extended community as well as within his family. I have, at times, experienced the oppressiveness of some of the expectations I have set for myself related to my identification with my maternal grandfather. I have often experienced myself as falling short of an expectation without being able to specify what that expectation was. Opening up this new root and gaining some sustenance from that part of my family has been, to some extent, freeing for me. It's hard to be really explicit about that but I think that there are some values that relate to community, laughter, and family that provide an important balance to those represented by my grandfather.

A: It is as if your grandfather's model and example was of striving, of going forward, achieving heroism and your other family provides a sense of survival and the heroism of simply being, of surviving at the most basic level, of the joy of living.

D: Yes, very much so, and that certainly has struck me from my vantage point as a therapist. I'm awed by the resources that people can muster up to respond to incredibly difficult circumstances. Within my family in Siberia I admired the heroism that was there in how they maintained a sense of self and direction in incredibly difficult circumstances. Throughout her ordeal my aunt seemed to provide her family with a model of nurturance and determination. She clearly did not give up her identity in spite of the cruel pressure to do so. For whatever reasons, the family continued to be highly connected throughout their ordeals.

A: It sounds as though it was their connectedness as family that was the key to their survival.

D: I believe so.

A: They were abandoned by the larger community, treated with horrifying cruelty and exploited by them, yet they bonded all the more strongly with each other.

D: I think that their focus on strong family bonds had a lot to to with their very receptive response to me. I was family and therefore I was part of them.

A: It seems that it was more than simply that they come from a more traditional and adamantly collective society, and therefore would have more of a family sense, but more that family is of the greatest value because of their own experience.

D: I think it goes well beyond the collectivist notion, where the bondedness is within the community rather than within the genetic families. The bondedness for them has certainly moved toward enmeshment in the way that Minuchin, for example, might view it. They drew me into those boundaries and I was very much a part of that unit while I was there. I also recognize that had I, for some reason, stayed there, this would have been quite uncomfortable for me.

A: I suppose that the changes that this experience and this connection will be making in you will continue and that it may be some time before they fully make themselves tangibly present, but can you talk at all, one year later, of how not only the experience but the sense of connection has affected you or changed you?

D: I think there are two issues there. One has to do with how it's affected me and the other is how it has changed me. I think that there is certainly a part of me that is now affected by those family members who want to become self-sufficient within a restructured Soviet Union. So I am strongly motivated to see what I can do to help them, financially, for example. There has been that effect on me. I can only speculate about ways in which I have changed. I think I'm becoming less focused on achieving career goals and probably more focused on what it is that I personally want to achieve. This may be as much a function of where I am developmentally as it is a function of my trip. Certainly, my aunt's quiet but profound model of heroism in some ways counterbalances the active public hero my maternal grandfather became for me. I think some of the oppressive expectations I have at times set for myself related to public performance may have lessened somewhat. As a therapist, counselor, and educator I have always focused on drawing out the resources that people bring to their experience rather than imposing solutions. During this past year, however, I have been even more focused on the incredible resources that people have to deal with difficult circumstances.

A: I could imagine that in your work, as people tell you their stories of being stuck and feeling helpless and powerless, you, connected as you now know you are to people who found resources where there didn't seem to be any, might be not only more encouraging to them but more persevering. You wouldn't easily be put off or set aside by protests of "We can't, we can't; how can we get out of here?" because you've been acquainted with and have been made part of a story of people who did persevere and prevail.

D: That's very true. Another level at which I work is with master's and doctoral students on both research projects and in clinical practice. Recently, my colleagues and I have submitted a paper for publication in which we looked at students learning from the perspective of facilitating a process of empowerment. Again, the focus is on utilizing and developing resources that students bring in. I think that my commitment to that approach has been strengthened.

A: You entered into and became part of your family's story, and they entered into your story. How do you think that you have impacted them?

D: Recently, I received a letter from one of my relatives there, and he indicated that two of my cousins have bought some land and are going to become farmers. A third relative is considering building a parking garage. Obviously, these decisions are a function of the changed political situation there. I also wondered, however, to what extent my having been there from a capitalist country might have influenced their dreams for themselves. The small amount of American money that I left there on behalf of my father may also have been a factor in that it now converts to a lot of buying power in rubles. I think that they may have been aware that there was some of what I had experienced that they wanted, and this related to achieving some material goals.

A: It sounds as though there is some movement on the part of those people to become landowners.

D: That's true. Another area where there has been an impact is that the grandchildren of several of my cousins are now learning English in school and they are highly motivated to learn English. They talk, in their letters to me, about watching television and being particularly interested in the figure skaters and the hockey team from Edmonton. So they've made a connection with where I live and that has, to some extent, broadened their perspective on who they are. They're not only these people living in Siberia but there is also a part of them living in a very different world.

A: It seems that the breaking down of the Iron Curtain and finding people of your own family who had experiences that you can only imagine enabled you and your family in Siberia to find new strength and inspiration and a further direction from each other.

D: The notion of the Iron Curtain really became a reality for me from the time I entered Leningrad. I felt as if I was entering a different world. My initial response was to dislike, feel repulsed by, and reject much of what I saw. It was an enlightening and moving experience for me to find within my own extended family there, many qualities that I highly valued.

A: Here is a story that up until a year ago hadn't been shared, and we see the power of joining that simply the sharing of the story can accomplish. They have shared their story with you, and in that sharing it has become part of your story and now part of your heritage, as yours seems to be in the process of becoming for them. So that what began as a silent story of a silenced family—a cruelly silenced family—a censored story, has through the power of sharing begun to weave its belated effect.

D: That's true. My view of my heritage has been enriched through my having been there. The fact that I viewed myself as connected with them by a genetic bond allowed me to join with their story. Even though I didn't know them previous to my spending time there I made a connection with them as part of my family. They look like me and I knew we had the same grandparents. So when they told their story, I accepted it as part of my story as well.

A: They ceased to be the mysterious other and became part of a "we," with "our" story.

D: Similarly, from their perspective I think that my siblings and I, as well as our children, have taken on a different kind of role for them. I think they now view us differently. They know more about who we are. They know we can laugh with them and cry with them. We are more than people out there; we are individuals who have a name and a face and with whom they have made a tangible connection.

A: So you have gained a new perspective and they have as well. One of the perspectives you gained was an appreciation for how they have managed to rise up after having been so cruelly beaten down.

D: That's true. I have a lot of respect for the way they were able to retain a sense of who they were throughout periods of incredible hardship. They managed to find meaning even when life looked black. It is my impression that they were able to find this meaning in what we would consider to be small things. One example was the colorful flowers in the meadow. Just as Victor Frankl maintained a sense of vitality in the prison camp, my family, I think, crystallized a set of values when things looked darkest. Even though they are now somewhat more secure economically, they continue to find meaning in nature and in relationships. They have certainly risen up from their home in the ground but have retained an earthy sense of humor and have cultivated very basic human values.

# 18

## Without a Net: Preparations for Postmodern Living

### THOMAS ALAN PARRY

*God save us from Single Vision and Newton's sleep.*
—WILLIAM BLAKE

*Each clue that comes is supposed to have its own clarity, its fine chances for permanence. But then she wondered if the gemlike "clues" were only some kind of compensation. To make up for her having lost the direct Word, the cry that might abolish the night.*
—THOMAS PYNCHON

The great accomplishment of modernity, the dominant mode of Western society since the 18th century, has been its imperfect success in making possible the liberation of individuals from the binding and defining claims on them of religion, state, social class, and more recently—in fact, the struggle for liberation continues—race and gender, indeed, from any claim that arbitrarily denies personal choice. I propose that modernity, culminating with the wholesale onslaught against all limits on personal preference, the "We want the world and we want it now" of the 1960s, has developed into postmodernity, a time forecast by Friedrich Nietzsche (1882) of weightlessness, the earth loosed from the sun, of the death of God, when all the foundations that have offered certainty—one God, one truth, one moral consensus, one best way of life, in short, all "single visions," all the grand unifying stories—have been shaken by challenges made with apparent impunity. At the same time that individuals have been freed to act on the basis of personal choice (even of unmitigated desire), they may never have felt—because of the massive perfecting of political and corporate bureaucracy; the capacity acquired by technology to serve people's wishes and whims; and the ability of the news and entertainment media to influence what we will know, what we will think, and even what we will want—more powerless or less aware of the forces that guide their choices.

It is important to distinguish modernity from modernism, on one hand, and postmodernity from postmodernism on the other. By modernity, I refer to that development in Western civilization which had its beginnings early in the 16th century with the growing realization there was a New World beyond the ocean to the west, hit is stride in the 18th century, dominated the 19th and exhausted itself in the 20th. It was characterized by a rapidly accelerating process of releasing the individual from the traditional constraints upon personal choice: established religion, fixed social class, the high risk of deadly disease, restricted geographical abode and limitations on economic opportunity. The exhaustion of modernity into postmodernity is, I propose, based on a growing perception that the *beliefs* that had upheld the constraints that modernity undid were now no longer regarded as unchallengable or even necessary. The postmodern condition could, therefore, be described as one in which these foundational beliefs—in such things as God, one objective reality, one truth—were themselves regarded as constraining, not only on individual behavior but on opportunities for expression and making choices by groups that have traditionally been marginalized—women, people of color, gays and lesbians—in part, at least, by some of those beliefs.

Modernism and postmodernism refer to more or less self-conscious movements in the arts, which attempt to hold a mirror to the time in which they have held sway. Modernism was a titanic movement in the history of the arts and literature as well as being itself an expression of modernity. It had a significant influence in altering the way people looked at the world and thought about themselves. However, the main value, as I see it, in examining an artistic or an intellectual movement has less to do with its capacity to influence the ways people live and much more to do with its success in holding a mirror to the times its works reflect. I especially think that such reflections are of great value for therapists, for we must be concerned with how people respond to one another, the assumptions that guide their responses, and the pervasive sociopolitical and cultural forces that, less tangibly though no less importantly, influence them. As practitioners of the art and science of therapy, the work that we do, whichever theoretical models we adopt, involves encouraging people to tell us their stories and helping them deconstruct and then reconstruct those stories in a way that empowers them. In such work it seems to me that we have an inescapable kinship with poets and story writers everywhere, even though, to be sure, we play more the role of editors. (The only stories we actually write are our own.) As with any writer, the question of voice is all important: How can persons find their own voice? How can they write/live their own story, describing their own experiences in their own words rather than mimicking the words of others to describe those experiences?

Whether we agree with him or not, we are heirs of Sigmund Freud, whose only Nobel Prize nomination was in literature and whose most cherished honor was his Goethe Prize in letters. Freud discovered that by listening nonjudgmentally to persons telling their story, their memory would begin to supply parts that had been forgotten through a survival-driven process of self-censorship. As patients became increasingly able to recount their own forgotten experiences in their own words, they began to find their own voice. Freud did not realize what he had discovered, partly because he believed in science and thought that he had to have a theory to explain what was *really* happening and partly because he was in the true succession of the modernist movement and thought that whatever was on the surface revealed a deeper, subterranean truth that would provide the clue to what was constraining the beset individual (Parry, 1991).

Freud, we know, was never modest about his discoveries, but he freely acknowledged that it was not he, but the poets and philosophers who preceded him, who had discovered the unconscious and its power. But if he was indebted to the Greek tragedians, to Shakespeare and Goethe, to Schopenhauer and Nietzsche, he in turn influenced a generation of writers and artists, much more than he was indebted to or influenced by the world of science. In our case today, in the midst of what is often called the postmodern period, it seems to me that if we wish to understand this unprecedented time, we can do as well by reading Thomas Pynchon as Michel Foucault, Salman Rushdie and Gabriel García Márquez as Jacques Derrida or Hans-Georg Gadamer. It is not so much that there is less value in the commentators, only, I suggest, that there is more for us in the story writers, the fellow therapists of the soul. Moreover, if the postmodern is a time of the crumbling of the foundations that have supported the great stories of Western tradition so that, as Kenneth Gergen (1991) suggests, the singular self as a foundation has also been a casualty, then all we have left are the stories themselves. Moreover, as Jean-François Lyotard (1984) proposes, if what he calls the "grand narratives" themselves have lost their traditional capacity to inspire us so, then, indeed, all we have now are our own stories and such new stories as we invent to encompass the clash between chaos and control that seems central to life in these days. If this is the case, we who work with people confused by a world of unrestricted desires and packaged choices need to understand it, and how better than by reading perhaps new grand narratives, stories by great postmodern writers?

## THE MODERNIST AGENDA AND ITS OUTCOME

It is impossible to understand the postmodern world without looking back at how we got here from there. If modernity has involved the concerted effort to liberate individuals from all forces that have restricted their capacity to make personal choices, I propose that modernism brought that agenda to the modern psyche. Its focus on the inner person left modernism largely indifferent to the massive social and technological forces that were imposing themselves on people at the same time that they were celebrating their increasing sense of inner as well as outer freedom. It is my argument that modernism's preoccupation with the inner person to the neglect of the outer has led to a state of affairs that we call postmodernity, which is characterized by a feeling in individuals of maximum freedom and minimum personal power. How did it come to this?

Modernism itself refers to that 100 years of "transgressive innovation," to use Stephanie Dudek's (1990) apposite term, from the 1860s and the emergence of Impressionism to the early 1960s, when the great shattering of that decade rendered its assumptions unequal to what was happening. At modernism's zenith, during the first quarter of the 20th century, the art of Picasso and the Cubists was changing Western society's very conception of the purpose and possibilities of art, from mirroring the beauty of the world to exposing its contemporary truth by holding to it the mirror of the fragmenting soul of the artist himself. In literature, at the same time, Thomas Mann, James Joyce, Marcel Proust, W. B. Yeats, T. S. Eliot, and others were describing the same crisis in Western society through the inner lives of questing souls. As much as these writers challenged and sought to subvert a society that had gained the world but was losing its soul in the process, they believed in the grand narratives of its tradition as the vehicle by which Western society could be rejuvenated. In the face of what they experienced as a spiritual emptiness accompanying this society's material conquest of the world, they saw in the realms of its imperial hegemony the furtherance of democratic rule and advances in scientific knowledge and medical technology, all of which made for a dramatic increase in the availability of the comforts and conveniences of life for more and more of its citizens. These advances gave people a sense of their own sufficiency, distancing death from its once ever-present Otherness. Meanwhile, the Weberian alliance between the Protestant ethic and the spirit of capitalism, which linked piety with worldly success, had effectively desacralized religion. As a result, Western society was seen by the modernists to be "progressing" toward its own disintegration. In order to communicate their message of the discrepancy they perceived between the pride and self-righteousness of the triumphant middle class, on one hand, and its spiritual emptiness, on the other, the great modernist artists and poets adopted the transgressive approach that quickly became the signature of the movement: art that sought to mirror the inner world of the artist rather than the outer world of man and nature and literature that abandoned conventional narrative forms in favor of the portrayal of inner torment and uncertainty, expressed symbolically, metaphorically, and (as with Joyce and Proust, for example) minutely.

As transgressive as their art was and as critical as their message of society's spiritual bankruptcy was, the modernists were staunchly optimistic in their vision of the sources and the possibilities of renewal. These would be found in the internalization—the psychologization, if you will—of the grand narratives: classical myths and archetypes, such as *The Odyssey* (Joyce's *Ulysses*) and Apollo and Dionysus (Mann's *Magic Mountain*); medieval myths, such as the Grail Quest (T. S. Eliot's *Waste Land*)—as well as the Christ story for the later Eliot—and the Celtic myths by W. B. Yeats. Thus, although critical in many ways of modernity, the modernists shared its utopian faith in the coming of a better world.

Modernity was characterized by a confident belief in Progress as a narrative of humanity's forward march by means of the fulfillment of its inventions or perfections, namely, democracy, human rights, science, and technology. Modernism would only add to these accomplishments the development of psychology, understood as the internalization of the grand narratives. Meanwhile, although by no means identifying himself as an artist—and still less, probably, as a modernist—Sigmund Freud may have done more than any of the poets or writers to carry forth the modernist program into the society at large. He happened upon the transgressive method of letting his neurological patients tell him their stories until they began to yield secrets hidden even from themselves. When he simply listened, with his famous "evenly hovering attention," to people whom others had dismissed as self-absorbed hysterics, shameful and terrifying memories returned to fill in gaps in these patients' stories so that their lives became coherent. They had been able to find their own voices, as we would say today. Like the modernists, Freud drew upon many of the grand narratives—the Oedipus myth most famously, of course—to help people make sense of their stories, and like them, he too believed that a complete narrative would make for a fuller life (though never a *fulfilled* life, for Freud, the stoic realist, suspected anything that smacked of the transcendent or the perfect, which to him was merely a problematic entity called the superego). His greatest legacy was probably that he made the examination of the inner life of the person respectable in its own right, rather than on moral or spiritual terms. He thereby stood in the great tradition of modernity, in encouraging a further step in the freeing of the individual from one more tyranny, that of the moral mystification by which parents influenced their children by convincing them that what they, the parents, desired was synonymous with goodness itself. C. G. Jung, Freud's student and later rival, took Freud's efforts a step further and virtually equated the inner quest with the sacred. Thus was the individual self encouraged to become even more autonomous and self-oriented, for the very wisdom of all significant human experience was deemed to be within that self.

Freud, Jung, and those who followed them in the emergence of the "science" they discovered could be credited with making the modernist agenda into a cultural institution. Their work succeeded in permeating the culture as that of the artists did not. The propositions of Freud and his successors also proliferated through a widespread process of oversimplification; stories spread of the harm parents could do by inhibiting the most fleeting of their children's "natural" impulses, and pronouncements were made of the necessity of sexual satisfaction and of the importance of certain measures, even of proper toilet training, as prerequisites of healthy adulthood. While Freud (1930) himself brooded upon the future of civilization and acknowledged that a slight lessening of the forces supporting the repression of sex and aggression might allow for a somewhat happier and healthier citizenry, in the hope that "eternal Eros will make an effort to assert himself in the struggle with his equally immortal adversary," few of his successors remained as mindful as he was of the wider social implications of the encouragement of greater self-expression. Yet Freud himself was a modernist and the Freudian case history concerned itself only with the inner life of the individual—notoriously so, as we now suspect, given Freud's decision to regard female reports of parental seduction as wish-fulfilling fantasies rather than interpersonal events.

As literate as Freud's case histories were—the creation of a new genre, in fact—they were very much in the antinarrative modernist tradition by concerning themselves only with the inner life of the protagonist while excluding the events of his or her outer life. Like other major works of modernist literature, Freud's stories further implied that even the individual's inner responses to events were secondary to a deeper struggle going on outside conscious awareness. Just as the stream of consciousness of Leopold Bloom was but an epiphenomenon of the living out of the myth of Ulysses in the life of a modern Everyman, so too was the individual as analyzed by Freud a largely passive, psychologically and neurologically determined instrument of a tempestuous conflict between the "seething cauldron" of biological demands (the id) and the equally irrational, internalized demands of the social world (the superego) for the soul of a person who had only the vaguest understanding of what led to his or her actions.

Paradoxically, then, in seeking nothing less than the regeneration of European civilization through the internalization of art and myth, the modernists left a strangely passive, acted-upon version of the self to contend with the spiritual and moral disintegration of a great civilization. They portrayed individuals as beings who, by implication, could not have been expected to know their own mind, who were essentially left having to seek out and rely on experts in psychological and mythological interpretation in order to understand themselves, not to mention change. Such change alone was supposed to save a Europe that was otherwise destroying itself.

By focusing on the psychological/spiritual health of individuals, yet managing to portray them as unwittingly passive, the modernist attitude played directly into two powerful forces at work in the 20th-century world: technology and popular culture. In addition, when modernism's largely inner focus was confronted by the disregard of the individual and the spiritual shown by the totalitarian response of fascism and communism to the challenges of modernity, this once-transgressive shock movement turned itself, by midcentury, into a defender of the status quo. Moreover, its very success now guaranteed that only an affluent elite could afford access to or appreciation of the art works that had so shocked and horrified their counterparts in the beginning of the movement. Of the writers, the most troubling had died—Joyce, Kafka, Proust—while Yeats became increasingly conservative, even reactionary, in the years leading up to his death; Mann, though a liberal, was always staunchly respectable, and Eliot's elegant poems on edifying Anglican themes suited the spiritual, and ignored the political, temper of Cold War America in the 1950s.

## MODERNITY: THE CHALLENGE FROM WITHIN

The influence of modernism in its own time and since has been considerable. It changed the way art, music, and literature reflect the world, namely, in terms of its inner truth, its spiritual estate, not its beauty. As such, I would go so far as to say that art has replaced institutional religion as the major source of transformative vision in the Western world, and I would date this change from the beginning of high modernism in the first quarter of the 20th century. The churches largely remain, sad to say, in "suburban captivity," to use the sociologist Gibson Winter's phrase from many years ago, and the Christian religion's most prophetic movement, liberation theology, and its most embracing, creation-centered spirituality remain under Vatican interdict. Yet, sadly, the penetrating diagnoses of the modern psyche and its times by the artists and writers of modernism have remained impenetrable to the general population, which prefers the shorter, sharper kick of the arts of popular culture.

There was an inescapable elitism about modernist art and literature, due probably to the departure it made from traditional canons of beauty in art and narration in literature. This elitism, as I have mentioned here and elsewhere (1991), had the effect of requiring the services of an expert interpreter to decipher the message behind the medium. This development put art, literature and its modernist cousin, psychoanalysis (and its therapeutic offshoots), alongside science and technology as provinces of the expert. This was particularly troubling in the case of the relational and psychotherapies, where, as a consequence, people seemed less and less prone to venture to understand themselves, their children, their spouses, or each other generally. That understanding was for experts in the appropriate disciplines to pronounce upon. What therapist has not heard the response of a client, when asked about his or her own experience: "I don't know, I'm not a psychologist."

In spite of the disposition of Freud and his early followers, including Jung and Otto Rank, to look to writers, mystics, and artists for intuitive support of their emerging theories and in spite of the remarkable influence these great pioneers had on the artistic, literary, and philosophical climate of the times, these therapists and those who followed in their wake were very intent on establishing scientific legitimacy. Indeed, such legitimacy was far more important to them than any reputation that might have implied something spiritual about their work, or even philosophical or literary. These could only diminish their claim to scientific status. Thus, if modernism could be said to have involved the joining of the arts to modernity's drive to ward individual freedom, psychotherapy, by adding creative self-expression to it, can be viewed as joining modernism in seeking the greater expression of the inner person—although as time went by this was increasingly through the application of technique to the inner life and behavior of persons.

After all, if any enterprise wanted to be considered truly modern and on the side of Progress, it had better ally itself with science and technology, the favored instruments of Progress. Anything that smacked of the spiritual was immediately suspect; the imaginative arts were not, because they belonged to the private realm of taste and preference. The only thing the arts might contribute to Progress was to help people become more broad-minded.

While, therefore, the modernist movement occupied itself with its transgressive vision, the population at large remained far more impressed by the apparently unlimited capacities of science and technology to perform what once would have been deemed miracles in making everyday life ever more comfortable, convenient, and safe from so much of the illness and premature death that once made it, in Hobbes's famous phrase, "nasty, brutish, and short." Enough can never be said regarding the effects of 20th-century technology on actually altering human consciousness wherever those effects have been felt, effects that have probably done little if anything to reduce human iniquity, malice, and greed appreciably—indeed, they may have increased them. Technical efficiency, after all, made the Holocaust possible. Thus, modernism served modernity by its encouragement that individuals exercise the freedom to express their innermost impulses, preferably creatively. This influence and the brilliant accomplishments of technology that made it possible to gratify personal wants came together explosively to make a world where less and less stood in the way of assuming that the point of life was the gratification of desire. Since, in addition, modernity in all of its forms had stressed freedom in such a way as to emphasize the rights of the individual self, it had less to say about mutual obligation or about the limit on personal rights to self-expression or gratification by the other. In a word, no provision had ever been made, within the agenda of modernity, for any inherent limitation on the exercise of individual freedom. With the decline of religion as a major societal force coupled with the emergence of an art that stressed the self as creative spirit, there was no vision arising out of modernity that included anything akin to an obligation to the other.

At the same time that the individual was being loosened from all traditional restraints and technology was creating a world that seemed to resemble more and more a source of gratification than of struggle, what Max Weber (1930) termed the principle of rationalization came increasingly to characterize the governmental and corporate life of the nations of the Western world. Weber used the term *rationalization* in a specific way to refer to "the organization of life through a division and coordination of activities on the basis of an exact study of men's relations with each other, with their tools and their environment, for the purpose of achieving greater efficiency and productivity" (Freund, 1968). Weber also described rationalization as pertaining to a striving for perfection in relation to the conduct of life and the pursuit of greater mastery of the external world. Thus, wherever this attitude was taken up, the analytical, the impersonal, and the abstract came to be the dominant modes of understanding and implementation.

For Weber, the steady process whereby more and more of human experience and endeavor is rationalized is synonymous with modernity. But if modernity is associated with the liberation of the individual from nonrational constraints, rationalization has more to do with the perfecting of efficiency, organization, and conceptualization as agents of mastery. Thus, governments and corporations came to be governed more and more by their bureaucracies and less and less by personal leadership. The effect of this has been to leave individuals feeling dwarfed by the massive, impersonal scale of corporate and governmental bureaucracy at the very same time that they are encouraged to believe that their every wish should be gratified. In short, the citizen of the modernist world is a powerless person with boundless desires.

Perhaps even greater, and more ominous, import has been the rise and influence of popular culture through the information and entertainment media and the application of what Jacques Ellul (1964) has called technique to its merchandising. Ellul's term is reminiscent of Weber's "rationalization." Technique is "the totality of methods rationally arrived at and having absolute efficiency (for a given stage of development) in every stage of human activity" (p. xxv). Its successful application means, for Ellul, that there is literally no human activity that cannot be brought under technical control, packaged, and then managed, a sure recipe for the dictatorship of the product.

Through technique it becomes possible not only to prepare and supply at a mass consumer level those goods and services that appear to gratify any desire but also to influence people into believing that what they desire is what has already been prepared and packaged for them. All people have to do, then, is purchase it or vote for it, as the case may be. Indeed, the merchandising techniques available to large corporations and political parties have become so sophisticated and specialized that such entities operate indefatigably, not ready to rest until they have obtained sufficient evidence of success, which is the convincing of large numbers of people that what they are being sold is what they most want.

This process becomes that much easier, I venture to say, because a paradox of living in the mode of desire is that people start becoming less and less certain about what they actually do want. It is only when there is a limit or a resistance before them that they are forced to stop and consider what they want. To the extent that they believe their desire can be gratified (indeed, that that is all the other is there for), any further reflection is unnecessary. Delay or denial is likely, then, to be greeted with impatience, anger, and "How dare you?" But without delay can there be a self that does the wanting?

A self, I say, comes about with enough experiences that have required delay of gratification that a person will have had to reflect on his or her options and come up against the desire of an other, who may or may not meet the person's desires because the other has requirements of his or her own. Enough of such experiences will force persons to come to terms with what they really do want, what priorities will govern the choices available to them, and how much of the other's agenda they are prepared to meet in order that their own will be met. If, however, persons have not had delays to frustrate them, have accepted choices made for them, and have regarded others primarily as means of gratification, they will not have or be a self. The self, in other words, is a product of spaces. Alas, I fear that modernity's project of the liberation of the individual from all nonrational impositions on his or her freedom has resulted in a steady erosion of such spaces. The prime casualty of the loss of spaces is awareness of and due regard for the other. Yet without the other there can be no self, however liberated.

## THE LOSS OF THE OTHER

There are three great Others in the grand narratives of the Western tradition: God, Death, and the marginalized. As the modern world has been disenchanted through the process of rationalization, God himself has become increasingly marginalized. The more the processes that brought the world into being and maintained it were shown to be rational and observable phenomena, the less need there was for God to account for the unexplainable. There were simply fewer instances of the unexplainable. This development, I argue, reached a critical point with the Holocaust. There, the unexplainable took on a different dimension. It's not that there was an adequate explanation, that this was one more event for which "the hypothesis of God" was no longer necessary; it was that an event had occurred of such horrifying magnitude that no explanation was adequate. That an effort was made as a matter of state policy in one of the great nations of Western culture, with silence even from the avowed enemies of that state at the time, to exterminate an entire race—the race, moreover, of the Chosen People of God in the dominant grand narrative of Western tradition—represented the death of God as an act of murder, as Nietzsche's madman had prophesied. For many, however, the great stumbling block in the face of this unspeakable event was the very silence of God. In explanation of the impunity with which modern man now felt free to act against everything the dominant Story had enjoined regarding the ultimate unity between God and humanity, God himself must be said to have been put to death with/as the six million.

As for Death, the great inescapable of human life, it has probably never fed more lustily than in the 20th century, at the same time as the miracles of medical technology were making it possible, within Western society at least, for most people to assume the likelihood of a full lifespan of upward of 70 years. This had the effect of at least postponing the encounter with that dread Other so that life could be lived for most with little thought of it. Yet the very massive scale of death in this century—millions here, millions there, killings featured on the news, killings featured as entertainment— seems to have made death grotesquely commonplace rather than the inescapable Other that might meet any one of us at any moment.

Following immediately upon the Holocaust and the silence of God in its wake, another remarkable phenomenon began to occur that we are all still struggling with: the increasing and spreading refusal of the third great Other in the Western tradition to accept what had been its lot. That third Other is composed of those groups of people, categorized as Other than those who sufficiently occupy the dominant social positions that they can confidently regard themselves as the Ones. Simone de Beauvoir, in her authoritative *The Second Sex* (1953) suggested that Otherness, in this third sense, is "a fundamental category of human thought." No group, she went on to say, sets itself up as the One without immediately setting an Other over against itself. History's first Other was woman, deemed secondary to the primacy of man. Wherever a group or community of people are relegated to some kind of secondary status simply by being members of that group, we have the phenomenon of the Other. Such people—whether as the "stranger," the "foreigner," the "Jew" to the anti-Semite, the "native" to the colonizer, "blacks" to all too many still, and male homosexuals (especially to men uncertain of their maleness)—are invariably placed into a less than fully human status and treated accordingly. Perhaps too no Other has been quite as marginalized and ravaged by this alienating phenomenon as has the Earth herself. Her story and those of all her marginalized Others are too sadly familiar to require illustration by examples.

Their stories have always been of bearing the unwanted sins of the Ones. However, the breakdown of the moral and spiritual consensus that had given the Western world its "single vision" has had this hopeful consequence: the marginalized Others, no longer mystified by the religions and ideologies of their "masters" into accepting their voiceless status as the will of God or fate, have been demarginalizing themselves. They demand to be accepted not as the Other but as other persons. Needless to say, the Earth as well has made her presence felt as the margins have collapsed. The conviction that the right to be regarded and treated as an individual be available to all is surely one of the great outcomes of modernity. The ideal had been widely disseminated and, as such, had pervaded the culture. Demarginalization began to occur only as the center no longer held and the margins began to cave in under pressure, the margins that were no longer able to hold in place women, daughters of Eve, as the instigators of the Fall; Africans and their descendants in America in place as the children of Ham destined for servitude; native peoples as benighted heathen in need of salvation; homosexuals as sinners who "burned with lust for one another" (Rom. 1:27); and the Earth as ours to be subdued. The challenge to post-moderns is of the extent to which we are willing to allow those who had played their designated roles for centuries as the marginalized Other to be accepted in every degree as persons to whom the modern Western ideal applies. For, after all, each of these groupings of people have played very convenient and serviceable roles, economically, socially, and psychologically. Given, moreover, the anxiety and uncertainty that a world without the security of an agreed-upon center strikes in many, the additional disadvantage of no longer having people subordinated to the margins to serve their allotted and historic roles may be more than people are willing to abide who were comforted by their assurance that they were among the Ones. If so, times lived in which not many are willing to serve as the Other will be interesting times indeed.

At the same time as the presence of the Other in its three historic forms wanes and the self, liberated from all traditional moral and social constraints, has only its desire to satisfy, we can only ask again, "What will be the limits of the self?" Modernity released the individual, modernism released the inner person, but the other as person was rarely addressed. This, I propose, is the great unanswered legacy of modernism and the make-or-break challenge of the postmodern world. By having to experience fewer and fewer obstacles against self-gratification, due precisely to the staggering success of the phenomenon of modernity, individuals have been left in a perilous predicament. They are taught, willy-nilly, that their rights are inviolable, that they are entitled to be happy, which comes to means gratified. Comforts, conveniences, and pleasures are ever dangled before them as temptations, the possession of which, they are reminded, give them worth and the envy and esteem of others. At the same time, they are accorded a growing list of rights and entitlements and are freed from such traditional expectations as courtesies toward and considerations of the other, implicit respect for parents only because they are parents, community pressures to behave in specific ways sexually, and certain moral and behavioral demands imposed as unquestioned obligations.

The effect of all of these freedoms for and freedoms from has unexpectedly left postmodern individuals in a position of assuming they are indeed free, believing they are or at least ought to be happy, but with few of the assurances and comforts that the bonds of shared obligations to others and the availability and even the expectation of various prescribed behaviors bring. At the same time that postmodern individuals may feel freer from obligation than any human being has ever felt before, they find themselves powerless in the face of massive social and economic forces that they are utterly unable to influence; that is, they may think that they are making free choices when, in fact, they are making choices that corporate, political, and entertainment bodies want them to make. Moreover, such "choices" are apt to have nothing to do with their own best interests and might even be inimical to them. Thus, as one side of modernity, the one associated with all those activities that have freed individuals from those political, religious, economic, and hygienic factors that confined them, has made it possible for them to assert themselves as agents of their own destiny as never before, another side, the one associated with the perfection of technique applied by the massive, impersonalized corporate structures that the rationalization process of modernity has made possible, has rendered them reactive to the agenda of the "corporate structures" and increasingly passive even to those desires of their own that they assume are evidence of their freedom.

## POSTMODERNITY: APOCALYPSE OR OPPORTUNITY?

I consider this coincidence of agency and passivity in the individual to be the central characteristic of the postmodern condition and, alongside the implacable reality of the Other, its major challenge. As such, it poses a challenge to all approaches to therapy, individual and relational alike. By the latter I mean therapies with groups, couples, and families. Furthermore, since psychotherapy was a child of modernity in the first place, especially by way of the modernist effort to liberate the creative resources of the inner person, it must be said to share some responsibility for the problem of both the self as passive agent and the self acting without regard for the other as an anchoring reference. Modernism was far removed from the forces of rationalization and technique that contributed so much to the emergence of the passivity of the postmodern individual. Nonetheless, it contributed to this passivity inadvertently by, I suggest, the role that it gave the expert in deciphering the "real" message of its nonrepresentational art and non-narrative literature. It did the same thing in psychotherapy through the power invested in the Freudian analyst to point out in various cryptic ways the "true" significance of the analysand's experiences. This was partly because the analyst—of whatever school—was, in effect, interpreting a text filled with myths, metaphors, and hidden meanings. At the same time, the analyst was constrained from adopting an approach that simply allowed the story to do the healing work. That would not have been rational, in the Weberian sense. For that there had to be a theory, an abstraction, rather than a narration of a person's experiences. Analysts were also constrained from adopting such an approach because they were busy trying to establish their scientific credentials. Those psychotherapies that later arose out of psychology and social work were driven by a similar urgency. Therapists had to present themselves, whatever they might also be, as scientists. Indeed, once we leave the world of the classically and humanistically educated early psychoanalysts and Jungian and Rankian schismatics, science and the technology of therapy reign supreme. There is not—there virtually dare not be—any serious recourse by therapists to their closest actual confreres (the fellow narratologists, the poets and novelists), who might have provided some balance for the virtually total reliance on technique that has come to characterize modern and relational psychotherapy. With the expert in charge, expected to know the clients better than they know themselves, and to introduce them to techniques that would free them up, the consequence has been a passivity similar to what was engendered by the application of technique to people's desires by the corporate merchandising world.

Psychotherapy also shares a great deal of responsibility, I must say, for the singularity of focus on the inner person and his or her personal satisfaction almost as life's *summum bonum*. This seems to me to be so obvious as to need no elaboration. The relational therapies represent, to some degree, an exception in that they address, by their very nature, matters pertaining to the self in relation to others. I would argue, however, that the theme of self-satisfaction has so pervaded the therapeutic milieu in all its forms, and through it the culture itself, that the relational therapies have not yet adequately capitalized on their own potentialities for addressing the full implications of coming to terms with the indispensable importance of the other for one's own well-being. As the challenge of the other cries out to be met, lest the postmodern be apocalypse rather than opportunity, the relational therapies (and family therapy particularly), are perhaps the best equipped, both theoretically and clinically, to meet that challenge.

Most forms of therapy—whether for individuals, groups, couples, or families—seek to enable persons to become agents of their own destinies, and therapists would not willingly choose to encourage or champion the kind of passivity that I have suggested so characterizes the all too frequently beleaguered postmodern individual and family. I would suggest, then, that we not make the same mistake so many of us have made in nailing our flag exclusively to the masthead of science and its technologies. Instead, I propose that this time around we who wish to better understand the challenge of the postmodern and assist our clients in living in it as agents of their own choices, look to see what those who also deal exclusively in stories as a way of understanding and shaping ourselves have identified as not only the challenges of the postmodern but also the ways of living in these pivotal and perplexing times.

## THOMAS PYNCHON'S CREATIVE PARANOIA

The novels of Thomas Pynchon are unrivaled, in my opinion, for describing the depth and complexities of life in a postmodern world and for offering some useful hints for meeting its challenges. Pynchon's output is limited thus far to four novels and a collection of his early short stories entitled *Slow Learner* (1984). The novels are *V.*, (1963), *The Crying of Lot 49* (1966), *Gravity's Rainbow* (1973), and *Vineland* (1990). These four novels could be said to represent a sequence of allegorical stories that cover the mythopoeic landscape of the Western world from the 1950s to the present.

I will focus my attention primarily on the themes of *The Crying of Lot 49* and *Gravity's Rainbow*. *V.* is a brilliant novel and a fascinating and absorbing read, and *Vineland,* Pynchon's most accessible novel, brings many of the themes of *Gravity's Rainbow* into the immediate present, but limitations of space and my conclusion that the challenges that I have suggested are particularly crucial in these postmodern times lead me to focus on the middle two. *The Crying of Lot 49* is a short, puzzling, but very readable novel that contains most of Pynchon's characteristic themes. It has become something of a classic text of postmodern literature in spite—or perhaps because—of its brevity and abundance of cartoonish characters. *Crying* tells the story of a postmodern quester, Oedipa Maas, who, like her classical namesake, is drawn to embark upon a mission in which she tries to decipher the meaning, significance, and even the reality of a series of signs that, she thinks, hint of the existence of an alternative mail service or communications network that has apparently been operating throughout modern Western society. It is known as the Tristero alternately spelled "Trystero," and its presence is announced by the symbol of a muted post horn. The means by which the Tristero conspiracy, for such it seems to be, sends messages is through mailboxes labeled w.a.s.t.e. Oedipa picks up on her quest by accident. She has been named, to her surprise and puzzlement, the executor of the estate of Pierce Inverarity, a mysterious figure of fabulous wealth who seems to own half of America. In the tradition of overdetermined naming, so characteristic of Pynchon's allegorical characters, Oedipa has been "pierced" or awakened out of the routine existence of an American suburban housewife of the early 1960s to embark upon a voyage of discovery. She is thrown into a series of meetings with an odd assortment of characters as she tries to find out what her role is in executing the vast estate of Pierce Inverarity. She starts coming across mysterious references, first of all to a message delivery or mail service referred to as WASTE and then to a small symbol of a muted horn. This is followed shortly thereafter by an equally cryptic and almost numinous reference to one "Who's once been set his tryst with Trystero" (p. 52).

More references and allusions follow, and Oedipa finds herself determined to find out what these signs mean:

> She could at this stage of things recognize signals like that, as the epileptic is said to—an odor, color, pure piercing grace note announcing his seizure. Afterward it is only this signal, really dross, this secular announcement,

and never what is revealed during the attack, that he remembers. Oedipa wondered whether, at the end of this (if it were supposed to end), she too might not be left with only compiled memories of clues, announcements, intimations, but never the central truth itself, which must somehow each time be too bright for her memory to hold; which must always blaze out, destroying its own message irreversibly, leaving an overexposed blank when the ordinary world came back. In the space of a sip of dandelion wine it came to her that she would never know how many times such a seizure may already have visited, or how to grasp it should it visit again. Perhaps even in this last second—but there was no way to tell. She glanced down the corridor of Cohen's rooms in the rain and saw, for the very first time, how far it might be possible to get lost in this. (p. 62)

At this early stage of her quest Oedipa awaits the customary blinding flash, a vision of a revealed truth even in this time—perhaps all the more especially in this time—of the death of God and the crumbling of those foundations that have for centuries guaranteed that there is One Truth. The more she searches, however, the more confused and uncertain she becomes, wondering whether Trystero does exist or was merely a figment of her own overworked imagination. She comes even to wonder whether the clues link themselves together in her mind as "only some kind of compensation. To make up for her having lost the direct, epileptic Word, the cry that might abolish the night" (p. 87). Is the search for meaning and the teasing hints that she might even be on to something simply a sad substitute for the inner experienced illumination that people perhaps once lived by?

Oedipa sees a group of children at play. "The night was empty of all terror for them, they had inside their circle an imaginary fire, and needed nothing but their own unpenetrated sense of community." As she further prowls the night streets of San Francisco, she becomes more and more aware of vast numbers of people who live their lives independently of the rules of the dominant system and its manner of communication that leads us customarily to believe that there is no alternative:

Last night she might have wondered what undergrounds apart from the couple she knew of communicated by WASTE system. By sunrise she could legitimately ask what undergrounds didn't. If miracles were . . . intrusions into this world from another, a kiss of cosmic pool balls, then so must be each of the night's post horns. For here were God knew how many citizens, deliberately choosing not to communicate by U.S. Mail. It was not an act of treason, nor possibly even of defiance. But it was a calculated withdrawal from the life of the Republic, from its machinery. Whatever else was being denied to them out of hate, indifference to the power of their vote, loopholes, simple ignorance, this withdrawal was their own, unpublicized, private. Since they could not have withdrawn into a vacuum (could they?), there had to exist the silent, unsuspected world. (p. 92)

There follows an immensely moving scene in which Oedipa comes upon one of the marginalized, "an old man huddled, shaking with grief she couldn't hear . . . On the back of the left hand she made out the post horn, tattooed in old ink now beginning to blur and spread. Fascinated, she came into the shadows and ascended creaking steps, hesitating on each one. When she was three steps from him the hands flew apart and his wrecked face, and the terror of eyes gloried in burst veins, stopped her" (p. 92). She asks if she can help. The old man, a sailor, has a letter for the wife that he left, Odysseus-like, "so long ago I don't remember." He wants Oedipa to post it for him, but to do so would be to acknowledge that there actually is a Tristero network linked by the WASTE system. She refuses at first, reluctant to commit herself to such a concrete step, even out of the compassion that she so obviously feels for the old sailor. She attempts to leave, but he follows her and persuades her finally to mail the letter. She actually finds one of the secret mailboxes, although it merely resembles a trash bin. On it are the telltale initials w. a. s. t. e. Is this objective evidence or what? Evidently not. Oedipa continues her quest; returning to her Berkeley hotel, she finds herself in the midst of a convention of left-wing deaf-mutes. She is swept into a ballroom where she is seized around the waist by a handsome young man who waltzes her round and round under a large, unlit chandelier.

> Each couple on the floor danced whatever was in the fellow's head: tango, two-step, bossa nova, slop. But how long, Oedipa thought, could it go on before collisions became a serious hindrance? There would have to be collisions. The only alternative was some unthinkable order of music, many rhythms, all keys at once, a choreography in which each couple meshed easy, predestined. Something they all heard with an extra sense atrophied in herself. She followed her partner's lead, limp in the young mute's clasp, waiting for the collisions to begin. But none came. She was danced for half an hour before, by mysterious consensus, everybody took a break, without having felt any touch but the touch of her partner. Jesus Arrabal would have called it an anarchist miracle. Oedipa, with no name for it, was only demoralized. She curtsied and fled. (p. 97)

The evidence of her senses followed by a miracle and Oedipa still cannot believe. She is forced to admit to herself that she wants Trystero, the supposed alternative mail service, to be a fantasy only or even that "she was some kind of a nut and needed a rest." But she also wants to know why the chance that Trystero was real should pose such a menace for her. She rushes to her never-far-from-demented therapist in hopes that he will talk her out of her fantasy. 'Cherish it!' cries Hilarius fiercely. 'What else do you have? Hold it tightly by its little tentacle, don't let the Freudians coax it away, or the pharmacists poison it out of you. Whatever it is, hold it dear, for when you lose it you go over by that much to the others. You begin to cease to be' " (p. 103). But on with the quest for Oedipa, to find out what, if anything, Trystero is, hoping still that it was only her fantasy.

Oedipa is introduced to evidence that Trystero has a long history as an alternative communications network that has been operating in the Western world alongside and divorced from the established systems of information, but whether this history is fictional or real still remains a question for her. One of her strange new acquaintances calls her to let her know that he has come upon an old U.S. stamp with the post horn and the motto *WE AWAIT SILENT TRISTERO'S EMPIRE.* Is the stamp genuine or a forgery? As Oedipa ponders the meaning and reality or otherwise, she checks her most "objective" sources and discovers that, indeed, they all trace back to the estate of Pierce Inverarity. What, she begins to wonder, does Inverarity not own? Was he playing an elaborate and inimaginably complex and costly trick on her? Yet what would it mean if there really were a Tristero, a world of the marginalized, of those who had not only been put into the margins but who had chosen freedom from the inviting oppression of the established organization and control of information to join instead "a network by which X number of Americans are truly communicating whilst reserving their lies, recitations of routine, arid betrayals of spiritual poverty, for the official government delivery system; maybe even onto a real alternative to the exitlessness, to the absence of surprise to life, that harrows the head of everybody American you know, and you too, sweetie" (p. 128).

Either there is, she is beginning at last to conclude, such an "other America" beyond appearances or this is just America as it is. Yet even if the latter is the case, "then it seemed the only way she could continue, and manage to be at all relevant to it, was as an alien, unfurrowed, assumed full circle into some paranoia" (p.137). Either way, then, Oedipa has to make a move, to recognize her oneness with the Other America, or simply recognize that she herself was Other to America itself. There is to be an auction of lot 49, which would include Pierce Inverarity's stamp collection, containing the Trystero stamps. She decides to pursue the mystery further by going to the auction to see who bids on that collection and see what clues that person offers. "The finest auctioneer in the West" Loren Passerine (pass her in) is to be there and so Oedipa Maas, open to whatever might reveal itself, goes to await "the crying of lot 49."

What are we to make of this story that reflexively awaits itself? We are left no wiser at the end than at the beginning as to the identity of Trystero. Is it a paranoid fantasy, reflecting the lengths to which a postmodern person will go to find some hint of meaning in a world that no longer has a single story that gives it meaning? Has Pierce Inverarity played a last trick on the earnest, befuddled Oedipa? Or is reality itself a trickster, clues dropped wherever one sees any connections at all? What of a historical conspiracy? Does Oedipa stand on the edge of something, needing only to take the leap of faith to find her answer? Take your pick, says Pynchon. There is nothing to verify any one of these or any other possible variations in interpretation according to any objective criterion. So choose and live accordingly; you will be as right or as wrong as the next person. No matter how proven or disproven any story may be shown to be, human beings will persist in seeking a pattern that gives meaning, "to make up for . . . having lost the direct, epileptic Word, the cry that might abolish the night."

But Pynchon is hinting at something more: not that there really is something out there to give us meaning but that there is something nonetheless. We can see it if we are prepared to, if we have eyes to see. For Pynchon, unlike the modernists, for whom the answer lay within, it lies out there, but in order to see it people must free themselves from the information overload of a world dominated by mass communication, represented in the novel by the dominant, government-owned postal system. Oedipa is so overwhelmed by the bombardment of information and multiple interpretations that all she is able to do is doggedly continue her pursuit of the "truth," grimly, humorlessly, passing up clues that take a different form from those involving the collection and collation of data. Thus, although she is immensely moved by the plight and the story of the old sailor who asks her to mail his letter to his wife through the Trystero system, and although she is then thrown into the experience of the "anarchist miracle," Oedipa can only continue on in her directed fashion. She passes by the Other order even as she pursues evidence of its truth.

Pynchon seems to be suggesting that in these times when the truth of something is so open to question, our own deep experience of events (what he later calls in *Gravity's Rainbow* the "penetration of the moment") is our best guide. Oedipa comes close to such pregnant moments, and when she does, she has glimpses into the reality, if not the truth, of the Trystero. There is, undeniably, an Other America of the marginalized, the disenfranchised, the wretched, those outside the system of ownership and information control represented by Pierce Inverarity, whose tentacles seem to reach everywhere. But as long as we continue questing, single-mindedly, we will keep missing what is also everywhere: the Other who seeks only to be met as an other person. Most importantly, we encounter the Other of the Trystero, the wretched, not only as obligation but as opportunity, perhaps the only opportunity for our own escape from the depersonalization of mass communication and corporate and government bureaucracy. Perhaps only by freely joining the Trystero are persons able to escape the domain of ownership and control, for then they will no longer want what the System wants them to want. This Trystero, moreover, is not to be found at the end of a dedicated search that we will reach by listening to the interpretations of those in the know; it is in our midst, discoverable when we pay attention, less to our own inner voices—they will only confuse us—than to the reality of the Other. This is a hint of Pynchon's "creative paranoia," one of the most important themes of *Gravity's Rainbow,* the novel that is to postmodernism what Joyce's *Ulysses* was to modernism. "Of course a well-developed They-system is necessary—but it's only half the story. For every They there ought to be a We. In our case there is. Creative Paranoia means developing at least as thorough a We-system as a They-system" (*Gravity's Rainbow,* p. 638).

## THE SONG OF THE PRETERITE[1]

Anything beyond the sketchiest summary of *Gravity's Rainbow* is imposs-ible within these confines. The story takes place during the closing months of World War II, when, Pynchon proposes, the shape of the world to come, the postmodern world as we know it, was being formed. Its plot revolves around the creation of the rocket as a human invention with the potential to become the means by which we either destroy ourselves or go to the stars—that is, death or transcendence. The title of the book suggests the Biblical covenant symbol of the rainbow as promise and gravity, as the claim the earth exerts on us and our pretensions to escape that claim. The rocket represents the human urge toward transcendence, its glory and its danger, while gravity reminds us that we both cannot and, if we know what is good for us, should not try to escape our earthiness. If there is any salvation, any hope for us, it is here rather than there. *Gravity's Rainbow* also returns, this time on a much wider and more penetrating scale, to the themes from *The Crying of Lot 49*: a world being overwhelmed by the scale of organization, control, and information-overload that is taking us to an entropic condition of chaotic dyscontrol. Against these massive forces that represent death Pynchon addresses the question (through various, some-times bizarre, always unusual characters) of what can be done for life in such a world.

Amidst a vast number of subplots and seemingly, but never entirely, unrelated incidents and episodes the main plot of *Gravity's Rainbow* con-cerns the German efforts to construct a series of superweapon rockets, culminating in the creation of an ultimate V2 rocket numbered 00000. The Allied side is determined both to stop the rockets from being launched or reaching their targets and, above all, to get the secrets of rocketry from the other side. Both sides are exposed as linked together in a gigantic military-industrial-scientific complex intent on making sure the world runs accord-ing to their interests and priorities:

> It means this War was never political at all, the politics was all theatre, all just to keep the people distracted . . . secretly, it was being dictated instead by the needs of technology . . . by a conspiracy between human beings and tech-niques, by something that needed the energy-burst of war, crying, "Money be damned, the very life of [insert name of Nation] is at stake," but meaning, most likely, dawn is nearly here, I need my night's blood, my funding, funding, ahh more, more. . . . The real crises were crises of allocation and priority, not among firms—it was only staged to look that way—but among the different Technologies, Plastics, Electronics, Aircraft, and their needs which are understood only by the ruling elite. . . .
>
> Yes but Technology only responds (how often this argument has been

---

[1]According to the Calvinist doctrine of double predestination, while a few—the Elect—are chosen by God for salvation and another few are chosen for eternal damnation, the rest are Preterite, simply, regrettably, passed over, all to God's greater Glory.

iterated, dogged and humorless as a Gaussian reduction, among the younger
Schwarzcommando especially), "All very well to talk about having a monster
by the tail, but do you think we'd've had the Rocket if someone, some specific
somebody with a name and a penis hadn't wanted to chuck a ton of Amatol
300 miles and blow up a block full of civilians? Go ahead, capitalize the T on
technology, deify it if it'll make you feel less responsible—but it puts you in
with the neutered, brother, in with the eunuchs keeping the harem of our
stolen Earth for the numb and joyless hardons of human sultans, human elite
with no right at all to be where they are. . . . (p. 521)

In other words, Pynchon shows us a gut-wrenching version of knowledge-as-power. The pursuit of the Rocket is a Grail Quest for supreme
knowledge-as-power. If there is a central adventure around which this quest
is organized, it is the exploitation of an amiable pleasure-seeker, Tyrone
Slothrop, by a ragtag assemblage who operate the White Visitation, a
bizarre parody of a wartime task force. Here, various kinds of occultists and
possessors of every kind of parapsychological power have been gathered to
uncover the secrets of the German rocket. The White Visitation is officially
led by a superannuated, well-intentioned, but senile veteran of World War I
named Brigadier Ernest Pudding. The dominant figure, however, and the
one most involved with the exploitation of a peculiar talent discovered to be
possessed by Slothrop, is a single-minded Pavlovian neurologist named
Edward Pointsman. Slothrop, as a small child, had been a subject of
conditioned learning experiments by a famed Pavlovian named Laszlo Jamf.
While Slothrop's conditioned response had long since been thought ex-
tinguished, it is discovered that the V2 rockets hitting London landed
according to a pattern that followed the places of Slothrop's sexual adventures. Perhaps Pavlov's ultraparadoxical response is operating. Pointsman,
who is the supreme embodiment of rationality, analysis, and control,
determines to use the talent Slothrop unwittingly possesses, his strange
connection with the Rocket. He arranges to send him on a mission to the
Zone in the hope that Slothrop will lead the Firm to the main sources of the
new rocket technology, the ultimate example of technological mastery and
power. Slothrop's adventures then serve as the skeleton upon which is hung
not only all the subplots and sidelong actions and characters but a powerful
and prophetic meditation on and exploration of the hope and necessity of
remaining human in an increasingly rationalized world dominated by
organization and technique.

By situating the action of the story at the time when the forces emerged
that, he believes, have come to dominate the modern world and threaten the
very existence or at least the humanity of our race, Pynchon is able to
portray their constituents through exaggeratedly representative figures for
whom mastery through analysis and control is synonymous with death.
Countering their quest for control are an odd assortment of characters and
images upon which stand the slender but real hope that life and humanity
will prevail. Pynchon's fictional world is seriously paranoid as a conscious

device employed to make clear the seriousness of the stakes. By interpreting in this fashion the magnitude and interlacing connections of the forces that exercise control by making available to us what we want and even convincing us to want what "They" want us to want, Pynchon asks us to realize that when the remarkable human capacity for rationality, analysis, and control is put to total use to master the world, even for the sake of our comfort and convenience, it cannot but kill the earth and destroy its principal beneficiaries.

Pynchon's paranoid strategy is not one of resignation to helpless victimhood. Quite the contrary. We are encouraged instead to consider various options that place us outside and beyond the reach of those—the System, Them, the Firm, the Man—who seek control. He calls them by many names, but most frequently, in paranoid fashion, as Them. Indeed, the labyrinthine plot with its dizzying cast of characters involves the exploration of possible options for freeing ourselves from Them. It is important to emphasize, however, that when Pynchon invokes the language and imagery of paranoid conspiracy, he does not mean that there is active conspiratorial plotting and planning by some power-lusting cabal but that when people take on the determination to control others, dominate their world, or exploit the earth, they come quickly to realize who their allies are and that they share vital interests with them. Whenever those interests are threatened, all who share them will close ranks. Sometimes, to be sure, They may appear to be on opposite sides, as in politics, business competition, or war, but if the System itself upon which the rivalry is based is challenged, They will come to each other's support, the ostensible rivalry being exposed as more of a game that keeps the System going.

In exploring and testing out possible strategies in battling for life, humanity, and the earth, Pynchon uses certain characters to represent the potential options. In doing so, he sets up a series of antinomies, though more by implication than declaration. The overarching antinomy is always between the Firm, all who avowedly work for it and represent it, on one hand, and those who purportedly work for it or are used by it but seek to escape it, on the other. The attempts of the would-be escapees, however, never involve escape as an end in itself; instead the escape is invariably undertaken in some kind of desperate search for a saving Word or transfiguring experience. It is, in its many forms, a search for a One, a spiritual quest. Nothing less than that is sufficient to save us from the Apocalypse, for the forces of technology, control, and the reordering of life, experience, and the earth itself in the image of technology is otherwise taking us inexorably toward the Zero of death and destruction:

> Kekule dreams the Great Serpent holding its own tail in its mouth, the dreaming Serpent which surrounds the World. But the meanness, the cynicism with which the dream is to be used. The Serpent that announces, "The World is a closed thing, cyclical, resonant, eternally-returning," is to be

delivered into a system whose only aim is to violate the Cycle. Taking and not giving back, demanding that "productivity" and "earnings" keep on increasing with time, the System removing from the rest of the World these vast quantities of energy to keep its own tiny desperate fraction showing a profit: and not only most of humanity—most of the World, animal, vegetable and mineral, is laid waste in the process. The System may or may not understand that it's only buying time. And that time is an artificial resource to begin with, of no value to anyone or anything but the System, which sooner or later must crash to its death, when its addiction to energy has become more than the rest of the World can supply, dragging with it innocent souls all along the chain of life. (p. 412)

Moreover, so pervasive and insidious is the power of the Firm, rooted as it is in its capacity to co-opt, giving us through technological packaging what we think we want and even what They want us to want, that all who would challenge the hold They have on us must first recognize, before we contend with Them, that we also work for the Firm. The question, then, becomes whether the image of this rainbow as the human pretension to transcend all earthly limitations, which Technology ultimately represents, will fall exploding to the earth or whether a self-transcending quest for the One will find its answer and its home on the Earth. These being the stakes, Apocalypse or Renewal and Return, how can we choose the latter and escape the fate of the former? Three of the pivotal antinomies that we must navigate between are the following: the One and the Zero, the Elect and the Preterite, History and Penetrating the Moment. Pynchon, consistent with his postmodern sensibility, appears to invite his readers to make their own interpretation by presenting a host of options and possibilities, but he does not imply that one is the definitive or favored choice.

Thus, the contradiction between the One and the Zero suggests the choices posed by all those antinomies that human consciousness seems bound to perceive—the closed and the open, definition and randomness, a mystical One and an inanimate void of facts and figures. An urge toward security and predictability seems to urge many of us toward one or the other of these, but the most difficult and risk-filled approach to navigate is, at the same time, the most life enhancing: the open space between the polarities:

> If ever the Antipointsman existed, Roger Mexico is the man. Not so much, the doctor admits, for the psychical research. The young statistician is devoted to number and to method, not table-rapping or wishful thinking. But in the domain of zero to one, not-something to something, Pointsman can only possess the zero and the one. He cannot, like Mexico, survive anyplace in between. Like his master I. P. Pavlov before him, he imagines the cortex of the brain as a mosaic of tiny on/off elements. Some are always in bright excitation, others darkly inhibited. The contours, bright and dark, keep changing. But each point is allowed only the two states: waking or sleep. One or zero. "Summation," "transition," "irradiation," "concentration," "recip-

rocal induction"—all Pavlovian brain-mechanics—assumes the presence of these bi-stable points. But to Mexico belongs the domain between zero and one—the middle Pointsman has excluded from his persuasion—the probabilities. (p. 55)

Roger's willingness to risk losing Jessica Swanlake to her official fiancé, an eminently respectable one-or-zero fellow named Beaver, but to abandon himself to their relationship while the circumstances of wartime give them the opportunity epitomizes the precarious humanity of the between option. It is assuredly not a comfortable choice but it is a vital choice, one that is at variance with the calculations of what motivates people, calculations upon which Pointsman and the technologists of power base their decisions on how to control the options from amongst which people make their supposedly free choices. Thus, the Roger Mexicos of the world are the ones whose courage and vitality keeps them free of the hold the Firm would otherwise have on them, free even while they do their own work within its structures.

One of the most arresting polarities that Pynchon presents in offering another option for life and freedom from the assumptions and control techniques exerted by the Man is that between the Elect and the Preterite. These are terms picked out from the Calvinist theology of Pynchon's own Puritan ancestors. The Elect are those specifically but arbitrarily chosen by God from eternity for salvation, while the Preterite are those who, through no fault of their own, were passed over. Pynchon makes Tyrone Slothrop's Puritan ancestor, William Slothrop (based, in fact, on Pynchon's own forefather, William Pynchon, himself an unorthodox Calvinist), the author of a theological treatise entitled *On Preterition*:

> Nobody wanted to hear about all the Preterite, the many God passes over when he chooses a few for salvation. William argued holiness for these "second Sheep," without whom there'd be no elect. You can bet the Elect in Boston were pissed off about that. And it got worse. William felt that what Jesus was for the Elect, Judas Iscariot was for the Preterite. Everything in the Creation has its equal and opposite counterpart. How can Jesus be an exception? Could we feel for him anything but horror in the face of the unnatural, the extracreational? Well, if he is the son of man, and if what we feel is not horror but love, then we have to love Judas too. Right? How William avoided being burned for heresy, nobody knows. . . .
>
> Could he have been the fork in the road America never took, the singular point she jumped the wrong way from? Suppose the Slothropite heresy had had the time to consolidate and prosper? Might there have been fewer crimes in the name of Jesus and more mercy in the name of Judas Iscariot? (pp. 555–556)

If there is a main character in *Gravity's Rainbow* it is Tyrone Slothrop, the lovable wildman, tarot fool, and pursuer of "mindless pleasures" (the original planned title), a Preterite if ever there was one. It is the planned use of his strange talent of getting erections in proximity to the V2 rockets that gets him sent to the Continent to find the secret of the ultimate Rocket, and it is his confounding of that mission that sets out the differences between the Elect (Them) and the Preterite (Us). The technological exploitation of Slothrop's peculiar talent, indicates both the determination and the capacity of *Technique* to turn everything into its own image and make it serve its own design. Slothrop, however, ever true to the humility of the Preterite that he is, does not take himself so seriously. Once in the Zone (ostensibly of Allied occupation but here represented as that space of chaotic openness where the postwar world was being shaped), Slothrop becomes immersed in a series of bizarre experiences in which he gradually begins to lose his ego. He takes on a series of make-believe roles that signify the shedding of his historic identity. He finally "disappears from history": ". . . and now in the Zone, later in the day he became a crossroad, after a heavy rain he doesn't recall, Slothrop sees a very thick rainbow here, a stout rainbow cock driven down out of the pubic clouds into Earth, green wet valleyed Earth, and his chest fills and he stands crying, not a thing in his head, just feeling natural. . . ." (p. 626). The cross-mandala image of redemption through self-abandonment suggests that in choosing to make himself unreachable by the allurements and techniques of the Man, Slothrop escapes the world of technological control of our desires by joining with the healing promises of a sacralized Earth—in which, Pynchon suggests, lies humankind's real hope.

The Preterite also represents, it seems to me, the perennially marginalized, exploited Other. Pynchon seems to be proposing, very much as he did in *The Crying of Lot 49,* that the longed-for healing Word is to be found not with the Elect, who serve the despot god of mastery and domination, but in responding in compassion to the Other as an other person. Through connecting with each other in the We-system of creative paranoia, the heart's real satisfactions will be found and we will not be so readily and easily controlled by those whose determination to exploit the Earth requires that we continually consume and continue to assume that our desires are being met when they are only being counterfeited.

The final option offered by Pynchon that I want to touch upon is his powerful image of "penetrating the moment," which stands in opposition to cause and effect, which he also describes as "secular history." He calls on us to surrender not only our demands for order (Levine, 1976) but also, I suggest, our postmodern passivity, our attitude of waiting for everything to be done for us, and to let ourselves instead be released into the "terror of the moment":

> She tried to explain to him about the level you reach, with both feet in, when
> you lose your fear, you lose it all, you've penetrated the moment, slipping
> perfectly into its grooves, metal-gray but soft as latex and now the figures are
> dancing, each pre-choreographed exactly where it is, the flash of knees under

pearl-colored frock as the girl in the babooshka stoops to pick up a cobble, the man in the black suitcoat and brown sleeveless sweater grabbed by policemen one on either arm trying to keep his head up, showing his teeth, the older liberal in the dirty beige overcoat, stepping back to avoid a careening demonstrator, looking back across his lapel how-dare-you or look-out-not me, his eyeglasses filled with the glare of the winter sky. There is the moment, and its possibilities. (pp. 158–159)

In this blur of images Pynchon is zooming in on the moment of passing from observer to agent, from purveyor of words to thrower of stones. Life in the realm of "secular history," of cause and effect, is the world of prudence, of calculation of interests, of fear for oneself. By encouraging caution and self-interest, the Firm is better able to keep people where it wants them. The Man stays in power by appealing to people's fear of violence. Yet all secular history is itself an act of violence, the turning of life into waste (Levine, 1976) by seeking to impose its order on things. These are times, however, when the attempts to maximize order lead to information overload: confusion, chaos, increasing disorder—in a word, entropy. To counteract these forces, which, as gigantic and monstrous as they are, are consuming themselves as they seek to consume the world, is Pynchon's penetration of the moment, which involves a degree of attention to what is happening around oneself—the very opposite of the modernist entry *into* oneself—attention, in other words, to the other, thereby breaking the prudence of the cause-and-effect pseudoconnection in order to experience one's very real, very concrete connectedness with all others in the ultimate, saving We-system:

On the last day, Pokler walked out the south end of the main tunnels . . .
The odors of shit, death, sweat, sickness, mildew, piss, the breating of Dora, wrapped him as he crept in staring at the naked corpses being carried out now that America was so close, to be stacked in front of the crematoriums, . . .
Where it was darkest and smelled the worst, Pokler found a woman lying, a random woman. He sat for half an hour holding her bony hand. She was breathing. Before he left, he took off his gold wedding ring and put it on the woman's thin finger, curling her hand to keep it from sliding off. If she lived, the ring would be good for a few meals, or a blanket, or a night indoors, or a ride home. . . . (pp. 432–433)

In the end all anyone has who goes with the way of the Preterite is one's song. It is one's "magic cape." Those who pursue noble and uplifting quests, those who remain single-minded in a world in which "single vision" keeps us from the humanity of the other, readily fall into the domain of the Man, for through the weapon of ideology he has become expert at covering his purposes with a cloak of high ideals and noble aims. "While the nobles are crying in their nights' chains, the squires sing. The terrible politics of the

Grail can never touch them. Song is their magic cape" (p. 701). So if there is a way to live in these postmodern times, in which unmitigated desire is loosed to give an illusion of complete freedom even as the Man promises us, with his colorful allurements, that he can fulfill those desires as long we work for him, it is the way of song. In marked contrast with the modernist, who hopes for societal rejuvenation through inner transformation, Pynchon, the preeminent postmodernist, calls on us to take the forces gathered against life and the Earth seriously and to take ourselves less seriously and with humor and lightheartedness dare to enter the terror of the moment, the reality of the other person, and in that connectedness find our heart's desire met, for true desire is for the other, not for the thing. Thus do we break the chain of cause and effect inasmuch as the hold the Man has over us is that he knows that he has what we want.

> [But] if the Counterforce knew better what those categories concealed, they might be in a better position to disarm, de-penis and dismantle the Man. But they don't. Actually they do, but they don't admit it. Sad but true. They are as schizoid, as double-minded in the massive presence of money, as any of the rest of us, and that's the hard fact. The Man has a branch office in each of our brains, his corporate emblem is a white albatross, each local rep has a cover known as the Ego, and their mission in this world is Bad Shit. We do know what's going on, and we let it go on. (pp. 712–713)

Through the crumbling of the old foundations that supported those single visions of God, Truth, or Reason (take your pick), the postmodern condition resembles that chaotic open space of Pynchon's Zone. It is a time, once again, when everything is up for grabs. All we have are our own and each other's stories; these are our magic capes. As long as we consider that we are not alone, that we have each other and the connectedness of stories that enter back and forth into one another's stories, then we can become a Counterforce against the forces that believe it is possible to control life but that, in trying to do so in the name of order, make waste. The time is short, however; the Preterite must make haste. Space does not permit us to look at Pynchon's most recent novel, Vineland, but its message is that the Man is so convinced he has won the majority over that it is no longer necessary for him to mask his intentions. Yet in a time of information overload, where events move so rapidly that no one can calculate or anticipate their direction, even he cannot be so sure. Such a time of chaotic openness is ready-made for the Preterite.

## OUR MAGIC CAPE

In a time when all we have are our own stories and such new stories as we now invent to identify the clash between control and chaos that so identifies these times, the job of the therapist involves, as never before, stories and their re-vision. When people go to see therapists, they do nothing and can do nothing other than tell their stories. Therapists, in turn, whatever else they do and however they do it, help their clients interpret the events and experiences of their lives in such a way that when they tell themselves or others what is happening to them, they begin to find that the story they are now telling is taking on a new plot. It might be said, in fact, that our job is to help people exchange old plots for new.

When I use the metaphor of a story to describe what a client is telling me, I sometimes hear the person insist, "This isn't a story, this is my life!" as if calling it a story somehow minimizes its reality and its significance. In an age so mesmerized with science and technology a story has come to suggest make-believe and fabrication, precisely the realm of the imaginary, the very opposite of anything real. For the former we use stories but for the latter, science and technology. This is a new development that is probably unique amongst the peoples of the world, who for countless millennia have resorted to stories whenever they have wanted to make an event more, not less, meaningful. However, in today's exceedingly complex and highly abstract society, the question might well be asked: "Of what use is a mere story, old or new, against the kinds of corporate and state forces that now dwarf the individual even as they encourage him to desire to his heart's content the goods that they offer?"

Modernity, furthermore, can be understood as a concerted effort to de-story the world. This was part of its project of liberating Europe from the literalizing and dogmatizing hold its grand narratives had come to have, which were also having the effect of keeping the people of Europe so ignorant and alienated from a world regarded as place of exile rather than as home that they had become locked in fear, ignorance, and pestilence, culminating in the despairing vacuum left by the century of the Black Plague. This necessary de-storying led to what Max Weber called the "disenchantment of the world," which followed in the wake of the increasing rationalization by the forces of science, economics, and technology. Enchantment and story have always gone together as the traditional ways of humanizing and enlivening the world. Story, in other words, was how people sought to understand the world of the living, which traditionally pertained to almost everything, while abstraction and technique pertained to (what there was of) the world of the nonliving—which later came to pertain to almost everything (Bateson, 1972). In the former, concepts and images become the currency in accounting for differences. Differences, in turn, provide information to "mind" or consciousness. For what the world regarded as nonliving, forces and impacts were the preferred language in the search for laws or predictable patterns in the movement of objects. There is no gainsaying that there is a vast middle area in which it is advantageous to treat some aspects of the living according to the methods and practices that typically pertain to the nonliving, as in the sciences and medical technologies of the human and animal body,—although even here, as we learn (or relearn) of the connections between mind and body, we can no longer be so certain. Nor can we cease to stand in awe before the accomplishments of Western science, which have been made possible by the steadfastness of its methods in investigating the world of the nonliving. However, perhaps it is time again, and the coast is sufficiently clear, to return wholeheartedly to the ancient approach when dealing with the world of the living, by replacing technique with story—but only if we can realize a story mode that truly empowers for coping with a world that disempowers in the name of wish fulfillment.

Yet there is no time like the postmodern present not only to return to the story as the chosen approach for dealing with matters pertaining to the world of the living but to regard therapy as an activity to be undertaken exclusively in this mode. In other words, even while tharapy's parent sciences of psychology and medicine may, at certain levels of activity, find it advantageous, even necessary, to use what Bruner (1986) calls the paradigmatic mode appropriate to the world of the nonliving, therapy should become a domain in which the language and approach used always pertain to the world of the living, that is, a domain in Bruner's narrative mode, which he defines as applicable wherever the subject matter has to do with "the vicissitudes of intention." Put another way, while there are occasions where it is all but unavoidable, expedient, and, at rare times, even helpful to treat a person as an object (certain aspects of surgery, for instance), therapy should be defined as that activity in which a person is always to be met as a subject and never as an object, the place where an I always meets a You.

The language of subject-to-subject encounter is that of conversation, which, however episodic, involves narration. One person is telling a portion of his or her story to another. Moreover, if the language is conversational between two subjects, it must involve a sharing of stories to the degree appropriate to the occasion. There will, as a matter of course, be a degree of one-sidedness to the story sharing of a therapeutic conversation. The client is there to tell his or her story in the service of changing its plot, not to hear the therapist's story, other than to the extent that it sheds some light on his or her own quest. The narrative mode is the discourse of choice for therapy not only because it happens to be best suited to its uniquely personal nature but also because, while not departing an iota from that imperative, it is so well suited to addressing the issue of the limits of perspective, which is likely to be at the heart of the impasse that has brought a person to therapy in the first place. Whatever persons tell about themselves, only will it be an account of events unavoidably perceived from their own perspective and theirs alone, but it cannot but be an abbreviated account, a summation that leaves out far more than it could possibly include. The very core of therapy, I propose, amounts to the deconstruction of what clients have chosen to include in relation to what they have, willy-nilly, excluded. Whether the therapy then goes on to inquire about the origins of the decisions of what experiences get included and what excluded the inclusions that went into the story represent clients' personal hermeneutic, their interpretation of themselves in relation to their world.

Many of what I would call the postmodern therapies address precisely this phenomenon of inclusion/exclusion by bringing to bear on clients' stories not the normative authority of the expert, the all-knowing interpreter of the subterranean realm, but simply the unexpected freshness of a different point of view that challenges the taken-for-grantedness of one person's perspectives. Thus, Steve de Shazer (1985) looks for "exceptions to the rule," Michael White stresses "unique outcomes" from the dominant story (Epston & White, 1989), and reflecting teams shower the family with alternative perspectives to the dominating either/or perspective that has them impaled (Andersen, 1987). In our "story re-vision" therapy (Parry & Doan, 1993) we build on the person's own experiences told in his or her own words, thereby questioning a story rooted in other people's descriptions of those experiences. In each of these therapies it is the neglected, passed-over experiences of strengths discounted by others that are brought forth to challenge an old story based on confused compliance. This process of newly emphasizing these neglected strengths makes for a story re-vision rooted in a renewed sense of personal agency. Moreover, it is this sense of finding one's own voice, describing one's own experiences in one's own words that, I propose, offers the means by which the postmodern person may be empowered to know what he or she wants. Our clients may, thereby, become less susceptible to wanting what They want them to want in order to keep the System going.

Released from those kinds of pressures, the postmodern world becomes a place of possibilities more than of personal powerlessness. It becomes a place and a time where "no story is the true story of God's anointed" and "all narratives are susceptible to being rewritten" (Edmondson, 1989), and as a consequence it presents us with the challenge of living in a democracy of stories. The loss of the overriding hold of the grand narratives as the stories that embody, more than other tales, the important truths and values of an entire culture need not result in Yeats's "mere anarchy" being "loosed upon the world." Far from being a mood that lacks a moral perspective, postmodernism offers a way of regarding the world in which we find ourselves today as one that challenges each of us to a new kind of strength, a strength rooted in simply acknowledging that one speaks of my perspective, my story, our perspective, our story—a story no "truer" than anyone else's, to be sure, but no less true either. When it comes to the truth, all of us are Preterite; no one any longer is Elect.

All each of us needs to seek, then, is our own story told in our own words and grounded in our personal experiences of the events that take place in our lives. "Song is their magic cape," says Pynchon, but a song is only a story set to music. The old story, derived from other people's words to describe one's own experiences, is embedded in "secular history," the chain of cause and effect. A new story can be sung, as it were, for each moment, freed from the the chains of the past, can now be penetrated to mine from it the uniqueness and richness it offers. It therefore behooves us to engage ourselves constantly in a process of story re-vision, according to which we expose our stories to the critical challenge of other stories, other perspectives, in an ongoing effort to "keep us from single vision and Newton's sleep," from a world in which we mistake our own perception for the only truth and our own story for the way things are, with our self, our nationality, our race, gender, sexual preference, or ideology at the center and with others there simply to support that story. If, however, we do live in that time spoken of in the rabbinical tale, when "there is only the story," then the only counterweight we have—and it is an essential one—to that most dangerous of follies is the connection of our story with the others and their stories. The other person's story, it is well to remember, is one in which I am no longer at the center but a player in the story. Since the other is also a player in mine, then neither of us can go forward until we both realize that the stories are connected, each of us having entered the world of the other. Such a sense of story calls for us to improvise constantly, like jazz musicians each playing off what the other introduces. If, too, our stories are our magic capes and we would give our lives a larger significance in order to make a difference, then we would do well to recognize that we have the choice as to which of the stories of our families, our communities, and of the Earth itself we will connect to our personal stories, whether those for life or those for death. And what a difference it might make to one's personal story if it is consciously offered to a happier outcome in the story of the "green, wet-valleyed Earth."

Psychoanalysis became not only the prototype but the popularizer of the modernist temper that sought to address a crisis of the spirit by empowering the individual from within. Family therapy, particularly through its emerging "therapies of possibility," stands ready to offer a comparable vision for the beleaguered postmodern temper, a vision of the self and the other connected through shared stories in preparation for living in a world in which no story has a singular claim on us save the story of those whom we encounter as persons full of possibilities, ours for their story, theirs for ours.

Now, everybody . . .

## ACKNOWLEDGMENT

I would like to acknowledge and indicate appreciation to the Grateful Dead, true postmodern Preterites, the name of whose recent album inspired the title of this chapter.

## REFERENCES

Andersen, T. (1987). The reflecting team: Dialogue and meta-dialogue in clinical work. *Family Process, 26*(1), 415–428.

Bateson, G. (1972). Form, substance and difference. In *Steps toward an ecology of mind* (pp. 456–457). New York: Ballantine Books.

Bruner, J. (1988). *Actual minds, possible worlds.* Cambridge: Harvard University Press (p. 39).

de Beavoir, S. (1953). *The second sex.* New York: Knopf.

de Shazer, S. (1985). *Keys to solution in brief therapy.* New York: Norton.

Dudek, S. (1990). Written in blood: 20th century art. *Canadian Psychology, 30*(2), 105–115.

Edmondson, M. (1989). Prophet of a new postmodernism: The greater challenge of Salman Rushdie. *Harper's Magazine, 279,* 62–71.

Ellul, J., (1964). *The technological society.* New York: Knopf.

Epston, D., & White, M. (1989). *Literate means to therapeutic ends.* Adelaide, Australia: Dulwich Centre Publications.

Freud, S., (1930). *Civilization and its discontents.* New York: Norton.

Freund, J. (1968). *The sociology of Max Weber.* New York: Pantheon Books.

Gergen, K. (1991). *The saturated self: Dilemmas of identity in contemporary life.* New York: Basic Books.

Levine, G. (1976). Risking the moment: Anarchy and possibility in Pynchon's fiction. In G. Levine & D. Leverenz (Eds.), *Mindful pleasures: Essays on Thomas Pynchon* (pp. 113–136). Boston: Little, Brown.

Lyotard, J. F. (1983). *The postmodern condition: A report on knowledge.* New York: Basic Books.

Nietzsche, F. (1882). *The gay science* (W. Kaufman, Trans.). New York: Vintage Books.

Parry, A. (1991). A universe of stories. *Family Process, 30*(1), 37–54.

Parry, A., & Doan, R. (1992). *Story re-visions: The art and craft of narrative family therapy.* Manuscript in preparation.

Pynchon, T. (1963). *V.* New York: Harper & Row.

Pynchon, T. (1966). *The Crying of Lot 49.* New York: Bantam.

Pynchon, T. (1973). *Gravity's Rainbow.* New York: Viking Penguin.

Pynchon, T. (1984). *Slow learner: Early Stories.* Boston: Little, Brown.

Pynchon, T. (1990). *Vineland.* Boston: Little, Brown.

Weber, M. (1930) *The Protestant ethics and the spirit of capitalism.* New York: Charles Scribner's Sons.

# Epilogue

" 'Remember only this one thing,' said Badger. 'The stories people tell have a way of taking care of them. If stories come to you, care for them. And learn to give them away where they are needed. Sometimes a person needs a story more than food to stay alive. That is why we put these stories in each other's memory. This is how people care for themselves' " (Lopez, 1990, p. 48).

## REFERENCE

Lopez, B. (1990). *Crow and weasel*. San Francisco: North Point Press.

# Index